COPYC

Recipes

200 MOUTHWATERING RECIPES TO EASILY RECREATE YOUR FAVORITE RESTAURANTS' DISHES AT HOME WITH QUALITY ON A BUDGET, EVEN IF YOU'RE NOT A FAMOUS CHEF

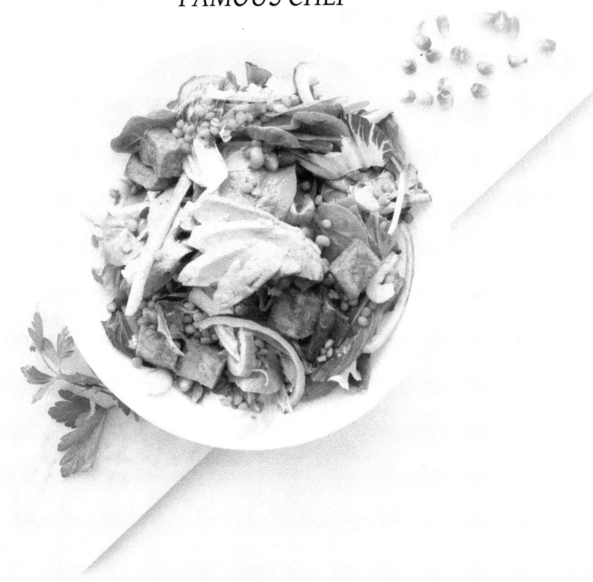

Elsie Lipsey

Table of Contents

Chapter 2
The perfect Mains 38

Introduction

Sooner or later, there is a need that every person cook their own food. Of course, lately, fast-food restaurants have been growing like mushrooms, and the freezers of all stores are littered with semi-finished products, but that doesn't solve the problem. Firstly, it's quite expensive, secondly, most often it's tasteless and, thirdly, it's certainly not useful. Therefore, the inexperienced in cooking novice raises a logical question: What is needed to learn how to cook recipes found in restaurants deliciously?

Using these copycat recipes has many advantages. You can save money and customize the recipes as well. You can reduce the amount of salt or butter and adjust the seasoning. You cannot only save money but provide nutritious meals for your family as well.

In using copycat recipes, you do not need to guess the ingredients that your favorite restaurant meals have. We provide it to you. The only thing you need to do is follow the steps to recreate the meal

Learning how to cook restaurant recipes is not really that difficult. Some people think that a degree in culinary is needed to be able to create secret recipes. The truth is that anyone can collect the ingredients themselves and cook a meal that tastes just like restaurant food.

But do top secret restaurant recipes really taste the way the chef served them? Perhaps. You can easily cook your favorite recipes with a little practice and patience. You would just want to cook the basic formula and start adding what you think would make the flavor of the recipe better after a while. But if you've ever badly prepared food of this kind on your own, it is not impossible! With a few and simple tricks and tips, you can also cook quality cuisine in your own kitchen. These tricks may not seem so strong on their own but can transform how you prepare and produce food when they are all used together. These tips help you cook at home like a pro from expired spices and how you use salt to literally arrange it before you start cooking.

When preparing desserts at home, you can tweak the recipes as you wish. As you sample the recipes, you will get to know the usual ingredients and techniques in making popular sweet treats. This could inspire you to create your very own recipes. You can substitute ingredients as your taste, health, or pocket dictates. You can come up, perhaps, not with a dessert that is the perfect clone of a restaurant's recipe, but with one that is exactly the way you want it to be. Most of all, the recipes here are meant for you to experience the fulfillment of seeing the smiles on the people with whom you share your creations. Keep trying and having fun with the recipes and you will soon be reaping your sweet rewards!

If prepared food arrives from outside the home you typically have limited knowledge about salt, sugar, and processed oils. In fact, we also apply more to our meal when it is served to the table. You will think about how much salt, sugar and oil are being used as you prepare meals at home.

Having said that, I think you are now ready to recreate your favorite restaurant dishes with the help of these 200 mouthwatering recipes!

Chapter 1
The Breakfast of Champion

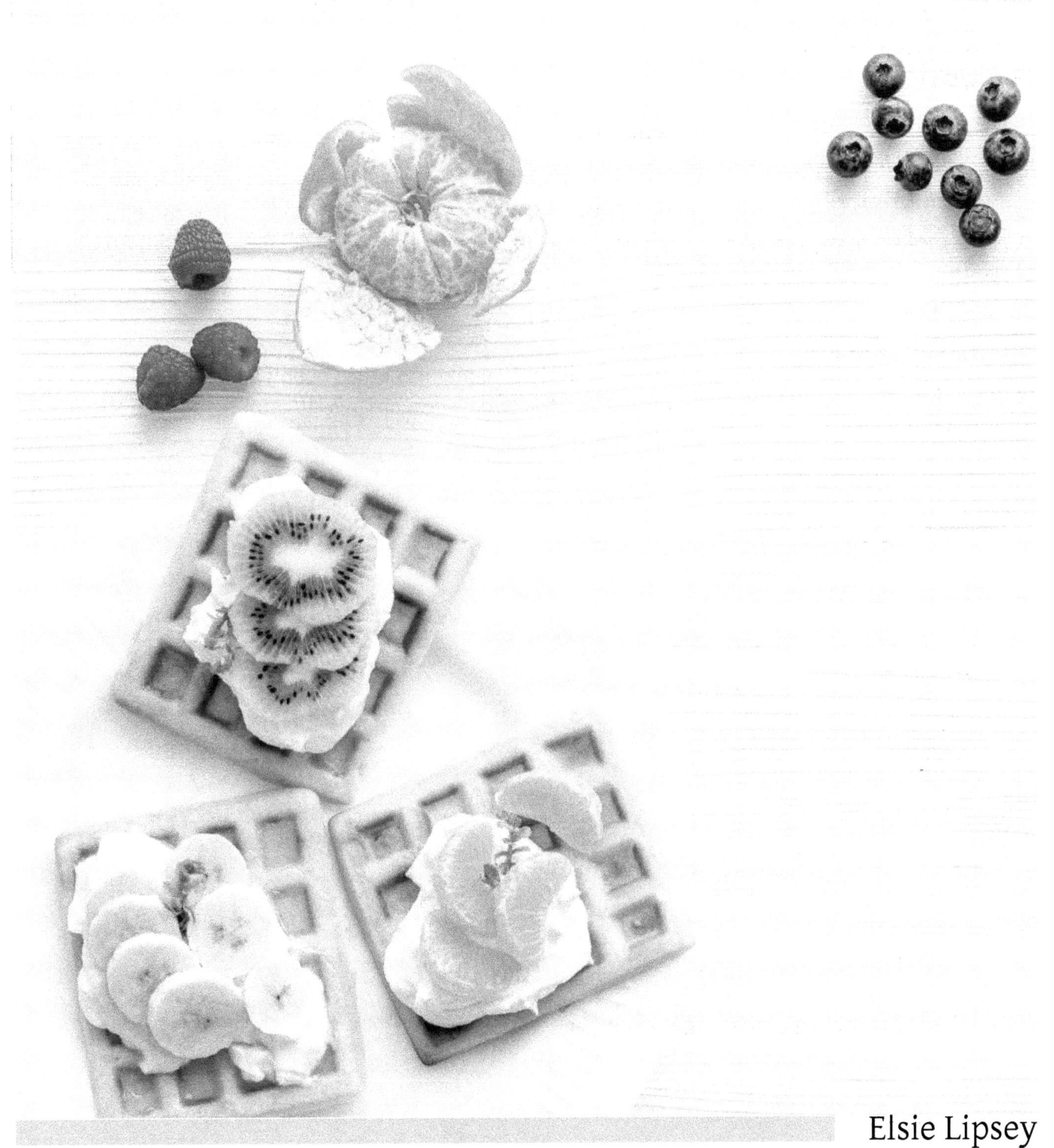

Preparation Time: 10' *Cooking Time: 45'* *Serves: 4-6*

1. Cracker Barrel's Hash Brown Casserole

Ingredients

- ***1 (30-ounce) bag frozen hash browns, thawed***
- ***½ cup butter, melted***
- ***1 can cream of fowl soup***
- ***1 small onion, chopped***
- ***1-pound cheddar cheese, shredded (divided)***
- ***1 teaspoon salt***
- ***½ teaspoon black pepper***
- ***1 cup butter cream***

Directions

1. Preheat oven to 350°F.
2. Prepare a baking dish either by using greasing the aspects or spraying with nonstick cooking spray.
3. Mix the onion, cream of hen soup, pepper, and all however 1 cup the shredded cheese in a massive bowl. When combined, combine in the bitter cream until it is well incorporated.
4. Add the melted butter and hash browns. Stir to combine. Pour into the greased baking dish.
5. Bake for forty-five minutes or till bubbly, then sprinkle the last cheese on top and bake again in 5–10 minutes or until the cheese is melted.

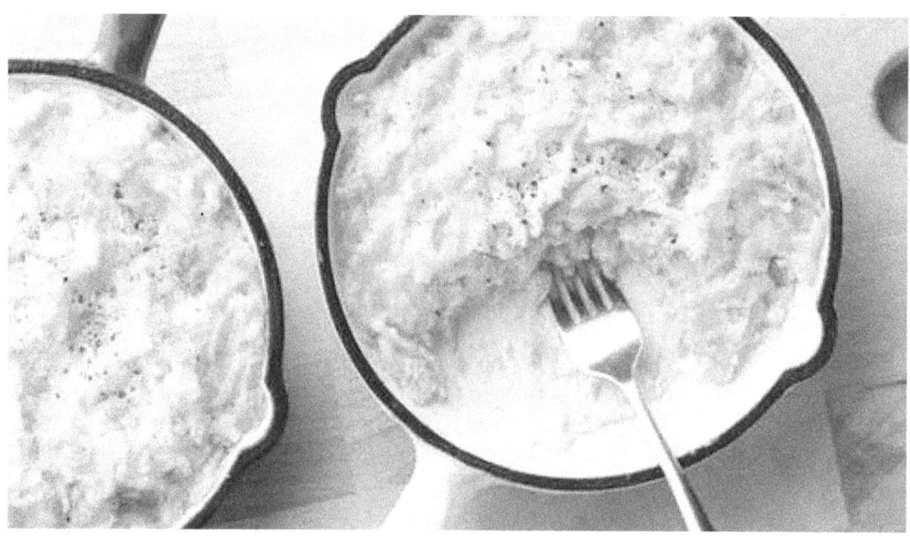

Nutrition

Calories: 112 Fat: 17g Carbs: 50g Protein: 7g

Preparation Time: 5' *Cooking Time: 15'* *Serves: 6*

2. Cracker Barrel's Buttermilk Pancakes

Ingredients

- ***2 cups un-sifted flour***
- ***2 teaspoons baking soda***
- ***1 teaspoon salt***
- ***3 tablespoons sugar***
- ***2 eggs***
- ***2 1/3 cups low-fat buttermilk***
- ***Butter for cooking***

Directions

1. Preheat a grill or massive skillet to 350°F.
2. Place a stick of butter after the skillet; you will butter it earlier than making ready every pancake.
3. In a medium bowl, put the eggs and buttermilk and whisk till they are properly combined. Whisk in the flour, baking soda, sugar, and salt. Whisk wholly till nicely combined.
4. Prepare the skillet with the aid of rubbing the butter in a circle in the center, then add about ½ cup batter. Spread the batter till its varieties an even circle.
5. When the pancake surface turns bubbly, flip and cook on the different aspects until you can't see moist spots on the sides.
6. Repeat with the last batter, making sure to butter the skillet earlier than you start each pancake.
7. Serve with your favorite syrup or fruit.

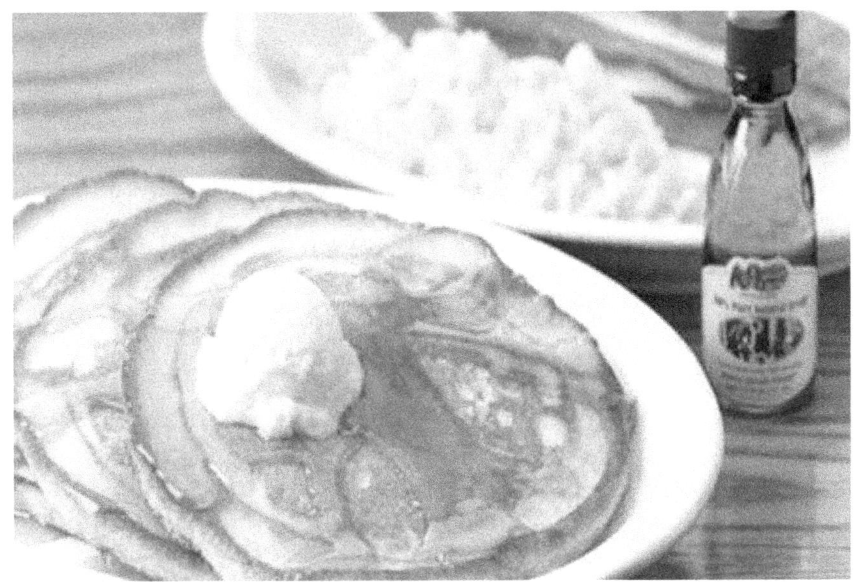

Nutrition

Calories: 80 Fat: 4g Carbs: 20g Sugars 2g Protein: 15g

Preparation Time: 10' *Cooking Time: 15'* *Serves: 4*

3. Cracker Barrel's Coleslaw

Ingredients

- ***2 cups shredded cabbage***
- ***½ cup shredded carrots***
- ***½ cup shredded red cabbage***
- ***1 cup miracle whip***
- ***1 teaspoon celery seeds***
- ***½ teaspoon salt***
- ***½ teaspoon pepper***
- ***1/3 cup sugar***
- ***¼ cup vinegar***
- ***¼ cup buttermilk***
- ***¼ cup milk***
- ***4 teaspoons lemon juice***

Directions

1. Toss the carrots and cabbages in a massive mixing bowl.
2. Stir in the Miracle Whip, celery seeds, salt, pepper, sugar, vinegar, buttermilk, milk, and lemon juice.
3. Toss once more to combine. Refrigerate for about three hours earlier than serving.

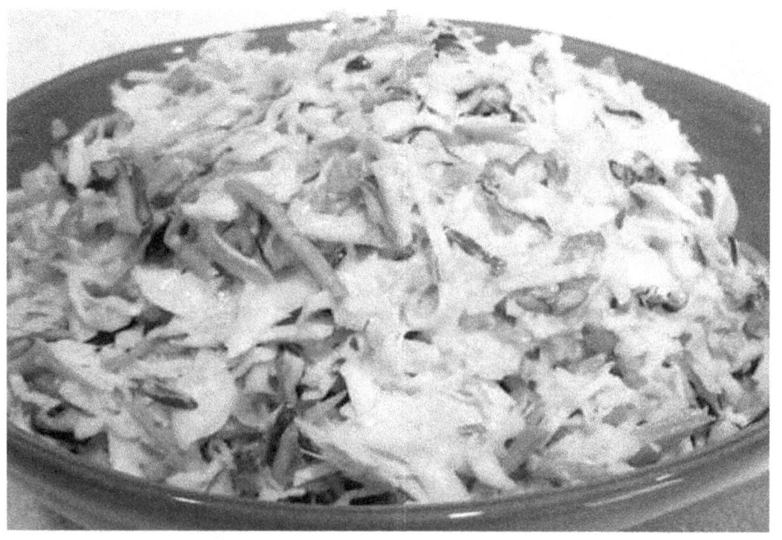

Nutrition

Calories: 178 Fat: 24g Carbs: 123g Protein: 27g

Preparation Time: 15' *Cooking Time: 10'* *Serves: 4*

4. Cracker Barrel's Breaded Fried Okra

Ingredients

- ***1-pound clean okra, rinsed and dried***
- ***1 cup self-rising cornmeal***
- ***½ cup self-rising flour***
- ***1 teaspoon salt***
- ***1 cup vegetable oil (for frying)***
- ***Salt and pepper to taste***

Directions

1. Put some oil in a giant skillet or deep fryer.
2. Cut the okra into ½-inch pieces.
3. Put together the cornmeal, flour, and salt in a large bowl.
4. Drop the okra portions into the bowl and toss to coat. Allow relaxing for a few minutes while the oil heats up.
5. Transfer the okra from the bowl into the warm oil using a slotted spoon.
6. Cook the okra until it has turned a nice golden color. Remove from oil and region on a plate lined with paper towels to drain. Season it to taste with salt and pepper.

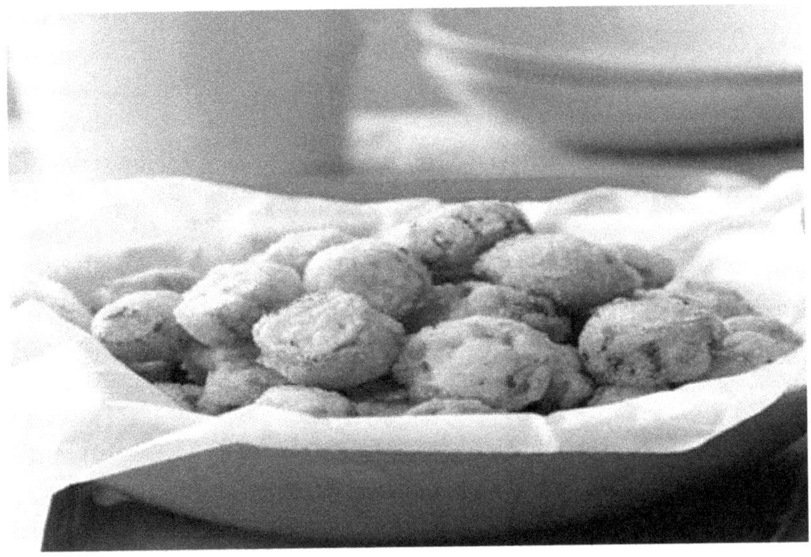

Nutrition

Calories: 119 Fat: 20g Carbs: 76g Protein: 10g

Preparation Time: 20' *Cooking Time: 30'* *Serves: 12*

5. Cracker Barrel's Corn Muffins

Ingredients

- ***¾ cup yellow cornmeal***
- ***1¼ cups self-rising flour***
- ***½ cup sugar***
- ***2 massive eggs***
- ***2 tablespoons honey***
- ***¾ cup buttermilk***
- ***½ cup unsalted butter, melted and cooled***

Directions

1. Preheat the oven to 350°F.
2. Put a line in a muffin pan using muffin liner or grease thoroughly.
3. Combine the cornmeal, flour, and sugar in a mixing bowl.
4. Beat the eggs in a medium bowl. Then, add the honey and buttermilk and whisk till nicely combined.
5. Slowly add the buttermilk to the cornmeal mixture, stirring as you add. There are some lumps, but don't over-mix.
6. Place the batter inside the muffin pan and fill holes to the ¾, and bake for 18–20 minutes or until set.
7. Remove from oven and enable to cool barely earlier than serving.

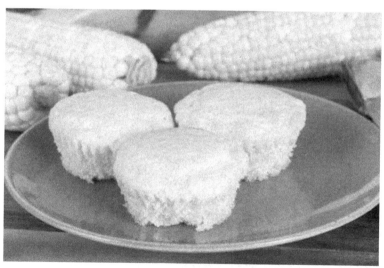

Nutrition

Calories: 184 Fat: 4g Carbs: 57g Protein: 12g

Preparation Time: 5' *Cooking Time: 15'* *Serves: 6*

6. Cracker Barrel's Apple-Cheddar Chicken

Ingredients

- *5 cooked skinless hen breasts, entire or cubed*
- *2 cans of apple pie filling with a cut of apples in 1/3*
- *1 bag extra-sharp cheddar cheese*
- *1 row Ritz crackers, beaten*
- *1 cup melted butter*

Directions

1. Preheat the oven to 350°F. Combine the chicken, apple pie filling, and cheddar cheese in a mixing bowl. Stir together. Pour the mixture in the casserole dish that has been greased.
2. Mix the Ritz crackers with the melted butter. Spread over the casserole. Bake for 45 minutes or till it starts evolved to bubble.

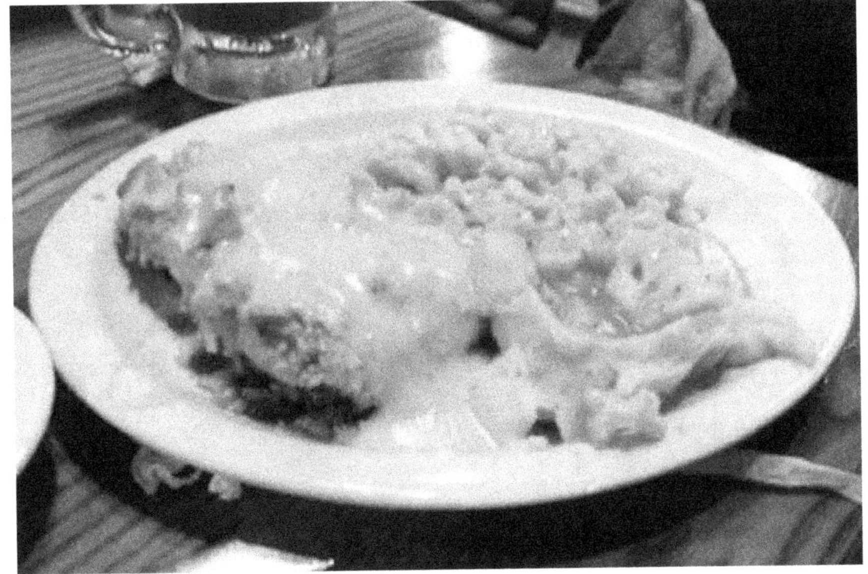

Nutrition

Calories: 158 Fat: 10g Carbs: 71g Protein: 7g

Preparation Time: 10’ *Cooking Time: 15’* *Serves: 4-5*

7. Cracker Barrel’s Lemon Pepper Trout

Ingredients

- *6 (4-ounce) trout fillets*
- *3 tablespoons butter, melted*
- *2 medium lemons, thinly sliced*
- *2 tablespoons lemon juice*
- *Sauce*
- *3 tablespoons butter*
- *¼ teaspoon pepper*
- *2 tablespoons lemon juice*

Directions

1. In a saucepan, it melts the butter over low warmness and enables it to cook until it starts to brown. Add the pepper and lemon juice. Brush the fish fillets with melted butter. Lay lemon slices on top of each.
2. If cooking on a grill, use a wire grilling basket sprayed with nonstick cooking spray. Grill for about 10 minutes or until the fish flakes effortlessly with a fork. Alternatively, you can bake in a 350°F oven for 10–15 minutes. Transfer to a serving platter and top with extra lemon slices.
3. Serve with the butter lemon sauce you made.

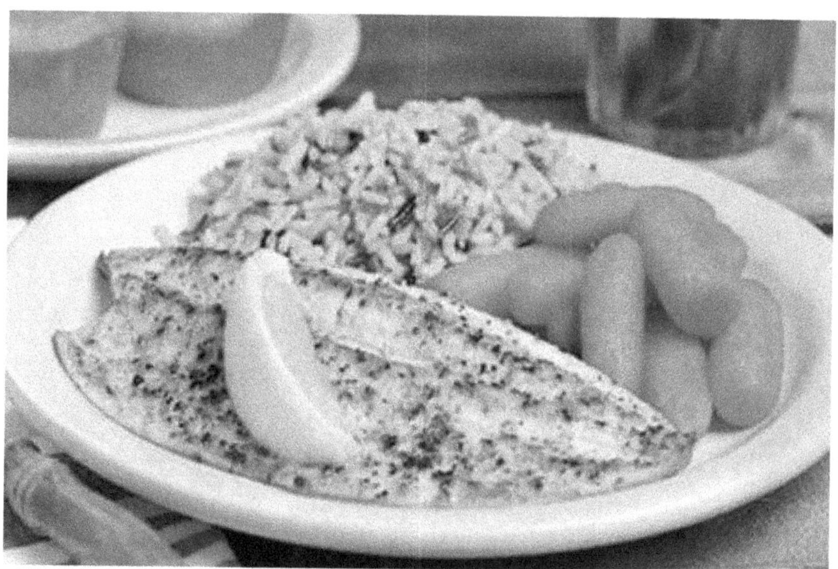

Nutrition

Calories: 242.8 Fat: 6.6g, Carbs: 38.4g Sugars: 3g Protein: 8.4g

Preparation Time: 5' *Cooking Time: 15'* *Serves: 6*

8. Cracker Barrel's Mushroom Swiss Chopped Steak

Ingredients

- ***1-pound floor sirloin, fashioned into four patties***
- ***1 tablespoon butter***
- ***Salt to taste***
- ***Pepper to taste***
- ***4 slices Swiss cheese***
- ***¼ small onion, sliced***
- ***1-pound mushrooms, sliced***
- ***1 (14 ½-ounce) can beef gravy (or equal package)***

Directions

1. Season the sirloin patties with salt and pepper, then cook to the favored temperature. You can grill, broil, fry, or even bake the ground meat; the choice is yours. Put the cooked patties to a plate and top everyone with a slice of Swiss cheese.
2. Sauté the mushroom and onion in a large pan. Add the red meat gravy. Top each patty with the onion, mushroom, and pork gravy mixture.

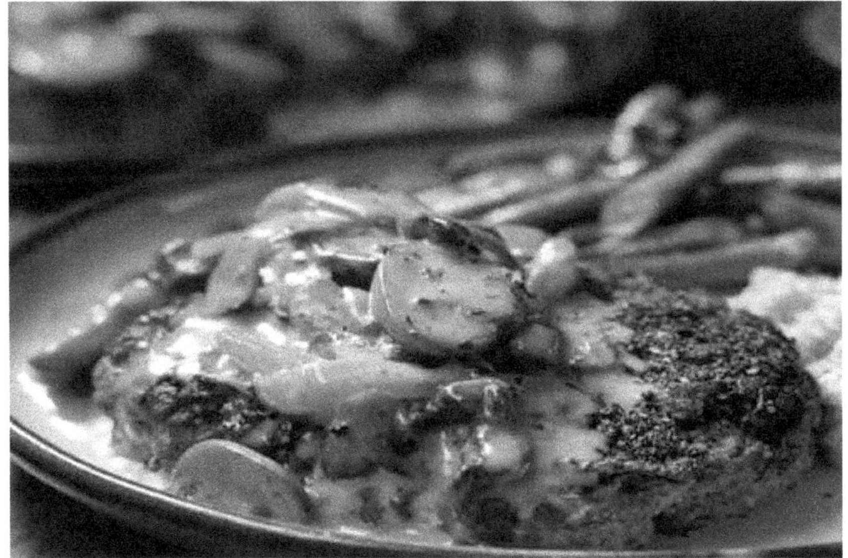

Nutrition

Calories: 150 Fat: 4.2g Carbs: 40g Sugars: 1g Protein: 9g

Preparation Time: 15' *Cooking Time: 10'* *Serves: 9*

9. Cracker Barrel's Campfire S'mores

Ingredients

- *Graham Cracker Crust*
- *2 cups graham cracker crumbs*
- *¼ cup sugar*
- *½ cup butter*
- *½ teaspoon cinnamon*
- *1 small package deal brownie combines or use the brownie ingredients listed below.*
- *Brownie Mix*
- *½ cup flour*
- *1/3 cup cocoa*
- *¼ teaspoon baking powder*
- *¼ teaspoon salt*
- *½ cup butter*
- *1 cup sugar*
- *1 teaspoon vanilla*
- *2 giant eggs*
- *S'mores Topping:*
- *9 massive marshmallows*
- *5 Hershey sweet bars*
- *4½ cups vanilla ice cream*
- *½ cup chocolate sauce*

Directions

1. Preheat the oven to 350°F
2. Put all together and mix the graham cracker crumbs, sugar, cinnamon, and melted butter in a medium bowl. Stir till the crumbs and sugar have blended with the butter.
3. Line the baking dish with parchment paper. Make positive to use adequate so that you'll be in a position to raise the baked brownies out of the dish easily. Press the graham cracker combination into the bottom of the lined pan.

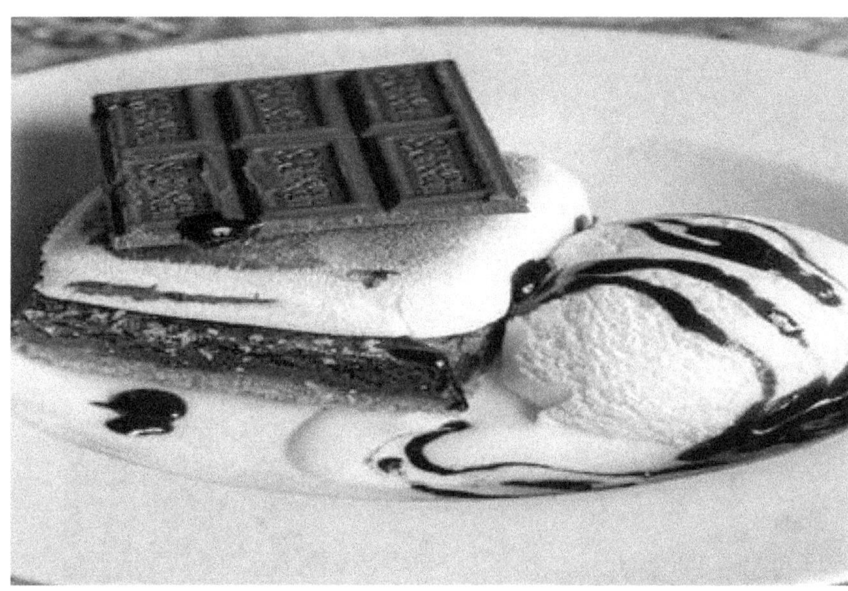

Nutrition

Calories: 100 Fat: 3g Carbs: 21g Sugars: 10g Protein: 5g

Preparation Time: 15’ *Cooking Time: 30’* *Serves: 4*

10. Paris’ Egg Bacon and Swiss Soufflé

Ingredients

- *Four slices bacon (thick cut)*
- *One container of croissants*
- *2 tablespoons flour*
- *5 large eggs*
- *4 tablespoons half and half*
- *½ tablespoon salt*
- *1/8 tablespoon black pepper (ground)*
- *¾ cup cheese (Swiss)*
- *1 cup onion (diced finely)*
- *1 tablespoon parmesan cheese (shredded)*

Directions

1. Microwave the bacon slices on a microwave-safe tray by placing between paper towels. Microwave it for 5 minutes. Let the bacon cool down and crumble. Preheat oven to 180ºC.
2. Spray cooking spray in 4 ramekins. Lay the croissants on a flat surface and flour the croissants lightly. Roll them in a square. Cut out four slices square. Lay each square in each of the greased ramekins. Press the squares to the base by using your fingers. Keep aside.
3. Take a bowl and combine half and half with the eggs. Add pepper and salt. Add the Swiss cheese to the mixture along with bacon crumbles, onion, and shredded parmesan cheese. Microwave the mixture on high settings for thirty seconds for reaching the consistency of runny scrambled egg.
4. Place the egg mixture in the four ramekins. Top the ramekins with cheese. Fold the croissant edges at the top properly for sealing. Brush the top with some eggs. Bake the ramekins for thirty minutes until puffy and golden in color. Serve with the ramekins or you can take out the soufflés as well.

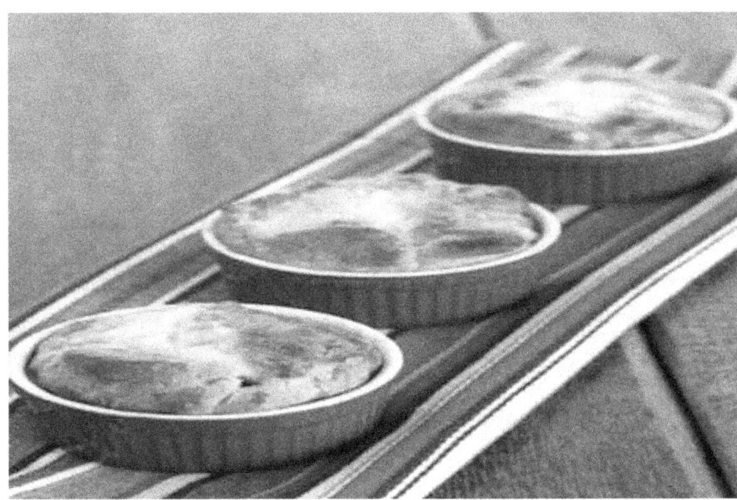

Nutrition

Calories: 575 Protein: 35g Carbs: 39g Fat: 28g Sugar: 3.9g

Preparation Time: 20' *Cooking Time: 30'* *Serves: 20*

11. Paris' Cheddar and Dill Puffs

Ingredients

- ***1 cup water***
- ***½ cup butter (unsalted)***
- ***½ tablespoon kosher salt***
- ***1 cup flour***
- ***5 large eggs***
- ***1 ½ cup cheddar cheese (grated)***
- ***2 tablespoons fresh dill (chopped)***

Directions

1. Preheat oven at 180ºC.
2. Take a saucepan and heat it over a medium flame. Add butter, water, and salt to the pan. Simmer the mixture and keep cooking until the butter melts. Mix the flour to the pan and stir continuously. Cook for two minutes.
3. Add the eggs to the batter. The mixture needs to be glossy and stiff enough for holding the peaks. In case the batter gets too stiff, you can add more eggs to the batter. Add the dill and cheese. Use parchment paper for lining two baking sheets. Use a scoop for dropping the batter on the trays. Bake the puffs until crispy and golden in color for thirty minutes.

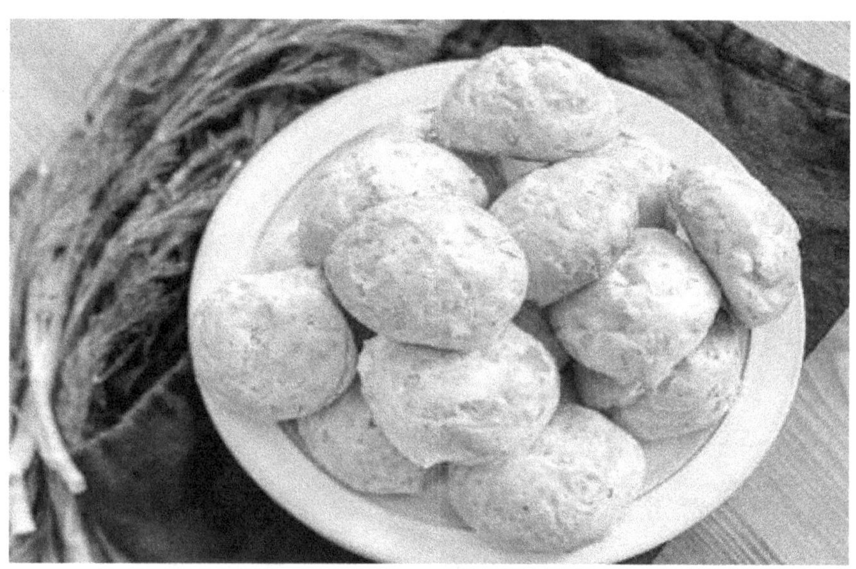

Nutrition

Calories: 103 Protein: 5g Carbs: 5.2g Fat: 6.8g Sugar: 1.1g

Preparation Time: 10' *Cooking Time: 35'* *Serves: 4*

12. Paris' Lyonnaise Potatoes

Ingredients

- ***2 pounds of russet potatoes (peeled, sliced in rounds of half an inch)***
- ***3 tablespoons butter***
- ***4 tablespoons vegetable oil***
- ***2 onions (sliced thinly)***
- ***½ cup parsley (chopped)***
- ***1 tablespoon kosher salt***

Directions

1. Boil the potatoes in water in a large pot. Cook for four minutes until the potatoes are crisp tender. Drain the water.
2. Take an iron skillet and heat one tablespoon butter in it. Add one tablespoon the vegetable oil. Put half of the onions and potatoes to the skillet. Cook the mixture for 5 minutes. Add the remaining oil, butter, onions, and potatoes to the skillet. Cook for fifteen minutes until the onions are browned.
3. Remove the skillet from heat and add parsley from the top. Serve with pepper and salt from the top.

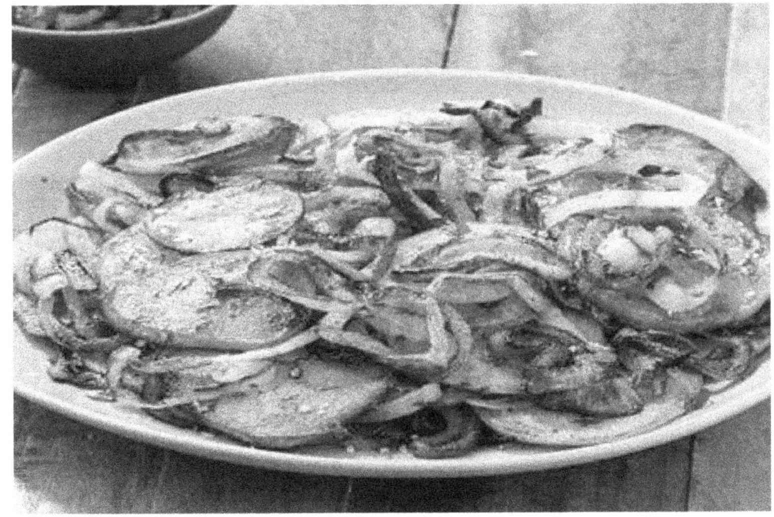

Nutrition

Calories: 320 Protein: 3.6g Carbs: 33g Fat: 19.2g Sugar: 4g

Preparation Time: 30' *Cooking Time: 1 hour* *Serves: 6*

13. Paris' Coq Au Vin

Ingredients

- ***3 pounds chicken drumsticks and thighs***
- ***2 tablespoons black pepper (ground)***
- ***6 bacon strips (cut in pieces of one inch)***
- ***8 ounces baby Bella mushrooms (sliced)***
- ***5 ounces onions (peeled)***
- ***1 carrot (chopped)***
- ***2 garlic cloves (minced)***
- ***1 tablespoon tomato paste***
- ***2 tablespoons flour***
- ***2 cups red wine***
- ***1 cup chicken stock***
- ***1 tablespoon brandy***
- ***1 bunch of thyme***
- ***3 tablespoons butter***
- ***Parsley (chopped, for garnishing)***

Directions

1. Preheat your oven to 180ºC.
2. Season the chicken with pepper and salt.
3. Take a skillet and cook the bacon until crispy. Cook for about eight minutes. Remove the bacon and keep aside.
4. Cook the chicken in the pot for 5 minutes on each side. Remove the chicken and keep aside.
5. Combine the onions, carrots, and mushrooms to the pot. Cook for 5 minutes until golden. Add the garlic and tomato paste. Give it a stir for coating the veggies. Add flour to the mixture and stir.
6. Slowly add the red wine, brandy, and chicken stock to the mixture. Return the cooked chicken to the pot along with half of the cooked bacon. Season with pepper and salt and add thyme. Boil the mixture.
7. When it is starting to boil, cover the pot and put it in the oven. Cook until the chicken gets evenly cooked for thirty minutes. Remove the chicken.
8. Return the mixture pot to the stove and add butter to it. Simmer the mixture for ten minutes until the sauce thickens.
9. Serve the chicken with sauce from the top. Add remaining bacon from the top along with parsley.

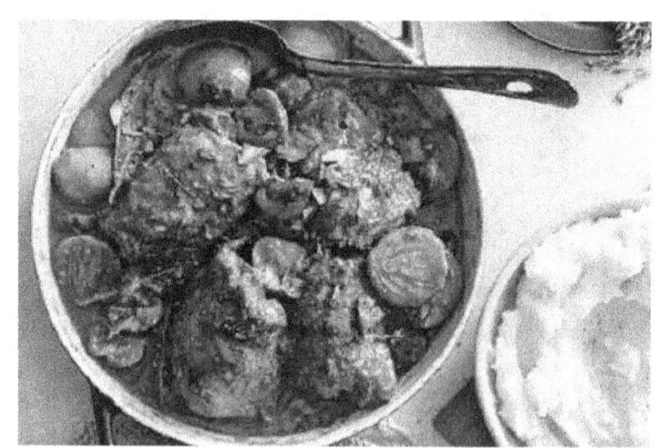

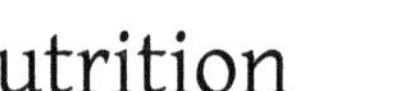

Nutrition

Calories: 265 Protein: 32g Carbs: 7.3g Fat: 7.8g Sugar: 2.1g

Preparation Time: 35' *Cooking Time: 20'* *Serves: 4*

14. Paris' Crepes

Ingredients

- ***1 cup flour***
- ***2 eggs***
- ***1 tablespoon sugar***
- ***¼ tablespoon kosher salt***
- ***2 cups milk (whole)***
- ***1 ½ tablespoon butter***
- ***Fresh fruits of your choice (for serving)***
- ***Powdered sugar (for serving)***

Directions

1. Combine and mix the flour together with sugar, and salt in a mixing bowl. Make a well in the center and start adding the eggs. Pour milk in the flour mix and whisk properly until combined. Allow the batter to sit at room temperature for twenty minutes.
2. Take a small skillet and heat the butter in it. Add one-fourth cup batter to the skillet. Swirl the skillet for coating properly.
3. Cook the crepes for two minutes and flip. Cook for 1 more minute. Repeat the same with the remaining batter.
4. Serve the hot crepes with powdered sugar and fruits from the top. Add chocolate syrup to the crepes if you want to.

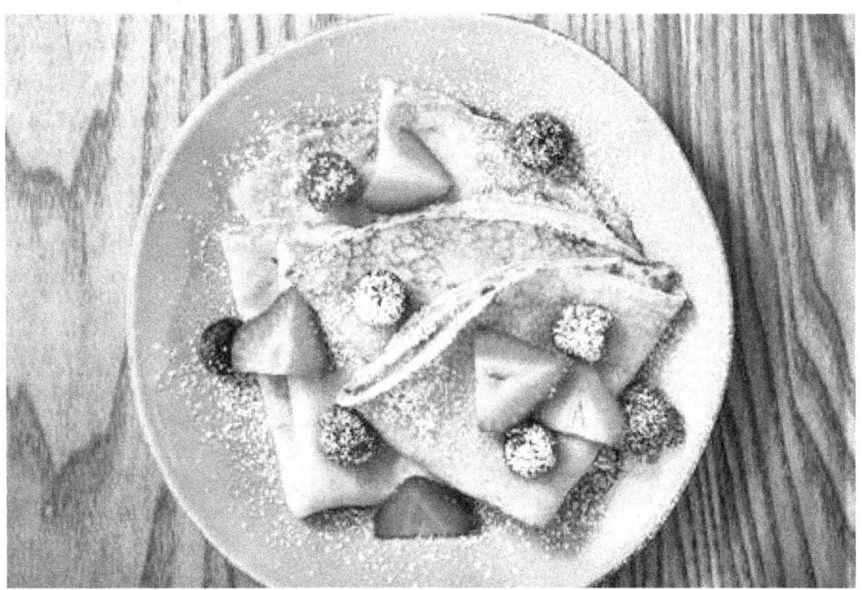

Nutrition

Calories: 162 Protein: 3.2g Carbs: 13g Fat: 4.6g Sugar: 0.9g

Preparation Time: 20' *Cooking Time: 1 h 10'* *Serves: 4*

15. Paris 'Onion Soup

Ingredients

- ***4 tablespoons butter***
- ***2 tablespoons flour***
- ***3 onions (sliced in half moons)***
- ***Kosher salt***
- ***½ cup white wine***
- ***Black pepper (ground)***
- ***2 cups chicken stock***
- ***4 cups beef stock***
- ***8 sprigs thyme***
- ***8 slices baguette***
- ***1 cup cheese (grated)***

Directions

1. Melt the butter in a pot. Add the onions and cook for twenty minutes until deep golden in color. Add the flour and stir for one minute. Add pepper and salt according to taste. Add the white wine and simmer the mixture for three minutes. Add the beef and chicken stock to the pot along with thyme and boil the mixture. Simmer the mixture for about fifteen minutes. Remove the thyme.
2. Preheat a broiler at high.
3. Place the slices baguette of a baking tray and add cheese from the top. Put the tray under the broiler to let the cheese turn into brown in color and is bubbling, for one minute.
4. Serve the onion soup with slices baguette.

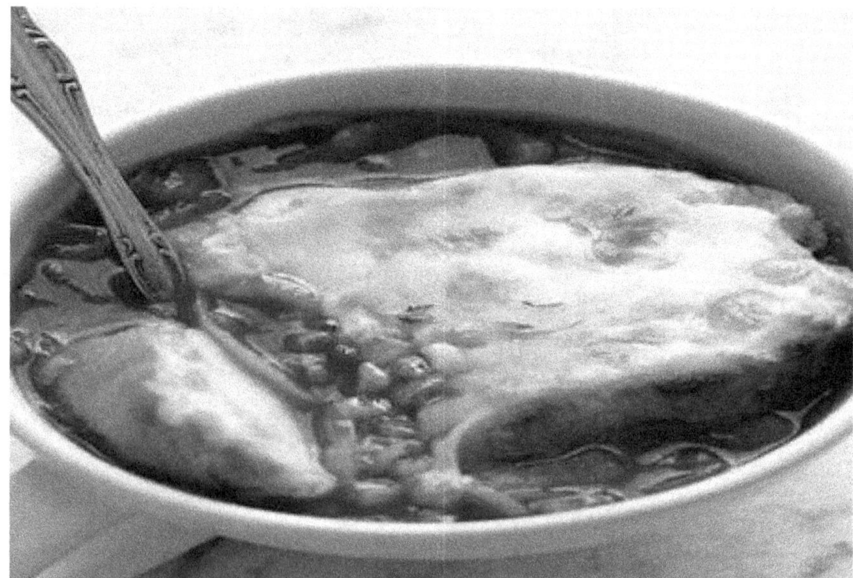

Nutrition

Calories: 275 Protein: 17g Carbs: 33g Fat: 9.4g Sugar: 0.6g

Preparation Time: 15' *Cooking Time: 20'* *Serves: 4*

16. Paris' Chicken Quesadillas

Ingredients

- ***3 chicken breasts (skinless)***
- ***1 tablespoon oregano (dried)***
- ***½ tablespoon garlic powder***
- ***Black pepper (ground)***
- ***Kosher salt***
- ***3 tablespoons olive oil (extra virgin)***
- ***1 cup Dijon mustard***
- ***8 tortillas (flour)***
- ***8 slices ham (deli)***
- ***2 cups Swiss cheese (shredded)***
- ***1 ½ cup moboarella cheese (shredded)***
- ***Parsley (chopped, to garnish)***

Directions

1. Season the chicken breasts with garlic powder, oregano, pepper, and salt. Take an iron skillet and heat two tablespoons oil in it. Add the seasoned chicken to the skillet and cook for ten minutes on each side. Let the chicken to sit for ten minutes. Slice into thin strips.

2. Spread the Dijon mustard on four tortillas and top them with two ham slices. Add the chicken strips, mozzarella, and Swiss cheese. Place the leftover tortillas on top.

3. Heat a skillet and add one tablespoon oil to it. Cook the quesadillas to the skillet until the tortillas are brown in color and the cheese melts, for three minutes on both sides.

4. Slice the quesadillas and serve with parsley from the top.

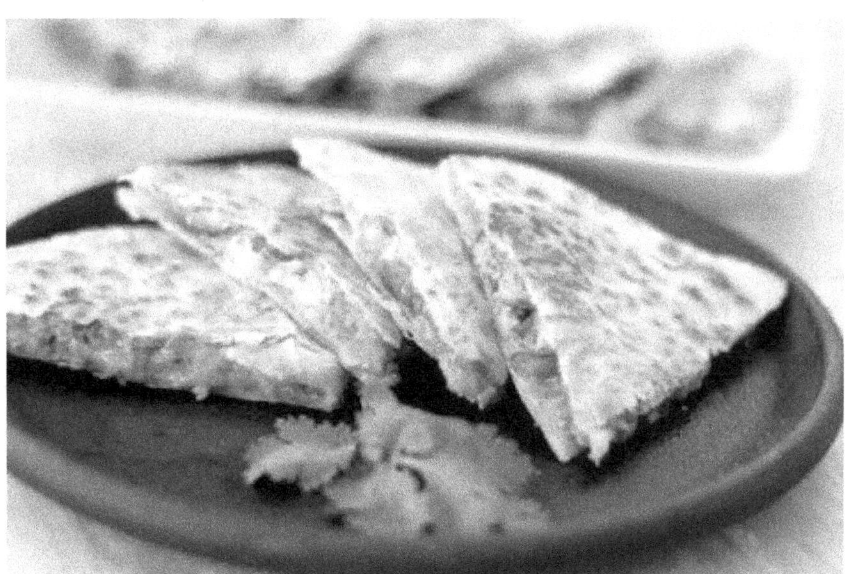

Nutrition

Calories: 340 Protein: 42g Carbs: 18.7g Fat: 11.3g Sugar: 10.3g

Preparation Time: 10’ *Cooking Time: 20’* *Serves: 6*

17. Paris’ Salad Nicoise

Ingredients

- *8 ounces green beans (halved)*
- *4 eggs*
- *2 tablespoons each*
- *Red wine vinegar*
- *Dijon mustard*
- *¼ cup olive oil (extra virgin)*
- *Black pepper (ground)*
- *Kosher salt*
- *2 sliced romaine hearts*
- *7 ounces canned tuna (drained)*
- *2 cups cherry tomatoes (halved)*
- *1 cup olives (sliced)*

Directions

1. Boil a pan of water with salt on medium heat. Add the green beans and cook for one minute. Wash the beans under cold water and pat dry them using a paper towel.
2. Again boil water in the pan and cook the eggs for ten minutes. Peel the boiled eggs and cut them lengthwise. Mix the mustard, oil, salt, pepper, and vinegar in a bowl. Add the sliced romaine for combining. Divide the salad among bowls and top it with tomatoes, tuna, green beans, olives, and sliced eggs.

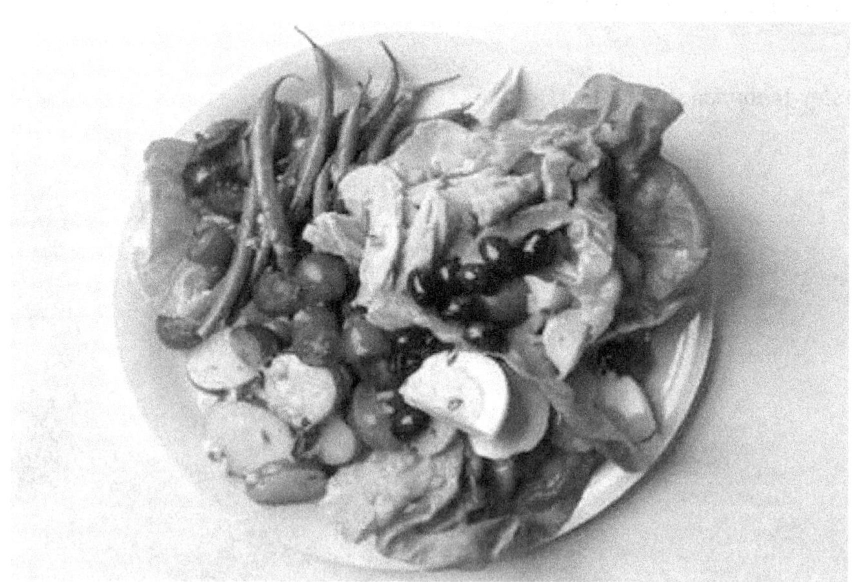

Nutrition

Calories: 382.2 Protein: 24g Carbs: 37.1g Fat: 17.8g

Preparation Time: 20' *Cooking Time: 0'* *Serves: 4*

18. BJ Restaurant's Fresh Mozzarella and Tomato Salad

Ingredients

- ***4 plum tomatoes, chopped***
- ***4 ounces fresh mozzarella cheese pearls, drained***
- ***¼ cup minced fresh basil***
- ***½ tablespoon minced fresh parsley***
- ***1 teaspoon minced fresh mint***
- ***2 tablespoons lemon juice***
- ***2 tablespoons olive oil***
- ***¼ teaspoon salt***
- ***1/8 Teaspoon black pepper***
- ***2 medium ripe avocados, peeled and chopped***

Directions

1. Prepare the veggies for the salad;
2. Take plum tomatoes and chop them;
3. Transfer the tomatoes to a salad bowl;
4. Spread a cheesecloth in a bowl and place the mozzarella cheese in this cheesecloth;
5. Hold the cheese in the cheesecloth and squeeze it to drain all the liquid out;
6. You can directly add the cheese pearls to the salad bowl or cut them in half to add to salad;
7. Take the mint and parsley sprigs and remove the stem from the leaves;
8. Chop the mint and parsley leaves then add to the salad bowl;
9. Toss in basil and mix all the veggies and cheese pearls well;
10. Refrigerate this salad for 15 minutes;
11. Meanwhile, prepare the salad dressing;
12. Take a small bowl, add lemon juice, black pepper, oil, and salt;
13. Mix these ingredients well then pour this dressing over the tomato salad;
14. Toss the salad again with the dressing to coat well;
15. Cover this mozzarella salad and refrigerate for 1 hour;
16. Cut the avocados in half and remove the pit;
17. Remove the avocado flesh and dice the flesh into cubes;
18. Add the avocado cubes to the tomato salad;
19. Serve fresh.

Nutrition

Calories: 178 Fat: 15g Carbs: 50g Sugars: 8g Protein: 9g

Preparation Time: 25' *Cooking Time: 5'* *Serves: 4*

19. BJ Restaurant's BJ's House Caesar Salad

Ingredients

- ***18 Cup grated Parmesan cheese***
- ***1/8 Cup mayonnaise***
- ***1 tablespoon milk***
- ***½ tablespoon lemon juice***
- ***½ tablespoon Dijon-mayonnaise***
- ***½ garlic clove, minced***
- ***Dash cayenne pepper***
- ***½ bunch romaine, torn***
- ***¼ cup croutons cubes***
- ***½ tablespoon olive oil***
- ***Grated Parmesan cheese, to serve***

Directions

1. Toss the croutons cubes with olive oil and spread these cubes in a baking sheet. Place the croutons in the oven and toast them for 5 minutes until golden brown in color. Allow the croutons to cool.

2. Meanwhile, prepare the remaining ingredients for the salad. Wash the romaine leaves in a colander and leave them to drain the excess liquid. Tear the romaine leaves and transfer them to a salad bowl. Shred the parmesan cheese with a grater and keep it ready aside;

3. Now prepare the salad dressing in a blender. Add mayonnaise, milk, lemon juice, Dijon mayonnaise, cayenne pepper and garlic to a blender jug. Hit the pulse button and blend the dressing until smooth and creamy. Pour half of this mayonnaise sauce into the salad and toss the romaine lettuce well. Refrigerate the salad for 30 minutes. Now remove the lettuce salad from the refrigerator. Add the shredded cheese to the Caesar salad and toss well. Top the Caesar salad with baked croutons. Garnish with extra parmesan cheese.

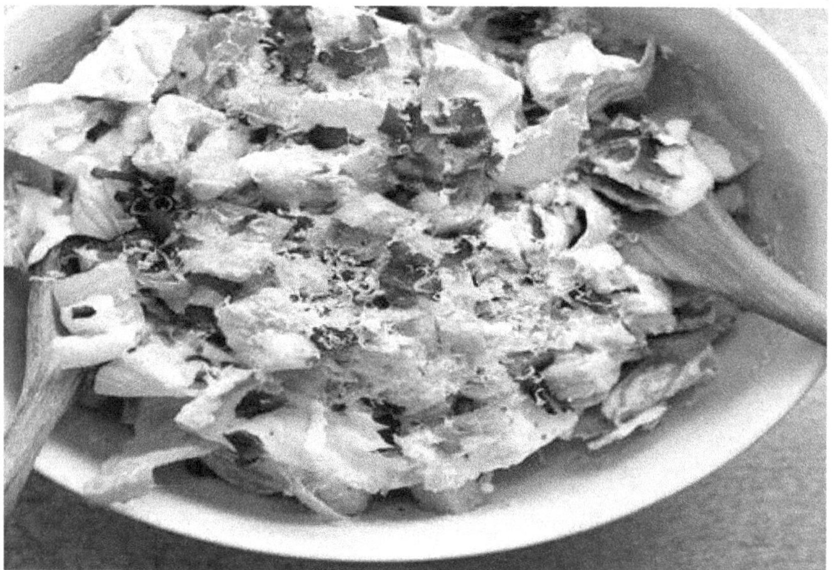

Nutrition

Calories: 150 Fat: 20g Carbs: 50g Sugars: 9g Protein: 15g

Preparation Time: 25' *Cooking Time: 42'* *Serves: 4*

20. BJ Restaurant's Tomato Bisque

Ingredients

- ***4 tablespoons unsalted butter***
- ***1 tablespoon minced bacon***
- ***1 Spanish onion, chopped***
- ***1 carrot, chopped***
- ***1 stalk celery, chopped***
- ***4 cloves garlic, minced***
- ***5 tablespoons all-purpose flour***
- ***5 cups chicken broth***
- ***1 (28-ounces) can whole tomatoes, chopped***
- ***3 parsley sprigs***
- ***3 fresh thyme sprigs***
- ***1 bay leaf***
- ***1 cup heavy cream***
- ***1 ¾ teaspoons kosher salt***
- ***Freshly ground black pepper***

Directions

1. Place a suitable soup pot over medium-high heat and add butter to melt; Stir in bacon and sauté until it turns crispy brown; Remove the sautéed bacon from the pot using a slotted spoon and place this bacon in a plate lined with a paper towel;

2. Reduce the stove's heat to medium-low and add carrots, celery, onion, and garlic; Sauté these veggies for 8 minutes with occasional stirring until the veggies turn soft; Slowly add the flour to the pot while mixing continuously;

3. Cook for 3 minutes then pour in broth; Mix until the cooked flour is thoroughly incorporated then add tomatoes. Cook this soup to a boil with occasional stirring; Tie thyme sprigs, parsley, and bay leaf together with kitchen twine;

4. Place the herbs bunch in the soup pot and reduce its heat to low. Cook this tomato soup on a simmer for 30 minutes. Now remove the cooked tomato soup from the heat and allow it to cool;

5. Discard the herb bundle from the soup. Puree the tomato soup in batches until smooth. When the tomato soup is finely pureed, pass it through a sieve placed over a soup bowl.

6. Return this soup puree to the soup pot and place it over medium heat. Stir in heavy cream and mix it until completely incorporated. Adjust seasoning with salt and black pepper. Divide the soup into the serving bowls. Garnish with crispy bacon.

7. Serve warm.

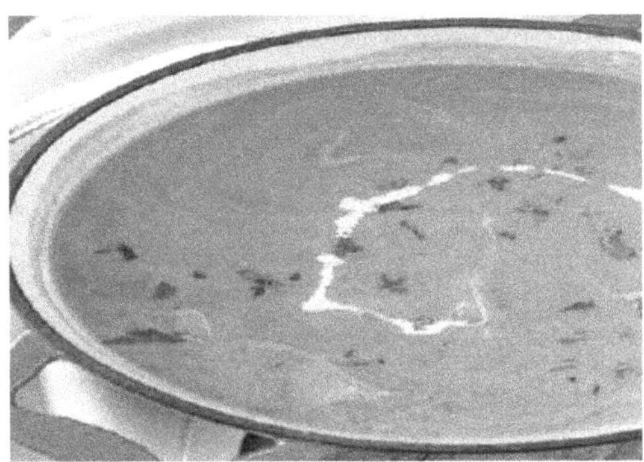

Nutrition

Calories: 160 Fat 10g Carbs: 50g Sugars: 6g Protein: 12g

Preparation Time: 10' *Cooking Time: 25'* *Serves: 5*

21. California Pizza's Cobb Salad with Ranch Dressing

Ingredients

For the Ranch Dressing:

- ***1 tablespoon ranch seasoning 3 tablespoons mayonnaise***
- ***2 tablespoons of water***

For the salad:

- ***½ pound roast chicken***
- ***3 ounces bacon, cooked***
- ***5 ounces chopped romaine lettuce***
- ***1 medium tomato, sliced***
- ***1 medium avocado, pitted, peeled, sliced***
- ***1 tablespoon chopped chives***
- ***½ teaspoon salt***
- ***1/3 teaspoon ground black pepper***
- ***2 hard-boiled eggs***
- ***2 ounces blue cheese, crumbled***

Directions

1. Prepare the dressing and for this, take a small bowl, put all your ingredients in it, then beat until well blended.
2. Assemble the salad and for this, cut the chicken into small pieces then divide it evenly between two bowls.
3. Peel the boiled eggs, cut them into slices and distribute them evenly in the salad bowls.
4. Add the vegetables, cheese and bacon, season the salad with salt and black pepper, then drizzle with the prepared vinaigrette.
5. Put some chives on top.

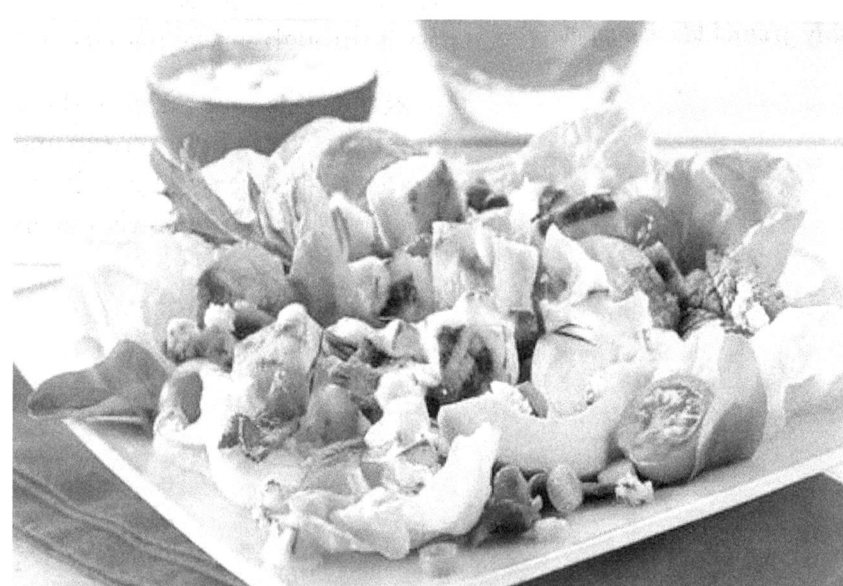

Nutrition

Calories: 100 Fat: 3g Carbs: 21g Sugars: 10g Protein: 5g

Preparation Time: 5' *Cooking Time: 10'* *Serves: 2*

22. Popeye's Parmesan Pork Chops

Ingredients

- ***4 boneless pork chops***
- ***½ teaspoon garlic powder***
- ***¼ teaspoon salt***
- ***¼ teaspoon ground white pepper***
- ***2 tablespoons avocado oil***
- ***1 egg***
- ***4 ounces grated parmesan***

Directions

1. Take a small bowl, place the garlic powder, add the salt and the black pepper and stir until everything is mixed.
2. Put some of the spice mixture on both sides of the pork chops, then press them.
3. Take a shallow dish, break the egg, and beat until it is frothy.
4. Take a separate shallow dish, place Parmesan cheese on top. Dip the slices pork in the egg, then garnish with cheese.
5. Take a skillet, place on medium-high heat, add oil and, when hot, add a prepared pork chop, then cook for 5 minutes on each side until golden and tender.
6. When finished, transfer the pork chops to a plate, then repeat with the remaining chops.
7. Serve immediately with cauliflower puree.

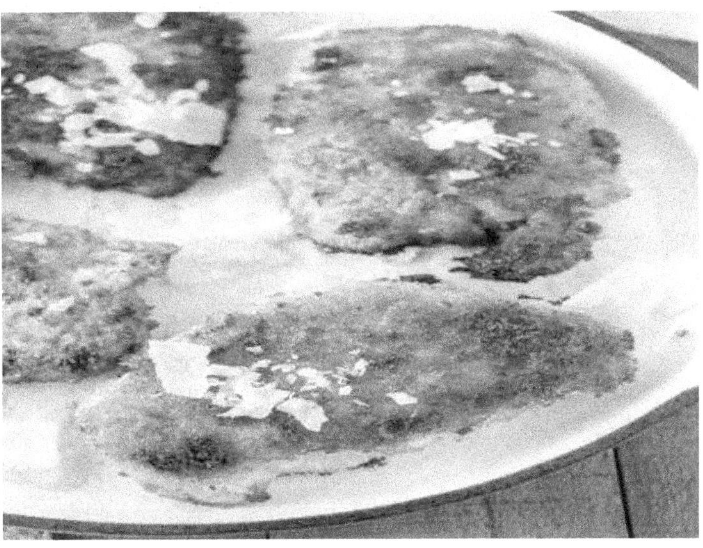

Nutrition

Calories: 147 Fat: 17g Carbs: 87g Sugars: 15g Protein: 14g

Preparation Time: 10' *Cooking Time: 20'* *Serves: 6*

23. Popeye's Chicken Strips

Ingredients

- ***2 pounds chicken breasts 2/3 cup almond flour***
- ***2 teaspoons of salt***
- ***1 teaspoon chipotle chili powder 2 teaspoons smoked paprika***
- ***1/3 cup low-carb Louisiana hot sauce***
- ***3 eggs***
- ***½ cup almond milk, sugar-free avocado oil as needed for frying***

Directions

1. Take a small bowl, pour the milk, and then beat the hot sauce.
2. Cut each chicken breast into four strips, place them in a large bowl, and pour half the milk mixture and leave to marinate for at least 1 hour.
3. Then take a shallow dish, place the flour and add the salt, paprika, and chipotle until they are combined.
4. Break the eggs with the rest of the milk mixture, then beat until they are frothy.
5. When the chicken is marinated, drain it well, fluff each chicken strip in the flour mixture, immerse it in the egg mixture and stir again in the flour mixture.
6. When you're ready to cook, take a large skillet, fill it with 2 ½ inches of oil, and bring the oil to 360 degrees F.
7. Then, lower the chicken pieces in the oil, do not overload them, then cook 5–7 minutes on each side. Do this until they are cooked and golden.
8. Transfer the chicken pieces to a plate lined with a paper towel, then repeat with the remaining chicken pieces.
9. Serve immediately.

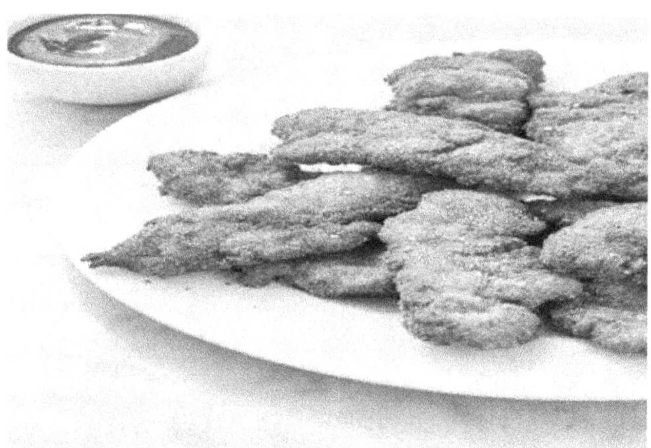

Nutrition

Calories: 242.8 Fat: 6.6g Carbs: 38.4g Sugars: 3g Protein: 8.4g

Preparation Time: 15' *Cooking Time: 25'* *Serves: 12*

24. Popeye's Zesty Coleslaw

Ingredients

- ***1 cup mayonnaise***
- ***1/3 cup sugar***
- ***3 tablespoons apple cider vinegar***
- ***1 teaspoon seasoned salt***
- ***¾ teaspoon pepper***
- ***½ teaspoon celery seeds***
- ***2 packages (14 ounces each) of coleslaw mix***
- ***1 small sweet red pepper, chopped***
- ***½ cup thinly sliced sweet onion***

Directions

1. Combine the first 6 ingredients and add the coleslaw, red pepper and onion mixture; set aside. Refrigerate at least 1 hour before serving.

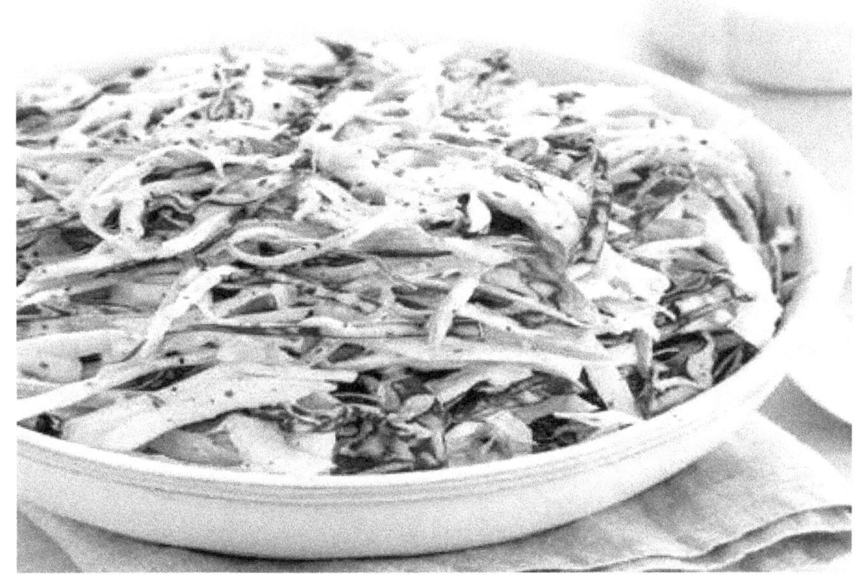

Nutrition

Calories: 150 Fat: 4.2g Carbs: 40g Sugars: 1g Protein: 9g

Chapter 2
The perfect Mains

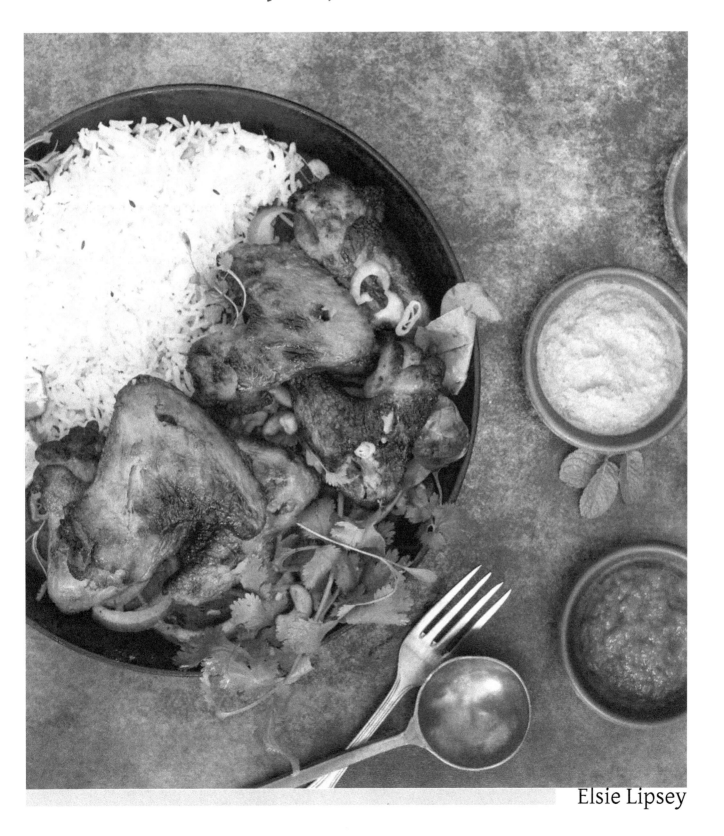

Preparation Time: 20' *Cooking Time: 10'* *Serves: 2*

25. Maggiano's Little Italy's Steamed Mussels

Ingredients

- ***1 tablespoon freshly squeezed lemon juice***
- ***20 mussels***
- ***½ teaspoon chopped basil***
- ***2 tablespoons cannellini beans***
- ***¾ cup chicken stock***
- ***½ tablespoon of minced garlic***
- ***½ cup white wine***
- ***2 tablespoons sun-dried tomatoes***
- ***2 tablespoons butter***
- ***½ tablespoon chopped parsley***
- ***Salt and pepper***

Directions

1. Combine the garlic and wine in a pan over medium heat.
2. Once hot, add the mussels and cook covered on high until the mussels open, about 5 minutes.
3. Put in the remaining ingredients, stir and allow to simmer over medium heat for 2-3 minutes. Put some pepper and salt to taste.
4. Serve the mussels in a bowl, drizzle with sauce, and then serve with 2-3 slices garlic toast.

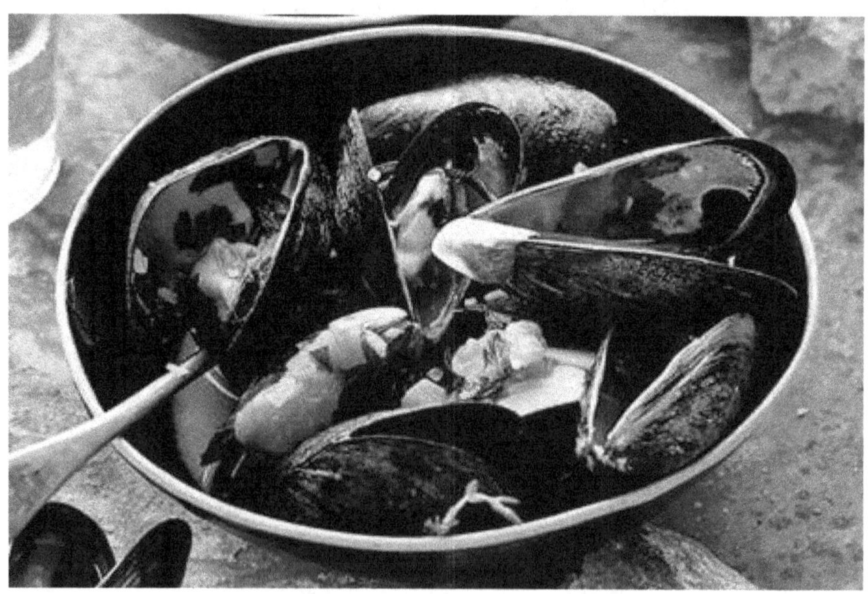

Nutrition

Calories: 178 Fat: 15g Carbs: 50g Sugars: 8g Protein: 9g

Preparation Time: 20' *Cooking Time: 20'* *Serves: 15*

26. Maggiano's Little Italy's Spinach and Artichoke Al Forno

Ingredients

- ***½ cup sliced scallions***
- ***2 cups canned artichokes (drained and rinsed)***
- ***1 cup heavy cream***
- ***2 cups shredded Asiago cheese***
- ***3 tablespoons olive oil***
- ***2 cups sautéed spinach (drained and sliced)***
- ***Pepper and salt to taste***
- ***1 tablespoon grated parmesan cheese***
- ***¼ cup chopped sun-dried tomatoes***

Directions

1. Preheat your oven to 350°F.
2. Put the scallions, heavy cream, spinach, Asiago cheese, olive oil, tomatoes, and artichokes in a bowl, then put some pepper and salt to taste.
3. Transfer the mixture into a greased oven friendly bowl, then top the mixture with the shredded parmesan cheese. Place the bowl in the middle tier of the oven and bake for 20 minutes at 350°F. Remove from the oven. Serve with slices Italian bread.

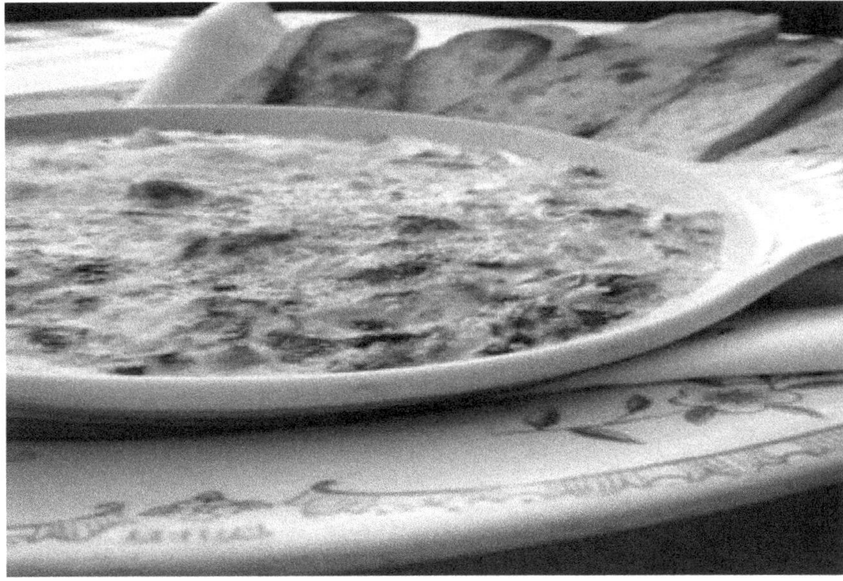

Nutrition

Calories: 150 Fat: 20g Carbs: 50g Protein: 15g

Preparation Time: 20' *Cooking Time: 50'* *Serves: 8*

27. Maggiano's Little Italy's Tuscan Sausage and Orzo Soup

Ingredients

- *1 tablespoon of Italian seasoning*
- *1 pound Italian sausage (casing removed)*
- *2 teaspoons fennel seeds (crushed)*
- *2 celery sticks (finely sliced)*
- *2 bay leaves*
- *4 cups chicken broth*
- *1 tablespoon of olive oil*
- *1 teaspoon red pepper flakes*
- *1 can of cannellini beans*
- *2 carrots*
- *1 ½ cups orzo*
- *1 can of stewed tomatoes with juice*
- *3 cloves garlic*
- *1 onion*
- *2 tablespoons ketchup*
- *Romano cheese for topping (optional)*

Directions

1. Cook the sausage over high heat until well browned, stirring frequently.
2. Add the celery, onions, garlic, crushed fennel seeds, carrots, Italian seasoning and pepper flakes.
3. Season salt and pepper to taste, then sauté until all the vegetables start to soften.
4. Add the broth, tomatoes, beans, ketchup and bay leaves, stir and bring to a boil, then allow to simmer for 25-30 minutes.
5. Cook the orzo separately. After this, drain and toss with olive oil to prevent it from sticking.
6. Add the orzo to the soup and cook for 1 minute.
7. Pour the soup into bowls and top it with grated Romano cheese.

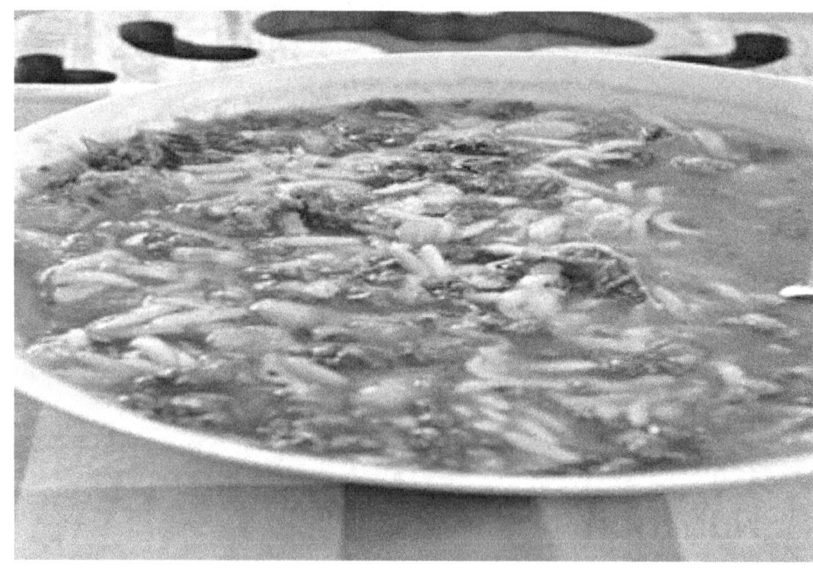

Nutrition

Calories: 160 Fat: 10g Carbs: 50g Sugars: 6g Protein: 12g

Preparation Time: 20' *Cooking Time: 0'* *Serves: 10*

28. Maggiano's Little Italy's Maggiano's Salad

Ingredients

- ***Corn oil (for frying)***
- ***5 cups chopped Romaine lettuce (cut into bite-sized pieces)***
- ***½ cup thinly sliced prosciutto***
- ***1 red onion (thinly sliced)***
- ***5 cups chopped iceberg lettuce (cut into bite-sized pieces)***
- ***½ cup crumbled blue cheese***

Dressing:

- ***1/8 teaspoon of dried oregano***
- ***1 tablespoon dijon mustard***
- ***2 cups vegetable oil***
- ***2 teaspoons of granulated sugar***
- ***Freshly ground pepper to taste***
- ***¾ cups water***
- ***1/3 cup red wine vinegar***
- ***Salt to taste***
- ***2 teaspoons minced garlic***

Directions

1. Put half a cup corn oil in a large skillet over medium heat, add prosciutto and cook for about 2-3 minutes.
2. After that, remove from heat and place on pieces of parchment paper to drain excess oil. Let it cool for 3–5 minutes, then crumble and set aside.
3. Combine the sugar, mustard, water, vinegar, and garlic in a medium mixing bowl, then season with salt to taste.
4. Slowly stir in the oil, then whisk until well combined and the sugar is completely dissolved.
5. Add the oregano and pepper and whisk again until well combined.
6. Toss the cheese, lettuce, prosciutto, and onion in a large salad bowl, drizzle some dressing over the salad and mix. Refrigerate any leftover dressing for later.

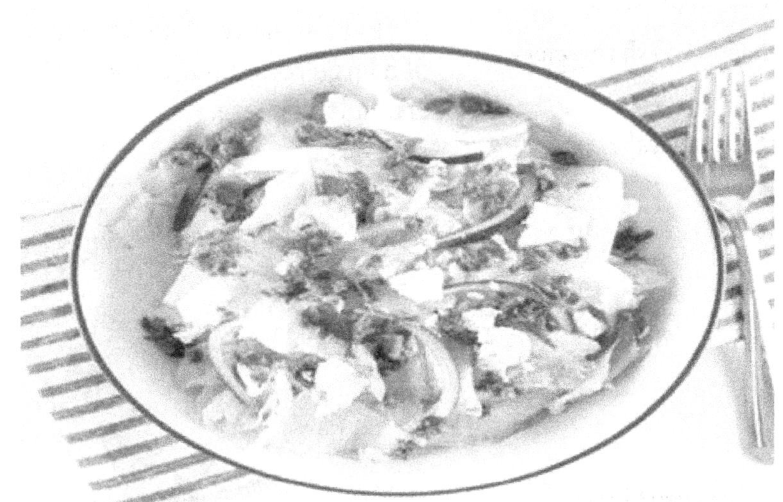

Nutrition

Calories: 140 Fat: 8g Carbs: 30 Sugars: 10g Protein: 25g

Preparation Time: 20' *Cooking Time: 15'* *Serves: 3*

29. Maggiano's Little Italy's New York Steak Al Forno

Ingredients

- ***Salt and pepper to taste***
- ***1 New York steak (large)***
- ***¼ cup sliced gorgonzola cheese***
- ***½ cup sliced red onion***
- ***1 tablespoon chopped parsley and basil***
- ***1 tablespoon softened butter***
- ***1 tablespoon garlic butter***
- ***¼ cup balsamic sauce***
- ***3 ounces roasted portabella mushrooms***
- ***Herb Marinade***
- ***¼ cup chopped fresh thyme leaves***
- ***½ cup olive oil***
- ***¼ cup minced garlic***
- ***1 tablespoon of freshly ground whole black peppercorns***
- ***¼ cup chopped fresh rosemary leaves***
- ***¼ cup chopped fresh sage leaves***

Directions

1. To make the herb marinade, put all the ingredients into a blender and pulse until smooth (add 2 tablespoons of water if difficult).

2. Rub the pepper and salt into the meat, add two tablespoons of the herb marinade and rub until the meat is coated with the mixture.

3. Put the meat in a broiler and cook for 3-4 minutes on one side over medium heat or until a brown crust forms, then flip and cook for the same amount of time or until the other side is well browned too.

4. Spread the garlic butter sauce on the steak halfway through the cooking time and let coat.

5. Sauté the mushrooms and onion in a pan over medium heat until they are both soft, add the balsamic glaze, stir and allow to cook for a minute or two.

6. Add the butter and chopped parsley/basil, stir and cook until butter is fully melted and well incorporated.

7. Put the sautéed mushrooms and onion mixture at the bottom of a large round plate, top with browned steak, then top with crumbled cheese.

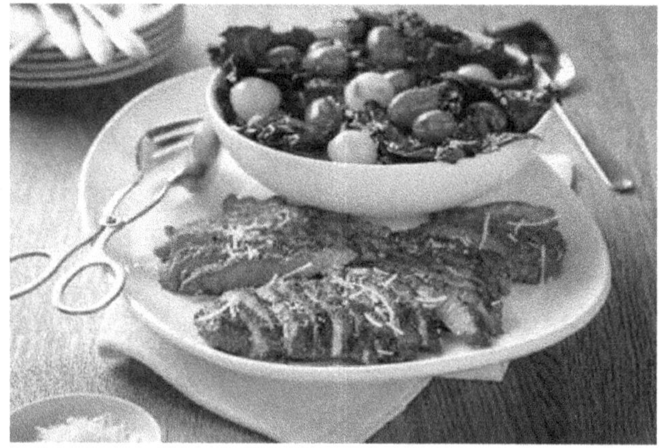

Nutrition

Calories: 115 Fat: 14g Carbs: 78g Sugars: 9g Protein: 8g

Preparation Time: 15' *Cooking Time: 30'* *Serves: 4*

30. Maggiano's Little Italy's Beef Medallion

Ingredients

- *¾ cup dry wine*
- *2 cups beef broth*
- *¼ teaspoon of freshly ground black pepper*
- *¾ cup whipping cream*
- *2 tablespoons of mixed dried wild mushrooms*
- *1 teaspoon of roasted garlic*
- *2 teaspoons of canola oil*
- *Salt to taste*
- *¼ cup diced shallots*
- *8 beef medallions*
- *1 tablespoon of softened butter*

Directions

1. Preheat your oven to 350°F.
2. Let the mushrooms be soaked in warm water for 20 minutes or until soft. Strain and reserve the liquid to be used later.
3. Heat one teaspoon of oil and the butter in a pan over medium heat, add shallots, mushrooms and roasted garlic, then cook until shallots start to brown, about 4 minutes, stirring frequently.
4. Pour in the wine and after for 2–3 minutes, add the broth and allow to simmer until the mixture loses half its moisture, about 8 minutes.
5. Rub the pepper and salt into the beef, heat the remaining oil into a large skillet over medium heat, then sear the meat for 2–3 minutes on each side.
6. Put into the oven and cook for 10–20 minutes until tender.
7. Serve it with some sauce on top.

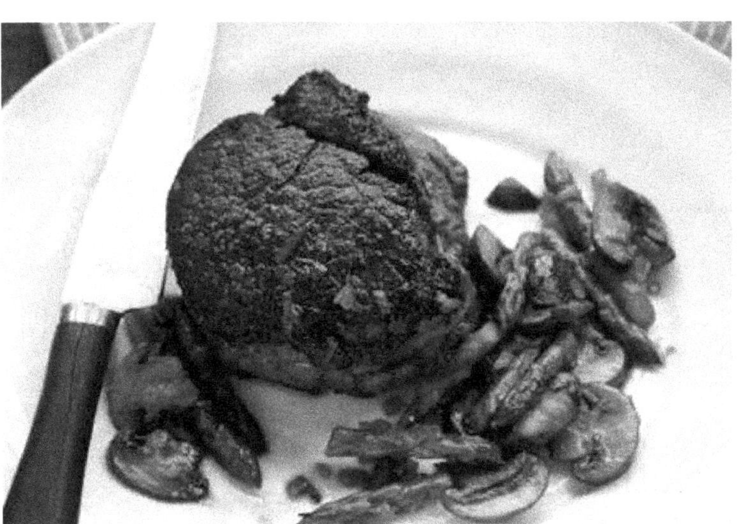

Nutrition

Calories: 112 Fat: 17g Carbs: 50g Sugars: 5g Protein: 7g

Preparation Time: 10' *Cooking Time: 20'* *Serves: 4*

31. Maggiano's Little Italy's Veal Marsala

Ingredients

- *¾ cup low sodium chicken broth*
- *8 veal cutlets*
- *2 ounces mixed mushrooms (sliced)*
- *Salt and pepper to taste*
- *½ cup sweet Marsala*
- *1 shallot (sliced)*
- *3 tablespoons unsalted butter*
- *1 tablespoon chopped fresh rosemary leaves*
- *3 cloves garlic (crushed)*
- *3 tablespoons olive oil*

Directions

1. Season salt and pepper all over the veal cutlets.
2. Heat two tablespoons of oil and butter in a large skillet over medium heat, add veal cutlets. Cook each side for 2-3 minutes or until browned, then remove and keep warm until ready to use.
3. Heat the oil in the skillet, add garlic and sauté until soft and fragrant, and then add the mushrooms.
4. Add some pepper and salt to season, then add the Marsala and cook for 2-3 minutes.
5. Add the rosemary leaves and broth, stir and cook for 4 minutes, then add the cutlets and cook for 1-2 minutes, pouring the sauce over the veal while stirring.
6. Stir in the last tablespoon of butter and cook for a minute or until the butter has completely melted.
7. Put the cutlets on plates and scoop the sauce over them.

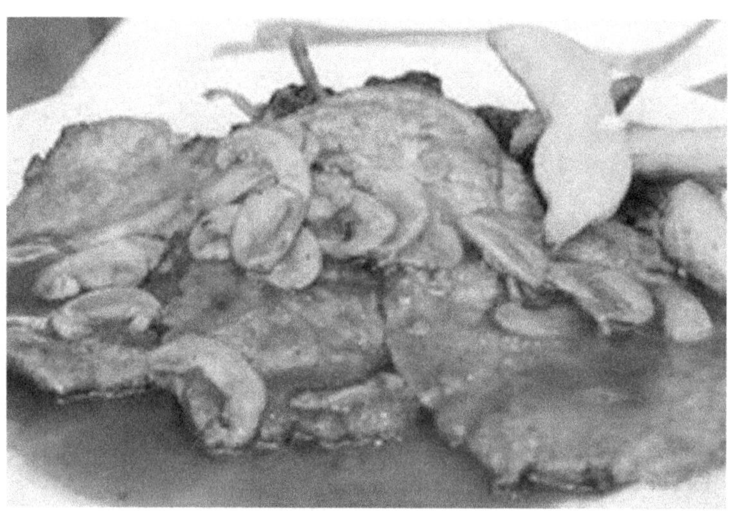

Nutrition

Calories: 80 Fat: 4g Carbs: 20g Sugars: 2g Protein: 15g

Preparation Time: 25' *Cooking Time: 1 hour* *Serves: 6*

32. Maggiano's Little Italy's Whole Roasted Chicken

Ingredients

- ***Salt and pepper to taste***
- ***1 whole chicken (washed and dried with a paper towel)***
- ***2 tablespoons lemon zest***
- ***½ cup softened butter***
- ***2 tablespoons olive oil***
- ***4 lemon wedges***
- ***¼ cup sliced onions***
- ***¼ cup chopped fresh rosemary leaves***
- ***2 ½ tablespoons freshly squeezed lemon juice***
- ***3 cloves garlic (minced)***

Directions

1. Preheat your oven to 425°F.
2. Put the olive oil, butter, lemon zest, garlic, and rosemary into a medium bowl, stir until well combined, then set aside.
3. Put some pepper and salt all over the chicken and inside the cavity.
4. Brush a generous amount of the butter mixture into the chicken, making sure it is properly coated.
5. Drizzle the lemon juice all over the chicken and stuff with chopped rosemary, two lemon wedges, and sliced onions.
6. Place the chicken on the pan and put into the oven. Bake for 40-45 minutes, remove from the oven and baste with more of the butter mixture.
7. Bake the chicken in the oven for another 10-15 minutes or until golden brown.
8. Remove the chicken from the oven and let it cool before serving.

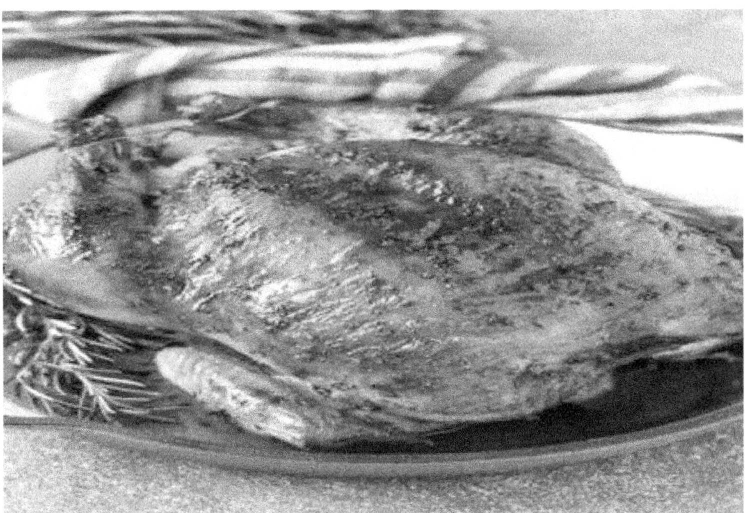

Nutrition

Calories: 178 Fat: 24g Carbs: 123g Sugars: 15g Protein: 27g

Preparation Time: 15' *Cooking Time: 10'* *Serves: 9*

33. Maggiano's Little Italy's Garlic Shrimp and Shells

Ingredients

- *¼ cup white wine*
- *¼ pound shrimp (peeled and deveined)*
- *½ pound cooked shell pasta*
- *¼ cup extra-virgin olive oil*
- *1 tablespoons garlic butter*
- *½ cup clam juice*
- *¼ teaspoon freshly ground black pepper*
- *Pepper and salt to taste*
- *1 cup fresh tomatoes (remove seeds, peel skin, and slice)*
- *4 fresh basil leaves (torn apart)*
- *¼ cup marinara sauce*
- *1 tablespoon minced garlic*

Directions

1. Marinate the shrimp with ground black pepper, salt to taste, and half of the olive oil.
2. Dip the shrimp in a bowl of hot water for less than a minute. Once the skin has softened, peel it off, then squeeze the tomatoes to remove the seeds before slicing into bits.
3. Put some oil in a pan and add the shrimp and sauté until they start to pinken about 3 minutes.
4. Add the minced garlic and sauté until fragrant, about 1 minute, then put in the tomatoes, clam juice and white wine, stir and bring to a boil.
5. Reduce the heat to medium, add garlic butter, marinara sauce, and basil, stir and allow to cook for 1-2 minutes.
6. Put in the pasta shells and simmer until al dente, then season with pepper and salt to taste.

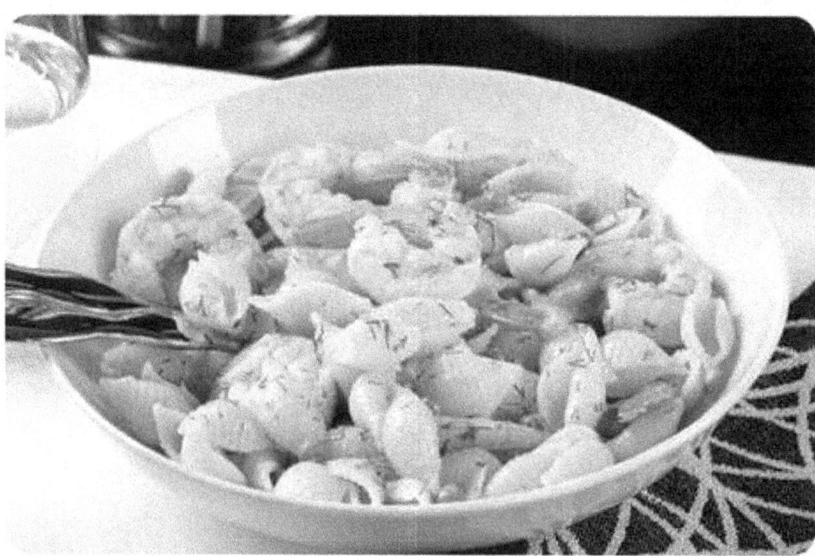

Nutrition

Calories: 119 Fat: 20g Carbs: 76g Sugars: 12g Protein: 10g

Preparation Time: 10' *Cooking Time: 15'* *Serves: 8*

34. Prudhomme's Poultry Magic

Ingredients

- ***½ teaspoons salt***
- ***¼ teaspoon cayenne pepper***
- ***½ teaspoon onion powder***
- ***¼ teaspoon granulated garlic***
- ***½ teaspoon paprika***
- ***¼ teaspoon ground dark pepper***
- ***¼ teaspoon scoured sage***
- ***¼ teaspoon dried thyme***
- ***¼ teaspoon dried oregano***
- ***1/8 teaspoon cumin***
- ***Red Lobster's Shrimp Diablo***
- ***3 lb. Huge Uncooked Shrimp in the Shells***
- ***Milk***
- ***½ lb. Unsalted Butter***
- ***BBQ Sauce (One jar Kraft)***
- ***½ cup Ketchup***
- ***1 tablespoon fresh ground pepper***
- ***¼ cup Frank's Red Hot Sauce***
- ***Chicken***
- ***Turkey***
- ***Water***

Directions

1. Combine all fixings and store in a sealed shut compartment. Use as a flavoring for chicken, turkey, or some other poultry.
2. Wash shrimp in cool water and expel heads if necessary.
3. Blend all sauce fixings in a sauce dish and mix until bubbling. Expel from warm and refrigerate for at any rate four hours. Channel milk from shrimp, place them in a heating skillet, and spread equitably with the sauce. Let stand 60 minutes. Heat in the preheated broiler (450ºF) for 15 minutes.

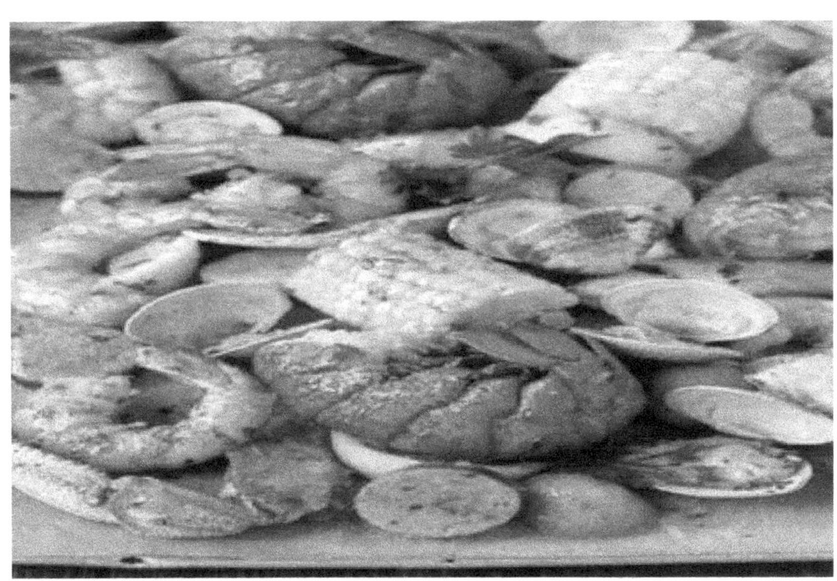

Nutrition

Calories: 184 Fat: 4g Carbs: 57g Sugars: 9g Protein: 12g

Preparation Time: 15' *Cooking Time: 30'* *Serves: 4*

35. Red Lobster's Ultimate Fondue

Ingredients

- ***1 cup Velveeta, cubed***
- ***1 cup swiss cheddar in little pieces***
- ***1 can Campbell's dense cream of shrimp soup 1 cup milk***
- ***½ teaspoon cayenne***
- ***½ teaspoon paprika***
- ***1 cooked lobster tail or ½ cups impersonation***

Directions

1. Slashed and Join everything except for the lobster in a medium pot and cook over low warmth until dissolved, blending sometimes. At the point when softened.
2. Mix in the lobster meat. Trimming with diced red pepper, whenever wanted, and present with French bread.

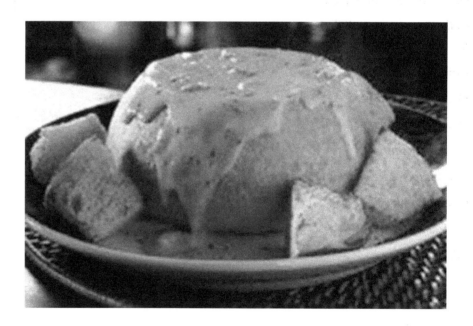

Nutrition

Calories: 147 Fat: 17g Carbs: 87g Sugars: 15g Protein: 14g

Preparation Time: 30' *Cooking Time: 1 hour* *Serves: 3*

36. Ruby Tuesday's White Chicken Chili

Ingredients

- ***6 cups chicken stock***
- ***1 lb. sack incredible northern beans (absorbed water for the time being)***
- ***2 medium onions, cleaved***
- ***6 cups diced cooked chicken***
- ***2 jalapeno peppers, seeded diced***
- ***2 diced stew peppers***
- ***½ teaspoons oregano 2 teaspoons cumin***
- ***¼ teaspoon cayenne pepper***
- ***2 garlic cloves, minced***
- ***1 cup salsa***
- ***1 tablespoon vegetable oil***
- ***Pinch salt (to taste)***

Directions

1. Heat beans, a large portion of the onions, and a large portion of the garlic for 2 hours in the chicken stock.
2. Include chicken and salsa. Sauté pepper, flavors, and the rest of the onions and garlic in the oil and add to the stew. Heat for one more hour.

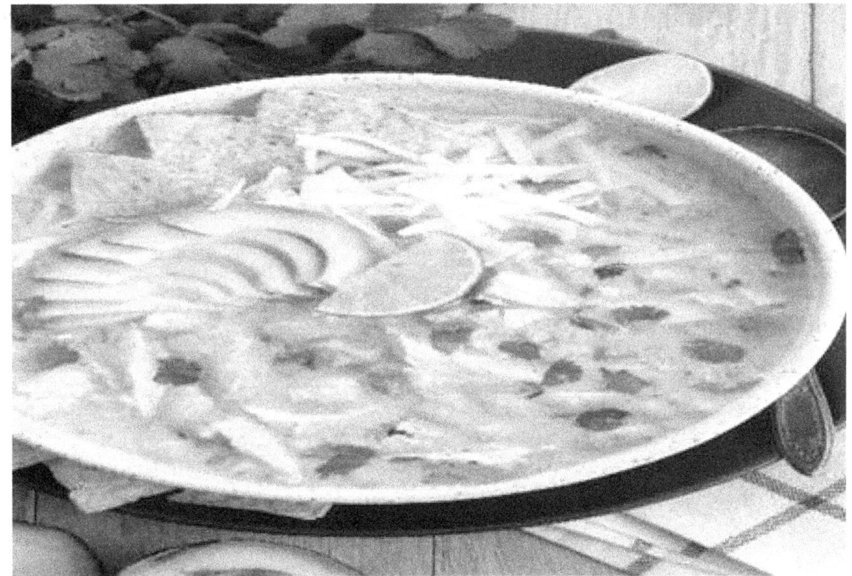

Nutrition

Calories: 158 Fat: 10g Carbs: 71g Sugars: 14g Protein: 7g

Preparation Time: 30' *Cooking Time: 45'* *Serves: 5*

37. Ruby Tuesday's Chicken Quesadillas

Ingredients

- ***5 ounces chicken bosom***
- ***Italian dressing***
- ***12-inch flour tortilla margarine***
- ***1 cup destroyed Monterey jack/ cheddar***
- ***1 tablespoon tomatoes, diced***
- ***1 tablespoon jalapeno peppers, diced***
- ***Cajun seasoning (to taste)***
- ***½ cup destroyed lettuce***
- ***¼ cup diced tomatoes sour cream***

Directions

1. Spot chicken bosom in a bowl with enough Italian dressing to cover; permit to marinate 30 minutes, refrigerated. Barbecue marinated chicken until done in a daintily oiled dish. Slice to three-quarter, (pieces) then keeps safe. Brush some margarine one side of tortilla and spot in a griddle over medium warmth. On one portion of tortilla, including cheddar, 1 tablespoon tomatoes, peppers, and Cajun preparing in a specific order. Try to spread to the edge of the half. Top with diced chicken, crease void tortilla side on top, and flip over in skillet with the goal that cheddar is on the head of the chicken. Cook until exceptionally warm all through.

2. Expel from skillet to serving plate and cut into six equivalent wedges on one side of the plate. On the opposite side put lettuce, finished off with ¼ cup tomatoes, and afterward finished off with acrid cream. Serve your preferred salsa in a little bowl as an afterthought.

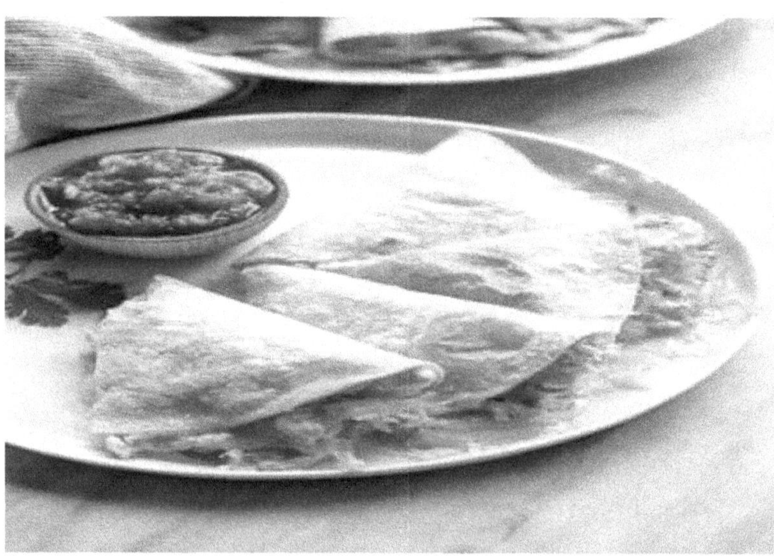

Nutrition

Calories: 242.8 Fat: 6.6g Carbs: 38.4g Sugars: 3g Protein: 8.4g

Preparation Time: 10' *Cooking Time: 30'* *Serves: 8*

38. Sbarro's Chicken Francese

Ingredients

- *5 (5-ounces) chicken bosoms*
- *5 eggs*
- *3 ounces Romano cheddar*
- *1 teaspoon of dehydrated parsley*
- *1 cup flour*
- *Pinch white pepper*
- *1 cup chicken stock*
- *½ pound spread juice from 2 lemons*
- *1.5 cups oil (10% olive oil, 90% vegetable oil)*

Directions

1. Lemon cuts and cleaved new parsley for embellish Pound chicken bosoms level and cut down the middle.
2. Put in a safe spot. Scramble eggs in the blending bowl. Include Romano cheddar, parsley, and white pepper. Blend and keep safe.
3. Put flour in a huge shallow bowl.
4. In a skillet, heat oil over medium warmth. Check the temperature by plunging an edge of a chicken piece in oil. On the off chance that it bubbles gradually, oil is prepared. Coat the two sides of a bit of chicken with flour. Dunk chicken in egg blend, ensuring all flour is secured with egg. Let abundance egg dribble off, at that point place chicken in hot oil. Rehash with 4 additional pieces. Fry each side of chicken until light fair shading. Expel from oil to a serving plate - keep warm. Rehash with other chicken pieces.
5. Carry chicken stock to a light bubble. Include spread, mixing consistently, until liquefied. Include lemon squeeze and cook for 1 moment while mixing persistently. Pour sauce over chicken and enhancement with lemon cuts and slashed new parsley.

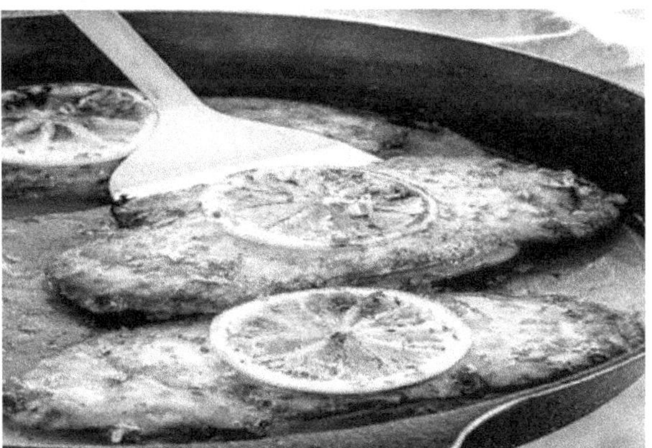

Nutrition

Calories: 150 Fat: 4.2g Carbs: 40g Sugars: 1g Protein: 9g

Preparation Time: 15' *Cooking Time: 30'* *Serves: 4*

39. Sbarro's Rigatoni Ala Vodka

Ingredients

- *2 lbs. rigatoni*
- *24 ounces canned pureed tomatoes (plain)*
- *2 tablespoons olive oil*
- *2 cloves new garlic, minced*
- *½ teaspoon split red pepper*
- *1 tablespoon salt*
- *½ teaspoon dark pepper*
- *1 teaspoon dried basil*
- *½ quart substantial cream*
- *½ ounces vodka*
- *1 ounces ground Romano Cheese*
- *1 ounces bacon bits*
- *½ ounces Italian parsley slashed*

Directions

1. In a medium sauce skillet, heat oil until hot. Include garlic and sauté until brilliant earthy colored. Include pureed tomatoes, salt, red pepper, dark pepper, and basil. Cook over medium warmth, mixing sometimes until completely warmed. Include substantial cream and vodka. Mix to blend and cook for a while.

2. Bubble rigatoni (don't overcook). In a blending bowl, join depleted pasta with cream sauce. Blend altogether. Place it to a bowl and top with ground cheddar, bacon, and parsley. Serve right away.

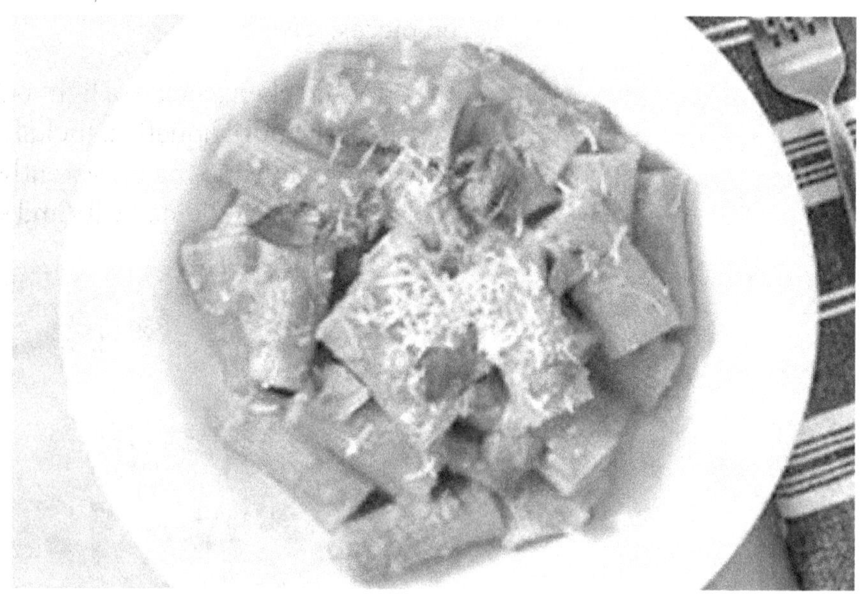

Nutrition

Calories: 100 Fat: 3g Carbs: 21g Sugars: 10g Protein: 5g

Preparation Time: 10' *Cooking Time: 20'* *Serves: 3*

40. Steak and Ale's Burgundy Mushrooms

Ingredients

- *¼ pounds mushrooms*
- *2 quarts water*
- *¼ cup lemon juice*
- *4 tablespoons margarine*
- *¾ cup yellow onions, diced*
- *½ cup Burgundy*
- *1 tablespoon hamburger bouillon granules*
- *¼ teaspoon garlic powder*
- *1/3 teaspoon ground white pepper*

Directions

1. Clean and dry the mushrooms. Join water and lemon juice in a secured saucepan. Bring to a bubble. In another pot, liquefy margarine and sauté onions until smooth (around 5 minutes).

2. In a bowl, add flavors and bouillon to Burgundy. Rush until bouillon is broken up. Add wine blend to onions. Stew over medium warmth around 10 minutes (until the liquor has vanished). Expel from heat. Add mushrooms to bubbling lemon water. Come back to the bubble. Expel whitened mushrooms from heat and altogether channel. Add mushrooms to wine sauce and mix until mixed.

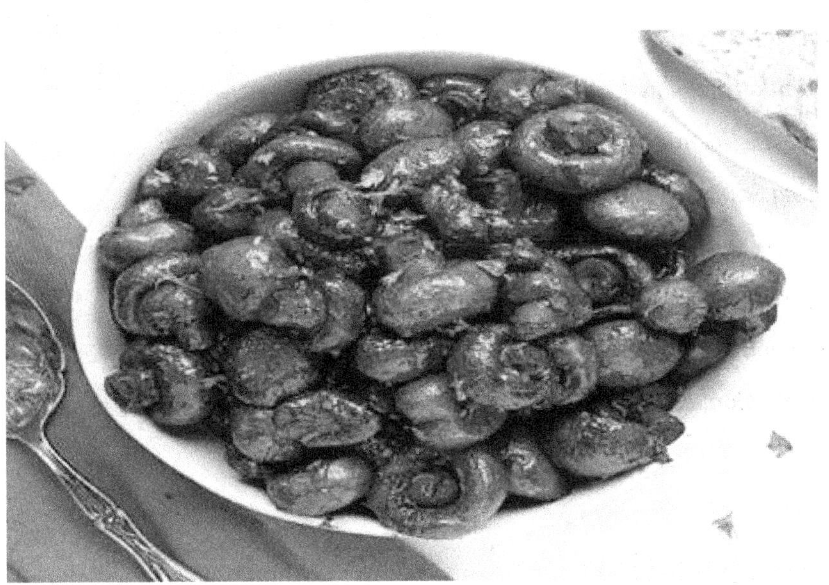

Nutrition

Calories: 178 Fat: 15g Carbs: 50g Sugars: 8g Protein: 9g

Preparation Time: 10' *Cooking Time: 30'* *Serves: 4*

41. T.G.I Friday's Pot Stickers

Ingredients

Batter:

- ***2 ½ cups flour***
- ***½ teaspoon salt***
- ***1 cup heated water***
- ***1 tablespoon oil***

Filling:

- ***1 pound ground pork***
- ***2 tablespoon soy sauce***
- ***1 tablespoon sesame oil***
- ***1 teaspoon ground ginger***
- ***Touch of sugar, salt, and pepper should be added to taste***
- ***3 green onions***
- ***1 egg***
- ***1 tablespoon corn starch***
- ***1 can water***
- ***Chestnuts finely hacked***
- ***1 clove garlic, minced***

Plunging Sauce:

- ***½ cup soy sauce***
- ***¼ cup white vinegar***
- ***1 teaspoon stew oil***
- ***1 green onion, cleaved***

Directions

1. Consolidate the flour, salt, high temp water, and oil in a bowl and fuse into a smooth batter.
2. Permit the mixture to rest for 20 minutes.
3. Consolidate the filling fixings. Join the plunging sauce fixings.
4. Turn the batter out around 1/8 thick.
5. Utilize a bread shaper or a glass to remove 3-inch circles.
6. Brush some water on the circles and add around 2 teaspoons of filling.
7. Overlay the circles into equal parts and press to seal, making a point to crush out any air.
8. Stand the dumplings up on the collapsed side and press marginally with the goal that they stand up pleasant.
9. To cook, carry a pot of salted water to bubble, and heat the dumplings until cooked through around 5 minutes. Channel well. The dumplings might be solidified now for some time later; this formula makes about 8 dozen. Warmth a skillet with around 2 tablespoon oil and fry the dumplings on one side just, until pleasantly seared.

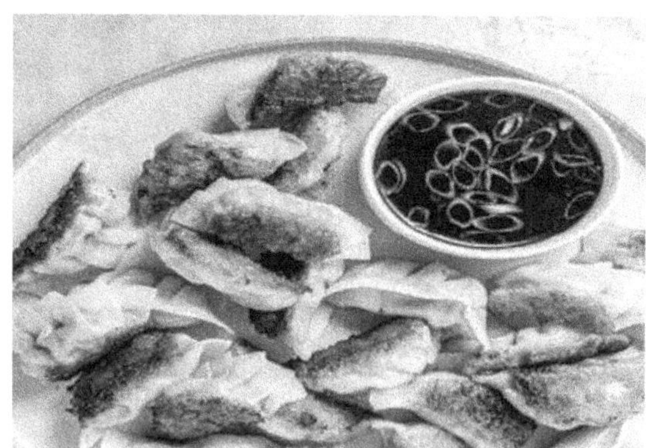

Nutrition

Calories: 150 Fat: 20g Carbs: 50g Sugars: 9g Protein: 15g

Preparation Time: 20' *Cooking Time: 6'* *Serves: 6*

42. Steak n' Shake's Chili

Ingredients

- ***1 tablespoon olive oil***
- ***2 pounds ground beef***
- ***½ teaspoon salt***
- ***2 tablespoons onion powder***
- ***1 tablespoon chili powder***
- ***2 teaspoons ground cumin***
- ***½ teaspoon ground black pepper***
- ***2 teaspoons cocoa powder***
- ***6 ounces canned tomato paste***
- ***13 ½ ounces canned tomato sauce***
- ***1 cup Pepsi***
- ***27 ounces canned kidney beans***
- ***Shredded cheese, sliced green onions for toppings, if you want***

Directions

1. Heat oil in a pan. Add beef and cook until brown, drain, then remove from heat.
2. In a bowl, add cooked meat, salt, onion powder, chili powder, cumin, pepper, cocoa powder, tomato paste, tomato sauce, and Pepsi. Mix until combined.
3. Put the mixture into a blender until well blended.
4. Add mixture into the slow cooker. Pour in beans. Cover cook for 6 hours.
5. Garnish with shredded cheese on top.

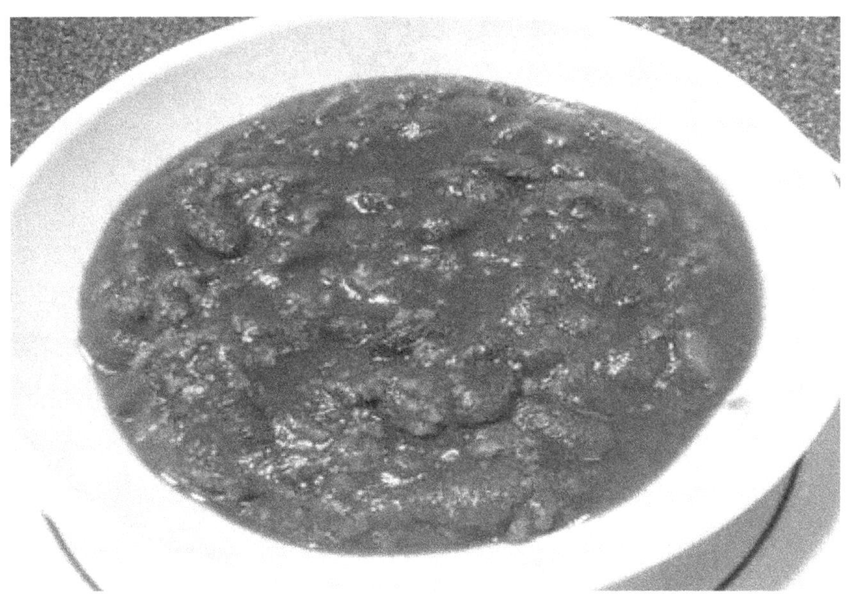

Nutrition

Calories: 653 Fat: 41g Carbs: 38g Sugar: 12g Protein: 35g Sodium: 1308mg

Preparation Time: 10' *Cooking Time: 1 h 10't* *Serves: 4*

43. Cracker Barrel's Meatloaf

Ingredients

- *1 pound ground beef*
- *1 onion, chopped*
- *1 green pepper, chopped*
- *1 can chopped tomatoes*
- *1 egg*
- *½ cup frozen biscuits, shredded*
- *1 teaspoon salt*
- *¼ cup ketchup (optional)*
- *Non-stick cooking spray*

Directions

1. Preheat oven to 350°F.
2. In a bowl, add beef, onion, green pepper, tomatoes, egg, biscuits, and salt. Mix well.
3. Using a non-stick cooking spray, coat bread pan. Then, pour the meatloaf mixture into the pan. Make sure the mixture is even and flat in the pan.
4. Bake for 1 hour and 5 minutes. Let it cool for about 10 minutes.
5. Drain excess juice, then invert cooked meatloaf onto a serving plate. Drizzle ketchup on top, if desired. Serve.

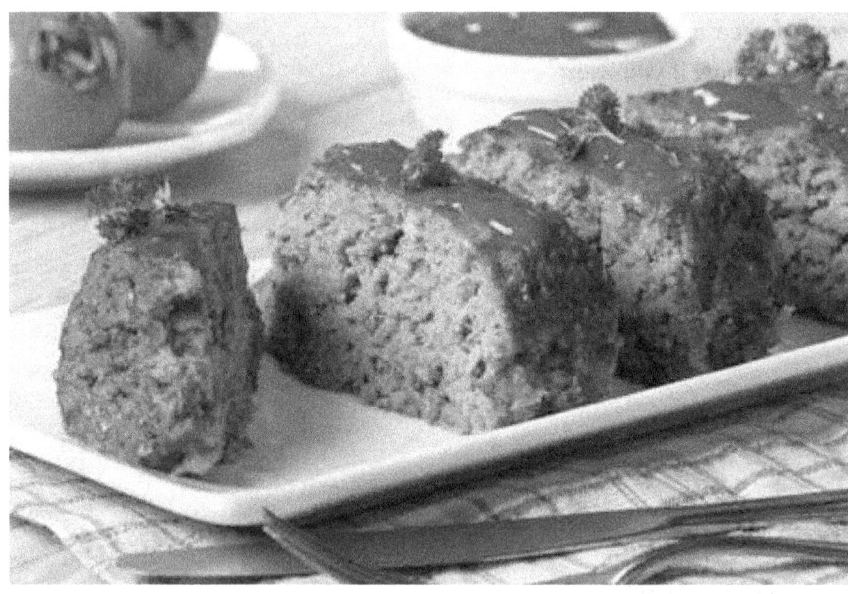

Nutrition

Calories: 485 Fat: 32g Carbs: 27g Protein: 23g

Preparation Time: 15' *Cooking Time: 1 h 35'* *Serves: 4*

44. Applebee's Sizzling Steak, Cheese, and Mushrooms Skillet

Ingredients

- *1 head garlic, cut crosswise*
- *2 tablespoons olive oil, divided*
- *Salt and pepper, to taste*
- *2 pounds Yukon Gold potatoes*
- *Water, for boiling*
- *2 tablespoons butter*
- *1 large yellow onion*
- *8 ounces cremini mushrooms*
- *Salt and pepper to taste*
- *½ cup milk*
- *¼ cup cream*
- *3 tablespoons butter*
- *2 ½ pounds 1-inch thick sirloin steak, cut into 4 large pieces*
- *8 slices mozzarella cheese*

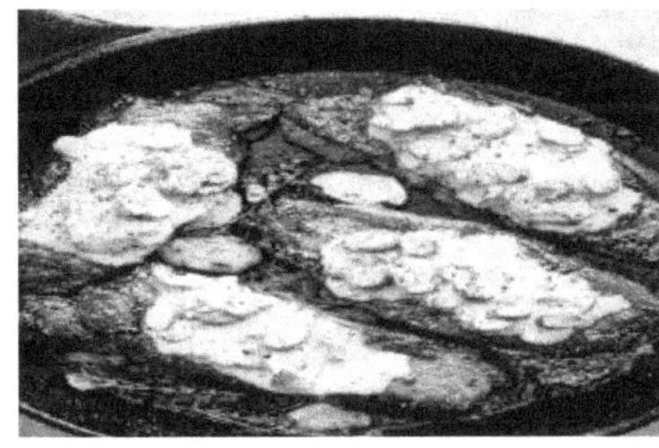

Directions

1. Preheat oven to 300°F.
2. Position garlic on the foil. Pour 1 tablespoon olive oil to the inner sides where the garlic was cut, then wrap foil around garlic.
3. Bake for 30 minutes. Remove from oven, and squeeze out the garlic from the head. Transfer to a bowl or mortar. Add salt and pepper, then mash together. Set aside.
4. In a pot, add potatoes. Pour enough water on top to cover potatoes. Bring to a boil. Once boiling, reduce heat to medium. Let it simmer for about 20-25 minutes or until potatoes become tender.
5. Melt butter on a non-stick pan over medium-low heat. Add onions and sauté for about 15 minutes until a bit tender. Toss in mushrooms and sauté, adjusting heat to medium. Season with salt and pepper. Cook for 10 minutes more. Set aside and keep warm.
6. Drain potatoes, then mash using an electric mixer on low speed. While mashing, gradually pour in milk, cream, butter, and mashed garlic with olive oil. Keep blending until everything is cream-like and smooth. Remove from the mixer and place a cover on top of the bowl. Set aside and keep warm.
7. Evenly coat steak pieces with remaining 1 tablespoon olive oil on all sides. Heat grill, then place the meat on the grill. Cook for 4 minutes. Flip and add mozzarella slices on top. Cook for another 4 minutes for medium-rare. Add additional minutes for increased doneness.
8. Transfer steaks to serving plates then top with onion/mushroom mixture. Place mashed potatoes on the side. Serve.

Nutrition

Calories: 1159 Fat: 60g Carbs: 47g Sugar: 4 g Protein: 107g Sodium: 1495mg

Preparation Time: 20' *Cooking Time: 40'* *Serves: 10*

45. Popeye's Red Beans and Rice

Ingredients

- ***3 (14-ounce) cans red beans***
- ***¾ pounds smoked ham hock***
- ***1¼ cups water***
- ***½ teaspoon onion powder***
- ***½ teaspoon garlic salt***
- ***¼ teaspoon red pepper flakes***
- ***½ teaspoon salt***
- ***3 tablespoons lard***
- ***Steamed long-grain rice***

Directions

1. Add 2 canned red beans, ham hock, and water to a pot. Cook on medium heat and let simmer for about 1 hour.
2. Remove from heat and wait until the meat is cool enough to handle. Then, remove meat from the bone.
3. In a food processor, add meat, cooked red beans and water mixture, onion powder, garlic salt, red pepper, salt, and lard. Pulse for 4 seconds. You want the beans to be cut and the liquid thickened. Drain remaining 1 can red beans and add to the food processor. Pulse for only 1 or 2 seconds.
4. Remove ingredients from the food processor and transfer to the pot from earlier. Cook on low heat, stirring frequently until mixture is heated through.
5. Serve over steamed rice.

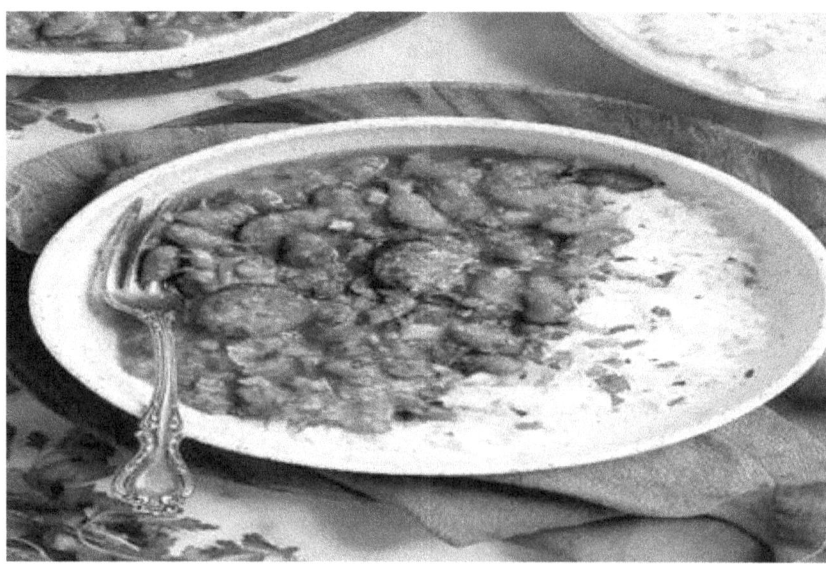

Nutrition

Calories: 445 Fat: 12g Carbs: 67g Sugar: 1g Protein: 17g Sodium: 670mg

Preparation Time: 10' *Cooking Time: 8'* *Serves: 8*

46. Café Rio's Sweet Pork Barbacoa Salad

Ingredients

- ***3 pounds pork loin***
- ***Garlic salt, to taste***
- ***1 can root beer***
- ***¼ cup water***
- ***¾ cup brown sugar***
- ***1 (10-ounce) can red enchilada sauce***
- ***1 (4-ounce) can green chilies***
- ***½ teaspoon chili powder***
- ***8 large burrito size tortillas***
- ***1½ serving Cilantro Lime Rice***
- ***1 can black beans, drained and heated***
- ***2 heads Romaine lettuce, shredded***
- ***1½ cups tortilla strips***
- ***1 cup Queso Fresco cheese***
- ***2 limes, cut in wedges***
- ***¼ cup cilantro***

Dressing:

- ***½ packet Hidden Valley Ranch Dressing Mix***
- ***1 cup mayonnaise***
- ***½ cup milk***
- ***½ cup cilantro leaves***
- ***¼ cup Salsa Verde***
- ***½ jalapeno pepper, deseeded***
- ***1 plump clove garlic***
- ***2 tablespoons fresh lime juice***

Directions

1. Sprinkle garlic salt on pork. Put in the slow cooker with the fat side facing down. Add ¼ cup root beer and water and cover. Cook on low setting for 6 hours.

2. To prepare sauce add the rest of the root beer, brown sugar, enchilada sauce, green chilies, and chili powder in a blender. Blend until smooth.

3. Remove meat from slow cooker then transfer onto a cutting board. Shred, discarding juices and fat. Return shredded pork to slow cooker with sauce. Cook on low setting for another 2 hours. When there is only about 15 to 20 minutes left to cook, remove the lid to thicken sauce.

4. Mix all dressing ingredients in a blender. Puree until smooth. Put into the fridge and chill for at least 1 hour.

5. To assemble salad, layer tortilla, rice, beans, pork, lettuce, tortilla strips, cheese, and dressing in a bowl. Serve with a lime wedge and cilantro leaves.

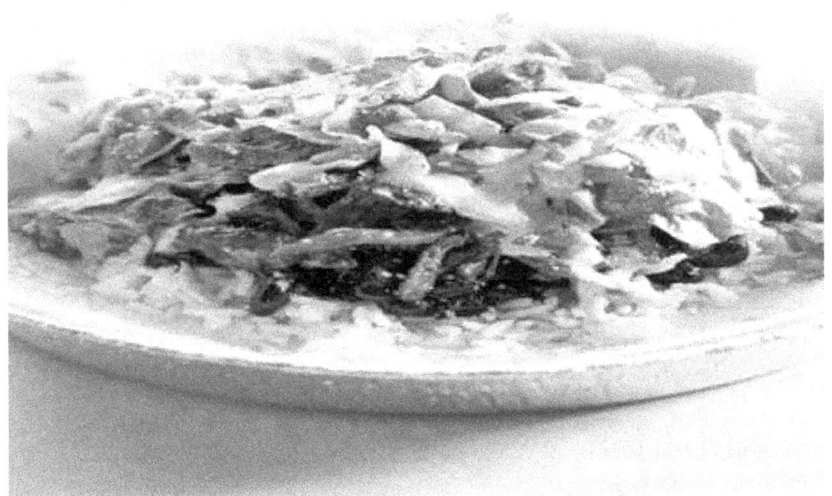

Nutrition

Calories: 756 Fat: 28g Carbs: 91gSugar: 31g Protein: 38g Sodium: 1389mg

Preparation Time: 15' *Cooking Time: 5-6'* *Serves: 2-4* *Marination: 20'*

47. Edo Japan's Sukiyaki Beef

Ingredients

- ***10 ounces sirloin steak, thinly sliced***
- ***½ carrot, thinly sliced***
- ***½ onion, sliced***
- ***1 green pepper, sliced***
- ***½ yellow bell pepper, sliced***
- ***½ cup sukiyaki sauce, divided***
- ***1 tablespoon oil***
- ***1 teaspoon chopped garlic***
- ***2 tablespoons ginger, finely chopped***
- ***2 teaspoons soy sauce***
- ***1 teaspoon sugar***
- ***1 tablespoon oyster sauce***

Directions

1. Pour half of the sukiyaki sauce into a medium bowl and add the sliced beef. Let the beef marinate for 20 minutes.
2. Pour some of the oil in a skillet and add the garlic and cook for a few seconds.
3. Add the beef, with the sauce. Cook in medium-high heat until the beef is cooked through.
4. Add the ginger, carrots, peppers, and onions and cook until the veggies have begun to soften.
5. Add the rest of the sukiyaki sauce along with the oyster sauce, soy sauce, and sugar. Cook for a few minutes. Serve over rice.

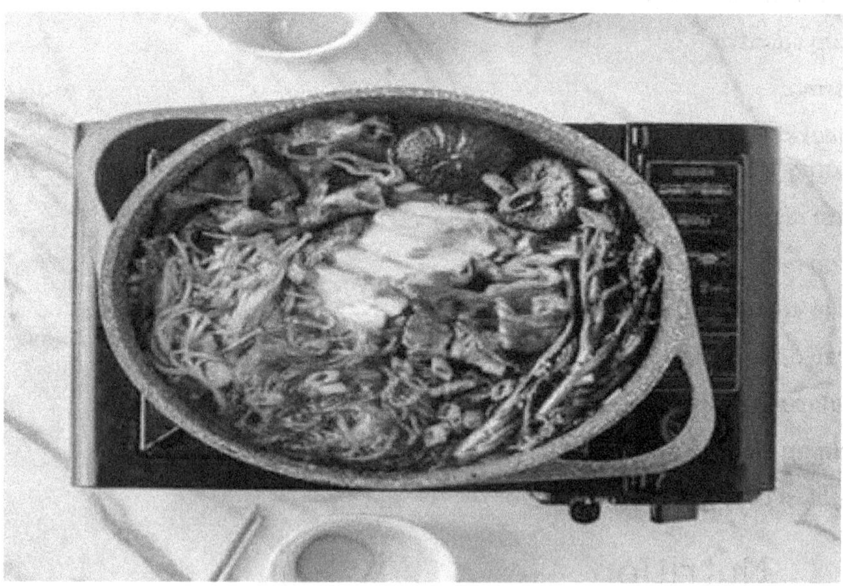

Nutrition

Calories: 152 Fat: 24g Carbs: 20g Protein: 5.6g Sodium: 627 mg

Preparation Time: 10' *Cooking Time: 20'* *Serves: 6*

48. Olive Garden's Steak Gorgonzola Alfredo

Ingredients

- ***18 ounces rib eye or sirloin steak, cut into 2–3-inch medallions***
- ***1 pound fettuccine***
- ***4 cups baby spinach***
- ***½ cup sun-dried tomatoes, chopped***
- ***½ cup gorgonzola cheese, crumbled***
- ***Balsamic glaze (or aged balsamic), as desired***
- ***Alfredo sauce***
- ***3 tablespoons butter***
- ***3 tablespoons all-purpose flour***
- ***2 cups heavy cream***
- ***½ cup pecorino Romano cheese, grated***

Directions

1. First, make the Alfredo sauce. Melt the butter over medium heat. Slowly add the flour, whisking frequently.
2. Add the heavy cream and grated cheese. Continue to whisk until thickened.
3. Cook fettuccine according to package directions. Drain and set aside.
4. Grill the steak to preference in a skillet. Set aside.
5. Place the Alfredo sauce in a pot and heat on low. Add the pasta and spinach. Continue to stir until the spinach wilts. Remove from heat.
6. Place the sun-dried tomatoes, gorgonzola cheese and steak on top of the pasta. Drizzle with balsamic glaze. Serve.

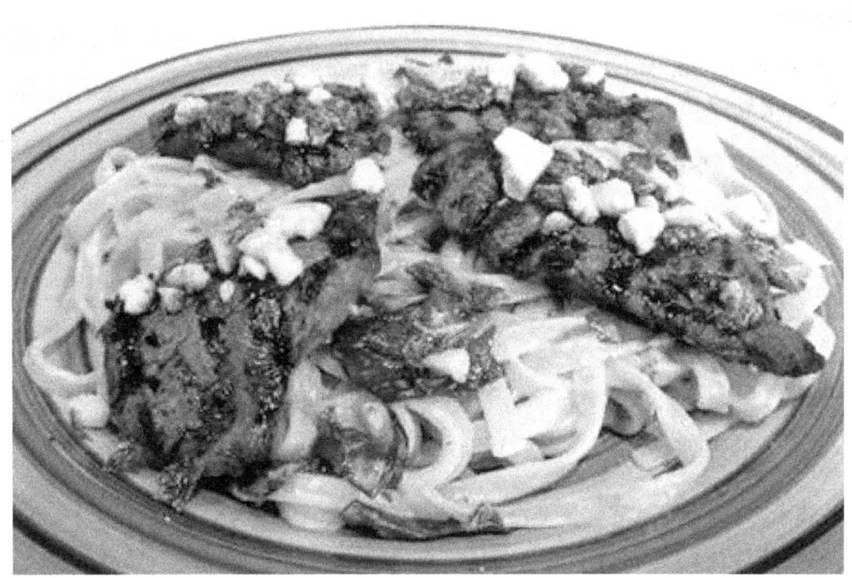

Nutrition

Calories: 150 Fat: 4.2g Carbs: 40g Sugars: 1g Protein: 9g

Preparation Time: 2h *Cooking Time: 2h* *Serves: 8*

49. Olive Garden's Pizza Bowl

Ingredients

- *Salt and pepper to taste*
- *Flour (for dusting)*
- *2 (1-pound) loaves frozen bread dough, thawed and brought to room temperature*
- *2 cups Alfredo sauce*
- *½ cup butter*
- *2 cups heavy cream*
- *Few dashes nutmeg*
- *½ teaspoon dry mustard*
- *¼ teaspoon salt*
- *¼ teaspoon white pepper*
- *1 teaspoon Italian seasoning (or ½ teaspoon dry oregano + ½ teaspoon dry basil)*
- *2 cups freshly grated parmesan cheese*
- *Meatballs*
- *½ cup milk*
- *1 cup coarse bread such as sourdough, crust removed and broken up into small pieces*
- *1 pound lean ground beef*
- *1 egg*
- *¾ cup whole milk ricotta, drained*
- *1/3 Cup onion, finely chopped*
- *2 tablespoons parmesan cheese, grated*
- *1 tablespoon fresh flat-leaf parsley*
- *Few dashes of nutmeg*
- *1 teaspoon salt*
- *¼ teaspoon black pepper*
- *¾ cup mozzarella, shredded*
- *¼ cup olive oil*
- *1½ quarts Italian tomato sauce*
- *Other:*
- *1 pound Italian sweet sausage, removed from casing*
- *1 pound lean ground beef*
- *1½ cups olive oil (divided)*
- *1 pound fontina cheese, shredded*
- *1 pound mozzarella, shredded*
- *2 cups freshly grated parmesan cheese, divided*

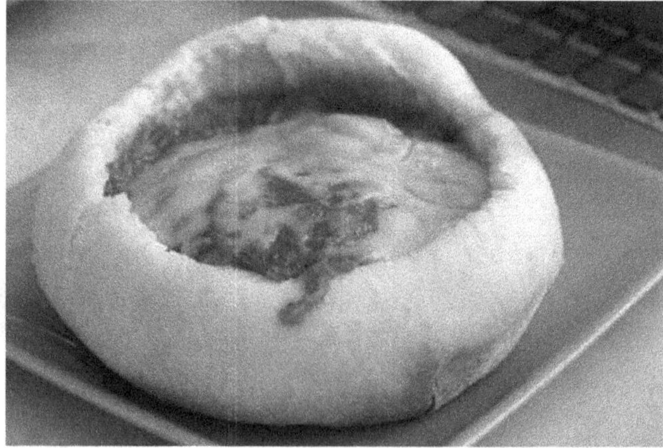

Nutrition

Calories: 242.8 Fat: 6.6g Carbs: 38.4gSugars: 3gProtein: 8.4g

Directions

1. Cut each bread dough in half to make 4 pieces. Dust the counter with flour. Roll the dough into balls.

2. Flatten into circles. Let the dough relax, then flatten again. Repeat until the dough is about 8 inches in diameter. Cover with a dish towel.

3. If using pre-made Alfredo, heat according to package directions. To make Alfredo sauce from scratch, melt butter over medium heat in a medium saucepan. Add the cream, nutmeg, mustard, salt, pepper, and Italian seasoning. Stir well, then add the parmesan cheese. Heat sauce until the cheese has melted. Remove from heat and set aside.

4. If using pre-made meatballs, cook according to package directions. To make the meatballs from scratch, preheat oven to 375°F. Pour milk into a medium bowl. Press bread into the milk and let soak.

5. In another bowl, combine the ground beef, egg, ricotta, onion, parmesan, parsley, nutmeg, salt, pepper, and mozzarella.

6. Squeeze the milk out of the bread. Discard milk. Combine the bread with the meat mixture. Mix well.

7. Put some parchment paper on the baking sheet and drizzle with olive oil. Make about 32–36 half-ounce meatballs and place them on the baking sheet.

8. Put some olive oil on top of the meatballs. Bake for 15 minutes or until completely cooked. Remove from the oven and set aside.

9. Dust off the flour from bread dough and place on a clean counter. Preheat oven to 450°F.

10. Find oven-safe bowls that are approximately 7 inches wide at the top, 3 inches wide at the bottom, and 4 inches deep for the perfect bowl shape. Dimensions can be slightly different as long as the dough holds its shape. Place the bowls upside down on a foil-lined baking sheet.

11. Put some olive oil on the dough and sprinkle with parmesan.

12. Brush the bowls with olive oil and drape the dough over them, cheese facing up.

13. Place in the oven. Bake for 5 minutes. Rotate the bowls and bake for another 5 minutes until golden brown. Lift off the dough and transfer to a cooling rack.

14. Cook the sausage and ground beef in a medium pan, then add the tomato sauce.

15. Assemble the pizza bowls by layering Alfredo sauce first, then fontina cheese. Pour the meat sauce over the cheese. Add the meatballs. Sprinkle shredded mozzarella. Add a layer of meat sauce and meatballs. Finish by topping with remaining parmesan cheese. Serve.

Preparation Time: 20' *Cooking Time: 10'* *Serves: 4*

50. Olive Garden's Beef Filet in Balsamic Sauce

Ingredients

- *¼ cup extra-virgin olive oil*
- *¼ cup butter*
- *1 yellow onion, medium and sliced thin*
- *Salt and pepper to taste*
- *½ cup dry white wine*
- *3 sprigs fresh rosemary, finely chopped*
- *½ cup Marsala wine*
- *½ cup beef broth*
- *2 tablespoons balsamic vinegar*
- *4 (6-ounce) beef tenderloin fillets*
- *1 dash parsley, finely chopped*
- *Rosemary sprigs (for garnish)*

Directions

1. In a large sauté pan, heat the oil and butter over medium heat. Cook the onion with salt and pepper for 10 minutes to caramelize it.
2. Pour the wine, broth, vinegar, and rosemary into the sauté pan. Bring to a boil, then reduce heat. Simmer for 10–15 minutes.
3. Marinate the beef fillets in oil, salt, and pepper. Grill to preference. Pour sauce over each fillet. Garnish with parsley and rosemary. Serve.

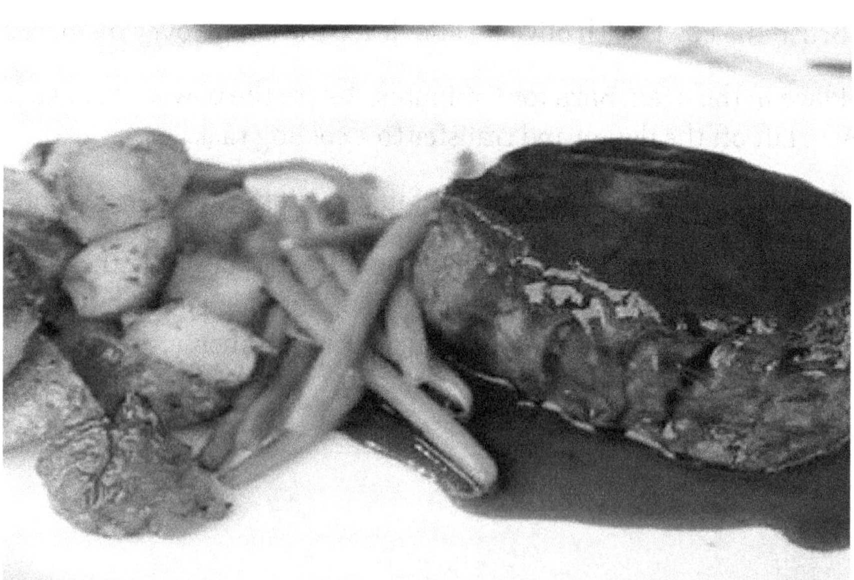

Nutrition

Calories: 150 Fat: 4.2g Carbs: 40g Sugars: 1g Protein: 9g

Preparation Time: 10' *Cooking Time: 45'* *Serves: 4*

51. Olive Garden's Rotini with Sausage and Asparagus

Ingredients

- ***½ pound sweet or hot Italian sausage***
- ***2 tablespoons extra-virgin olive oil***
- ***1 pound fresh asparagus***
- ***½ cup heavy cream***
- ***1 pound rotini pasta***
- ***2 tablespoons butter***
- ***Parmesan cheese, grated***
- ***Salt and pepper to taste***

Directions

1. In a sauté pan, heat the oil over medium heat. Completely cook the sausage while breaking it into pieces. Drain the liquid.

2. Remove 2 inches off the bottom of the asparagus and cut the remaining stems into 1-inch pieces. Boil until tender. Remove the tips and set aside.

3. Heat the heavy cream and asparagus stems together over medium heat. Cover and simmer for 10–12 minutes.

4. Cook the rotini according to package instructions. Drain, then add to the cream sauce. Add parmesan, butter, salt and pepper, and cooked sausage. Simmer.

5. Transfer to a platter. Garnish with asparagus tips. Serve.

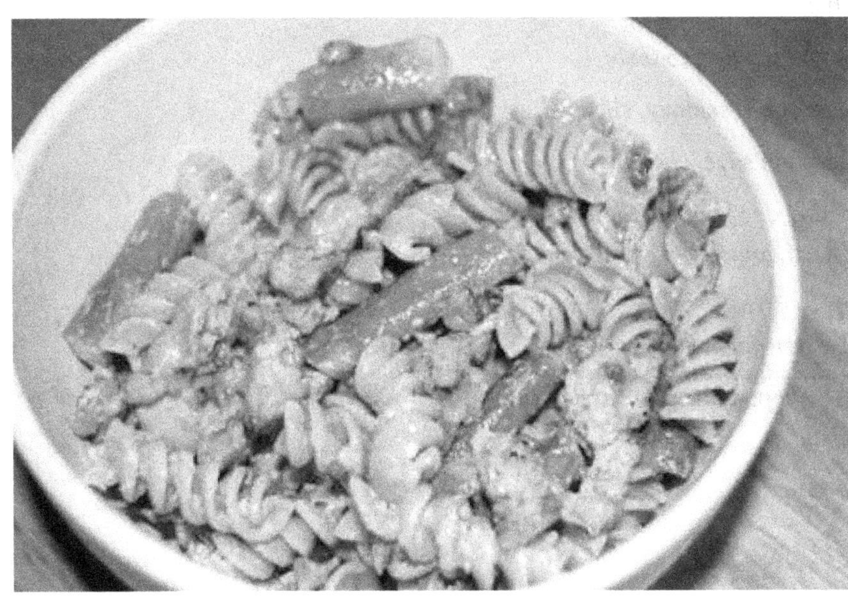

Nutrition

Calories: 178 Fat: 15 g Carbs: 50g Sugars: 8g Protein: 9g

Preparation Time: 10' *Cooking Time: 1h 15'* *Serves: 4*

52. Olive Garden's Beef Bolognese

Ingredients

- ***2 tablespoons olive oil***
- ***1 onion, finely chopped***
- ***1 carrot, finely chopped***
- ***1 celery stick, finely chopped***
- ***2 cloves garlic, finely chopped***
- ***½ pound ground beef***
- ***6 ounces Italian sausage, hot or mild according to preference, skinned***
- ***1 cup red wine***
- ***1 (28-ounce) can Italian tomatoes, crushed***
- ***Salt and pepper, to taste***
- ***1 teaspoon rosemary, chopped***
- ***1 teaspoon sage, chopped***
- ***¾ pound dry long pasta such as spaghetti, angel hair, or fettuccini***
- ***Freshly shredded parmesan cheese, for garnish.***
- ***Fresh chopped Italian parsley for garnish***

Directions

1. Heat the oil over medium heat. Add the celery, carrot, onion, and garlic. Cook for 5 minutes.
2. Put the meat and cook for 10 minutes while stirring.
3. Pour the red wine and let it simmer.
4. Add the tomatoes and other remaining ingredients. Simmer for 1 hour.
5. Cook pasta in boiling water and drain. Serve with a generous amount of sauce and sprinkle with chopped parsley. Top with freshly shredded parmesan cheese. If desired.

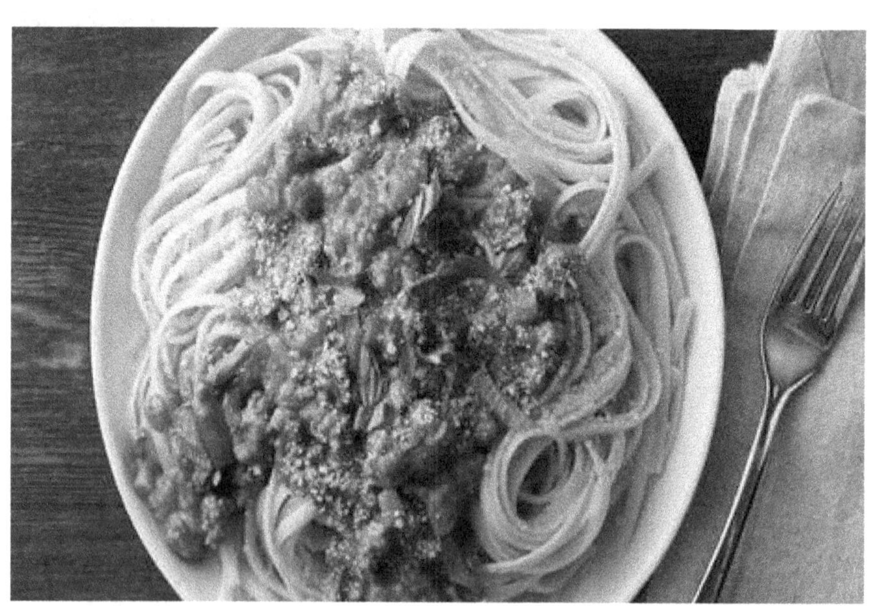

Nutrition

Calories: 150 Fat: 20g Carbs: 50g Sugars: 9g Protein: 15g

Chapter 3
Sides and Appetizer

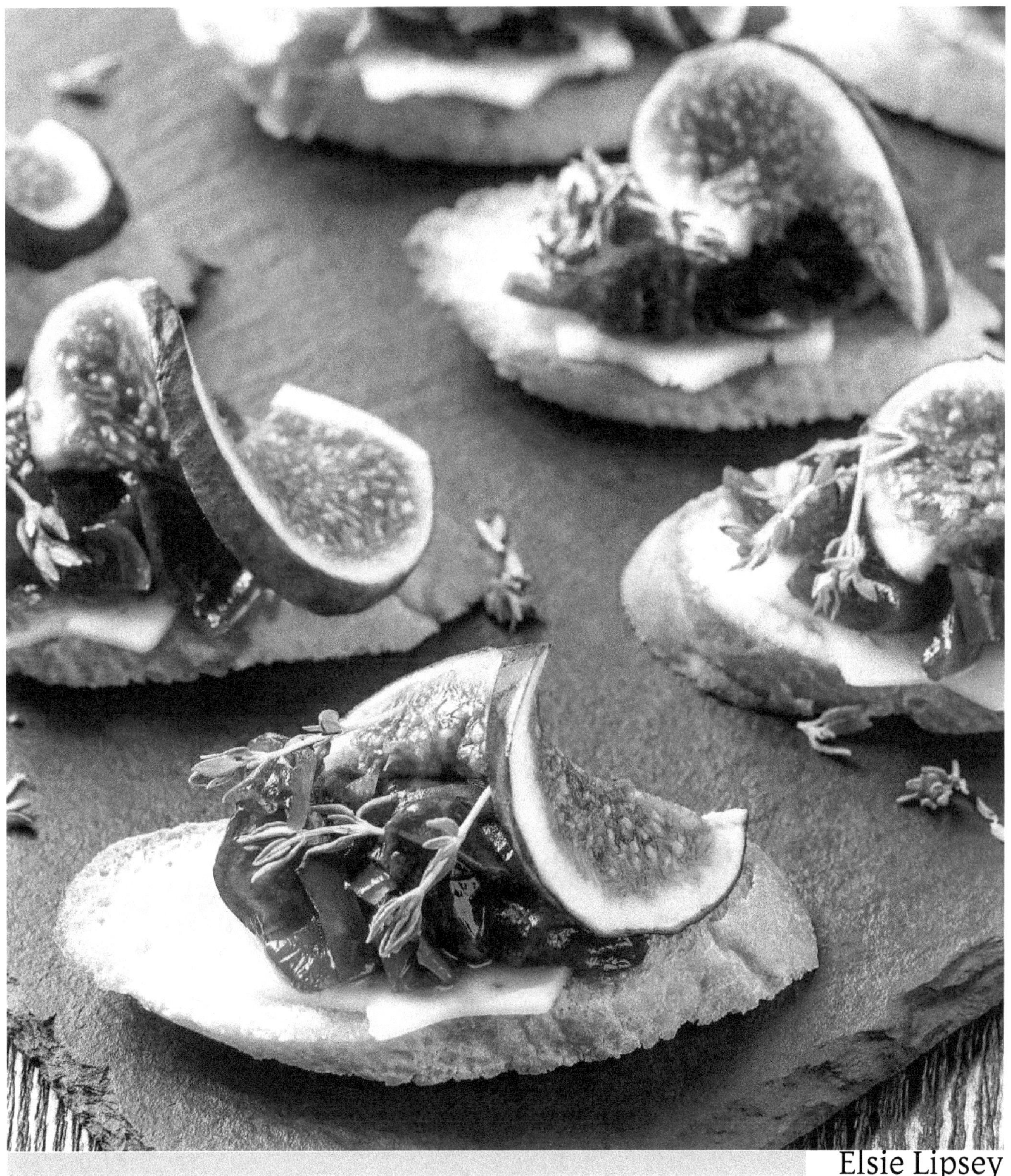

Elsie Lipsey

Preparation Time: 3h 5' *Cooking Time: 15'* *Serves: 4-6*

53. Stakehouse'sFried Mac and Cheese Balls

Ingredients

- *Sauce:*
- *1 ¾ cups marinara sauce*
- *1 ¾ cups Alfredo Sauce*
- *¼ cup heavy whipping cream*
- *1 teaspoon garlic powder*
- *½ cup ricotta cheese*
- *1 cup Italian blend shredded Cheese*
- *¼ cup red wine*
- *Balls:*
- *16 ounces grated white sharp cheddar, grated*
- *16 ounces smoked gouda cheese, grated*
- *3 tablespoons butter*
- *2 tablespoons flour*
- *2 cups whole milk, warmed*
- *1 pound large elbow macaroni, cooked*
- *Salt and pepper, to taste*
- *3 eggs*
- *3 tablespoons milk*
- *3 cups panko bread crumbs*
- *Fresh Parmesan cheese for garnish only*
- *Vegetable oil for frying*

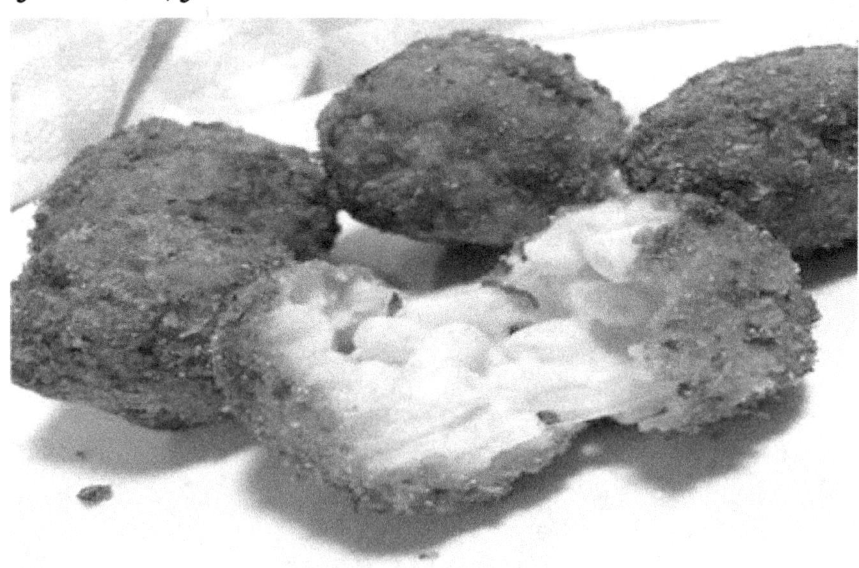

Nutrition

Calories 115 Fat: 14g Carbs: 78g Sugars: 9g Protein: 8g

Directions

1. Make the balls. In a mixing bowl, combine the shredded cheddar and shredded Gouda.

2. In a large saucepan, melt the butter. Add the flour slowly, whisking until there are no lumps. Gradually add the 2 cups warm milk. Whisk until smooth, and continue cooking until the sauce begins to thicken.

3. Wait until the sauce has thickened and take it off from the heat and gradually mix in the cheddar and Gouda cheeses and stir well.

4. Add the cooked macaroni and salt and pepper into the cheese sauce and stir well.

5. Butter a large cake pan spread the mac and cheese mixture evenly into the pan, put in the refrigerator for at least two hours. You want the mixture to set and make it easier to form into balls.

6. After 2 hours, get the tray from the refrigerator and form the mac and Cheese into evenly sized balls about 2 inches in diameter. Cover, and put them in the freezer for at least an hour.

7. Beat the eggs and 3 tablespoons of milk together.

8. Place the bread crumbs in a shallow dish.

9. Heat enough vegetable oil so that the balls will be covered when you fry them.

10. When the oil is heated to 350°F, dip each ball in the egg mixture, then the panko crumbs, and drop them into the oil. Work in batches, and cook until the balls are a nice golden brown color, about 3–4 minutes. Transfer to the paper towel as they finish cooking to drain.

11. Make your cheese sauce by combining the marinara and Alfredo sauce in a small saucepan. Heat over medium and when warm, add the ricotta, Italian cheese blend, and wine. Stir to combine.

12. When the cheeses have melted, remove the pot from the heat and add the garlic powder and heavy cream. Stir well.

13. Serve the macaroni balls with the cheese sauce and a sprinkle of Parmesan.

Preparation Time: 2' *Cooking Time: 3'* *Serves: 8*

54. ChikFil-A's Raspberry Lemonade

Ingredients

- ***1 cup water***
- ***1 cup sugar***
- ***1 cup freshly squeezed lemon juice***
- ***1 ½ cups fresh raspberries***
- ***Added sugar for the rim of your glass***

Directions

1. In a small saucepan, heat the water and sugar until the sugar completely dissolves.
2. Meanwhile, purée the raspberries in a blender. Add the contents of the saucepan and the cup lemon juice.
3. Soaked the rim of your glass and dip it into a bit of sugar to coat the side before pouring the lemonade into the glass.
4. Serve.

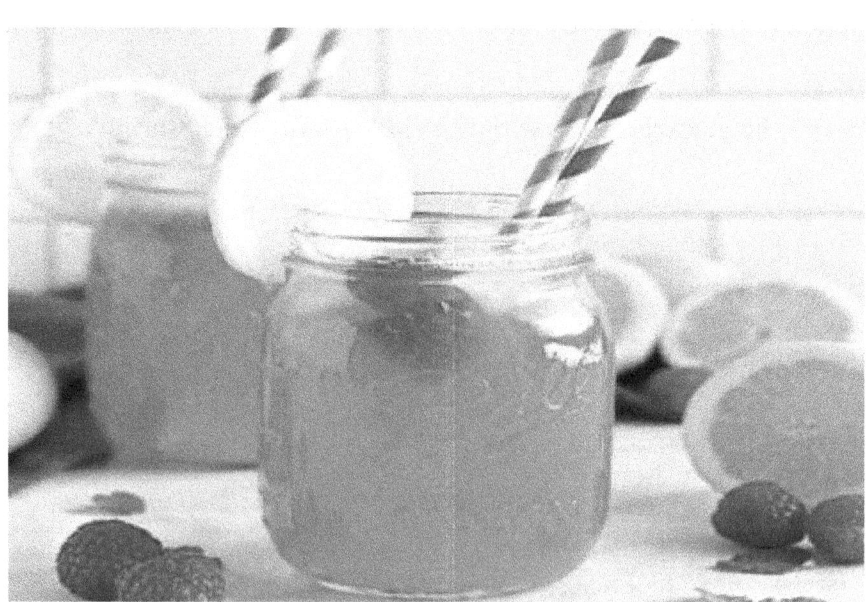

Nutrition

Calories: 112 Fat: 17 Carbs: 50g Sugars: 5g Protein: 7g

Preparation Time: 20' *Cooking Time: 4'* *Serves: 14*

55. Olive Garden's Lasagna Fritta

Ingredients

- ***2/3 + ¼ cup milk (divided)***
- ***1 cup grated parmesan cheese, plus some more for serving***
- ***¾ cup feta cheese***
- ***¼ teaspoon white pepper***
- ***1 tablespoon butter***
- ***7 lasagna noodles***
- ***1 egg***
- ***Breadcrumbs***
- ***Oil for frying***
- ***2 tablespoons marinara sauce***
- ***Alfredo Sauce, for serving***

Directions

1. Place the butter, white pepper, □ cup milk, parmesan, and feta cheese in a pot. Stir and boil.
2. Prepare lasagna noodles according to instructions on the package.
3. Spread a thin layer of the cheese and milk mixture on each noodle. Fold into 2-inch pieces and place something substantial on top to keep them folded. Place in the freezer for at least 1 hour, then cut each noodle in half lengthwise.
4. In a small bowl, mix the ¼ cup milk and egg in another bowl, place breadcrumbs.
5. Dip each piece into the egg wash then the breadcrumbs. Fry the noodles at 350°F for 4 minutes.
6. Serve by spreading some alfredo sauce at the bottom of the plate, placing the lasagna on top, and then drizzling with marinara sauce. Put some grated parmesan cheese on top.

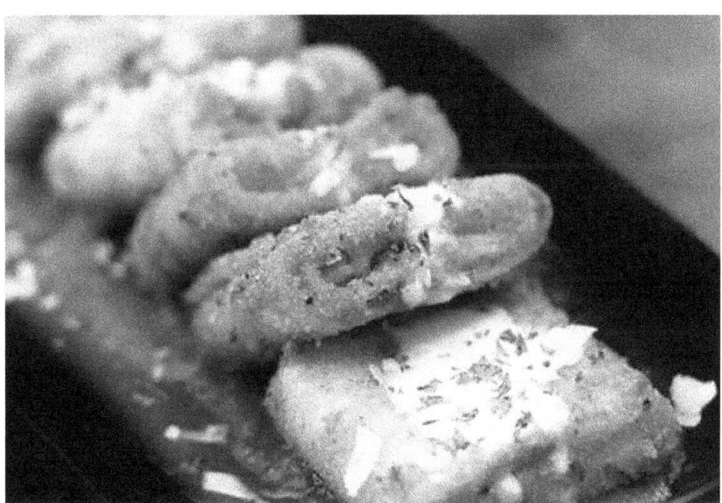

Nutrition

Calories: 103 Fat: 21g Sodium: 1590mg Total Carbohydrate: 82g Protein: 9g

Preparation Time: 20' *Cooking Time: 10'* *Serves: 4-6*

56. PF Chang's Shrimp Dumplings

Ingredients

- ***1 pound medium shrimp, peeled, deveined, washed and dried, divided***
- ***2 tablespoons carrot, finely minced***
- ***2 tablespoons green onion, finely minced***
- ***1 teaspoon ginger, freshly minced***
- ***2 tablespoons oyster sauce***
- ***¼ teaspoon sesame oil***
- ***1 package wonton wrappers***
- ***Sauce***
- ***1 cup soy sauce***
- ***2 tablespoons white vinegar***
- ***½ teaspoon chili paste***
- ***2 tablespoons granulated sugar***
- ***½ teaspoon ginger, freshly minced***
- ***Sesame oil to taste***
- ***1 cup water***
- ***1 tablespoon cilantro leaves***

Directions

1. Finely mince ½ pound of the shrimp.
2. Dice the other ½ pound of shrimp.
3. In a mixing bowl, combine both the minced and diced shrimp with the remaining ingredients.
4. Spoon about 1 teaspoon of the mixture into each wonton wrapper and wet the edges of the wrapper, then fold up and seal tightly.
5. Cover and refrigerate for an hour.
6. In a medium bowl, put all together with the ingredients for the sauce and stir until well combined.
7. When ready to serve, boil water in a saucepan and cover it with a steamer. Put a light oil on the steamer to keep the dumplings from sticking. Steam the dumplings for 7–10 minutes.
8. Serve with sauce.

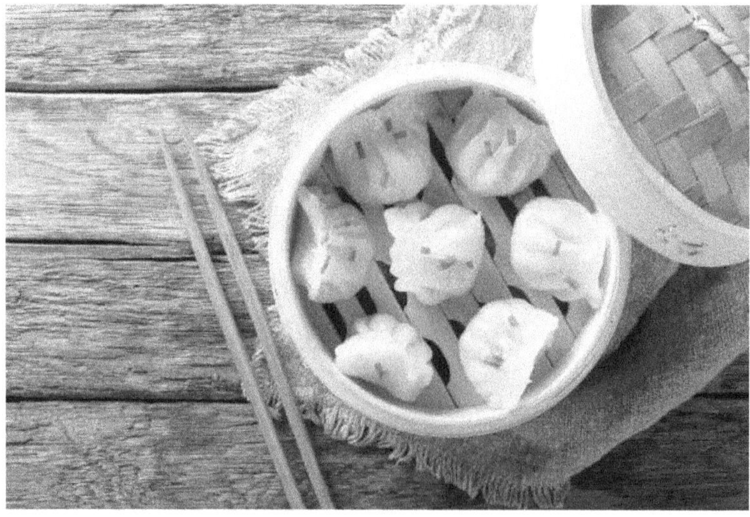

Nutrition

Calories: 137.1 Sodium: 1801.5mg Total Carbohydrate: 21.1g Protein: 10.5g

Preparation Time: 10' *Cooking Time: 1'* *Serves: 4-6*

57. Pei Wei's Vietnamese Chicken Salad Spring Roll

Ingredients

- ***Salad***
- ***Rice Wrappers***
- ***Green leaf lettuce like Boston Bibb lettuce***
- ***Napa cabbage, shredded***
- ***Green onions, chopped***
- ***Mint, chopped***
- ***Carrots, cut into 1-inch match-sticks***
- ***Peanuts***
- ***Chicken, diced and cooked, about 6 chicken tenders drizzled with soy sauce, honey, garlic powder, and red pepper flakes***
- ***Lime dressing***
- ***2 tablespoons lime juice, about 1 lime***
- ***1½ teaspoons water***
- ***1 tablespoon sugar***
- ***1 teaspoon salt***
- ***Dash of pepper***
- ***3 tablespoons oil***
- ***Peanut dipping sauce***
- ***2 tablespoons soy sauce***
- ***1 tablespoon rice wine vinegar***
- ***2 tablespoons brown sugar***
- ***¼ cup peanut butter***
- ***1 teaspoon chipotle Tabasco***
- ***1 teaspoon honey***
- ***1 teaspoon sweet chili sauce***
- ***1 teaspoon lime vinaigrette***

Directions

1. In a large bowl, mix all of the salad ingredients except for the rice wrappers and lettuce.

2. Place the rice wrappers in warm water for about 1 minute to soften.

3. Transfer the wrappers to a plate and top each with 2 pieces of lettuce.

4. Top the lettuce with the salad mixture and drizzle with the lime dressing. Fold the wrapper by tucking in the ends and then rolling.

5. Serve with lime dressing and peanut dipping sauce.

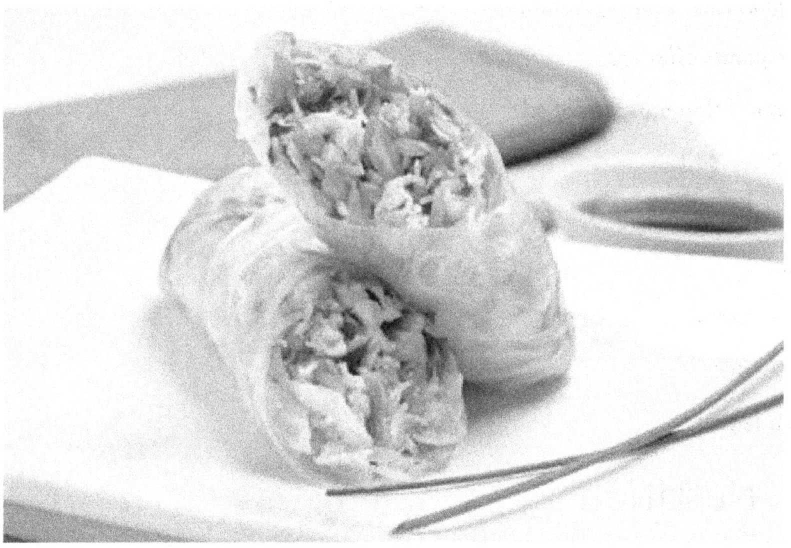

Nutrition

Calories: 80 Fat: 4g Carbs: 20g Sugars: 2g Protein: 15g

Preparation Time: 10' *Cooking Time: 1'* *Serves: 24*

58. Mexican's Shrimp Taco Bites

Ingredients

- ***24 wonton wrappers***
- ***Oil to coat***
- ***Guacamole***

Shrimp:

- ***½ pound shrimp, peeled and deveined***
- ***1 lime, juiced***
- ***2 Tablespoons cilantro, coarsely chopped***
- ***¼ cup olive oil***
- ***½ teaspoon sea salt***
- ***½ teaspoon black pepper***
- ***¼ teaspoon cayenne***

Cabbage slaw:

- ***¼ cup mayonnaise***
- ***1 ½ Tablespoons lime juice***
- ***¼ teaspoon lime zest (optional)***
- ***2 Tablespoons cilantro***
- ***1 teaspoon jalapeños, chopped***
- ***Pinch of sea salt***
- ***2 cups red cabbage, shredded***

Toppings:

- ***Jalapeno slices***
- ***Cotija cheese***
- ***Cilantro leaves***

Directions

1. Mix the lime juice, shrimp, and cilantro together with the olive oils, salt, and pepper to taste and cayenne. Marinade it for 15-20 minutes.
2. Preheat your oven to 350°F.
3. Put some wonton wrapper on the mini muffin tin and gently push down the middle to line the cup with wonton. Brush the wrappers with olive oil then bake it for 10 minutes until it turns golden brown and set aside.
4. In the meantime, whisk the mayonnaise, zest, lime juice, salt, and jalapenos together and add the cabbage to the mixture.
5. Heat a pan in medium-high heat then add the shrimp and marinade. Let it cook for 1-2 minutes each side. Once done, set it aside to let it cool slightly. Then, slice the shrimps into halves of thirds and put it into the cabbage slaw.
6. Put one teaspoon on guacamole on the bottom of each wonton cup. Put in some of the shrimp mixture and cabbage slaw. Do this for all of the cups. Top them with cilantro, jalapeno slices, and cotija cheese.

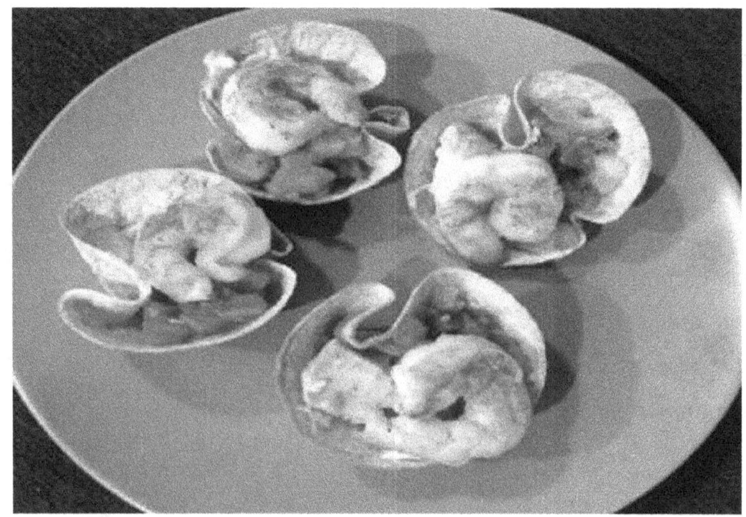

Nutrition

Calories: 140 Fat: 8g Carbs: 30 Sugars: 10g Protein: 25g

Preparation Time: 10' *Cooking Time: 35'* *Serves: 4-6*

59. Moe's Southwestern Grill's Taco Pie

Ingredients

- ***1 ½ cups crushed tortilla chips***
- ***2 teaspoons taco seasoning***
- ***3 tablespoons butter, melted***
- ***3 cups leftover taco beef***
- ***1 ½ cups refried beans***
- ***1 cup spicy salsa***
- ***1 cup grated cheddar cheese***
- ***Cherry tomatoes, halved***

Toppings:

- ***Salsa***
- ***Sour cream or crema***
- ***Chopped salad***

Directions

1. Preheat the oven to 450°F.
2. In a mixing bowl, combine the crushed tortilla chips, taco seasoning, and melted butter. Mix well and press the crust into a 9-inch pie plate. Bake for 10 minutes.
3. Reduce the oven temperature to 375°F.
4. Spoon the taco beef into the crust and spread the refried beans on it. Layer the salsa on top, and then the grated cheddar. Scatter the tomatoes on top.
5. Bake for 20 minutes, switching to broil in the final few minutes to ensure the cheese is melted and lightly browned.
6. Let the pie cool down before slicing. Serve with favorite toppings.

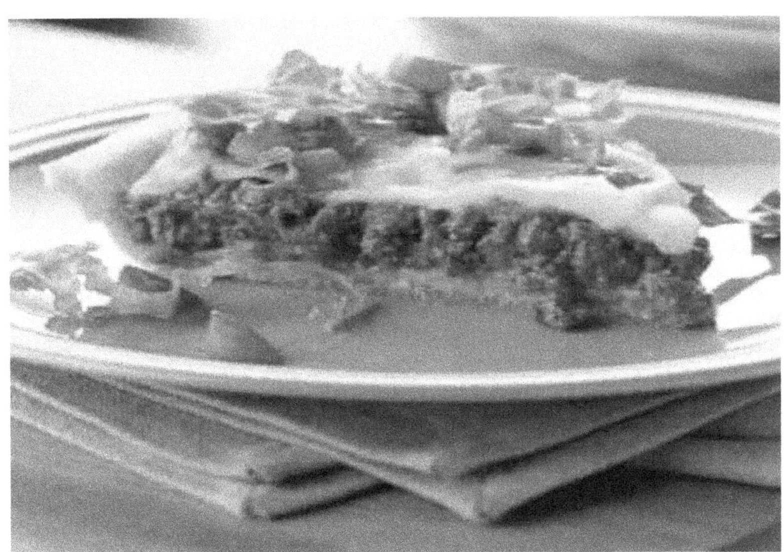

Nutrition

Calories: 140 Fat: 8g Carbs: 3 Sugars: 10g Protein: 25g

Preparation Time: 15' *Cooking Time: 40'* *Serves: 6*

60. Chi Chi's Chili Cheese Enchiladas

Ingredients

- ***1 ½ cups shredded Cheddar cheese, divided***
- ***1 cup shredded Monterey Jack cheese***
- ***¼ cup diced green chilies, drained***
- ***2 (15-ounce) cans chili with beans, excess liquid drained***
- ***12 (6-inch) tortillas, heated***
- ***1 cup enchilada sauce***

Directions

1. Preheat the oven to 350°F. Grease a 9x13 baking dish.
2. Combine a cup shredded cheddar with the green chilies and the chili. Stir.
3. Scoop about half a cup the chili mixture into each tortilla and roll them up. Place them in the prepared pan.
4. Pour the enchilada sauce over, and top with the remaining cheese.
5. Bake for 35–40 minutes.

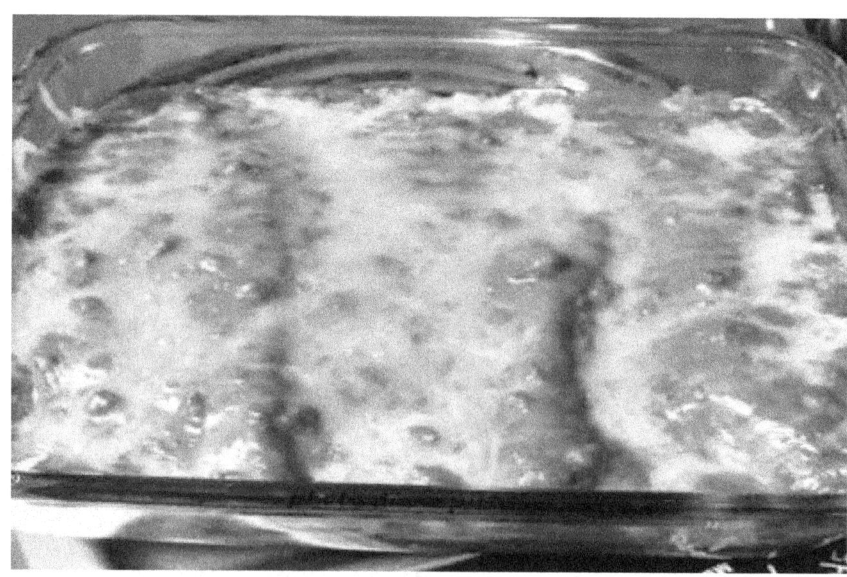

Nutrition

Calories: 115 Fat: 14g Carbs: 78g Sugars: 9g Protein: 8g

Preparation Time: 20' *Cooking Time: 1 hour* *Serves: 6*

61. El Chico's Albondiga Soup

Ingredients

For the Meatballs (albondigas):
- *2 slices white bread*
- *½ cup milk*
- *1 ½ pounds ground beef*
- *1/3 Cup dry long-grain rice*
- *2 eggs*
- *1 ½ teaspoons salt*
- *2 teaspoons black pepper*

For the Soup (sopa):
- *2 tablespoons vegetable oil*
- *1 onion, diced*
- *1 small bell pepper, diced*
- *3 cloves garlic, chopped*
- *3 quarts water*
- *3 tomatoes, diced*
- *1 cup dry rice*
- *2 tablespoons salt*
- *1 tablespoon cumin*
- *1 tablespoon black pepper*
- *3 carrots, thinly sliced*
- *1 small zucchini, thinly sliced*

Other Ingredients:
- *Cilantro*
- *Corn tortilla strips*
- *Fresh limes, cut in wedges*

Directions

1. Prepare the meatballs. Preheat the oven to 400°F. After this, line a baking tray with foil.
2. Soak the bread slices in the milk for 5–10 minutes. Add the remaining of the meatball ingredients and mix to incorporate.
3. Roll the meat mixture into 1-inch balls and arrange them on the baking tray.
4. Bake for 20 minutes and drain on paper towels.
5. Prepare the soup. Put some oil in a pot or Dutch oven to heat. Sauté the onion and pepper until they begin to sweat and soften, about 5 minutes. Add the garlic and cook 1 more minute.
6. Add the water, tomatoes, rice, and seasonings. Let it boil, and then carefully add the meatballs, carrots, and zucchini.
7. Let the mixture simmer for thirty minutes or until the rice turns soft.
8. To serve, garnish with cilantro and tortilla strips. Squeeze lime juice over the bowls.

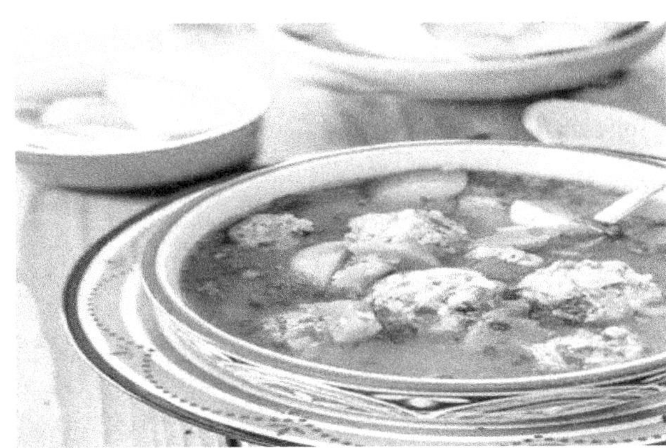

Nutrition

Calories: 112 Fat: 17 Carbs: 50g Sugars: 5g Protein: 7g

Preparation Time: 20' *Cooking Time: 25'* *Serves: 6-8*

62. Taco Bell's Beef Chalupa

Ingredients

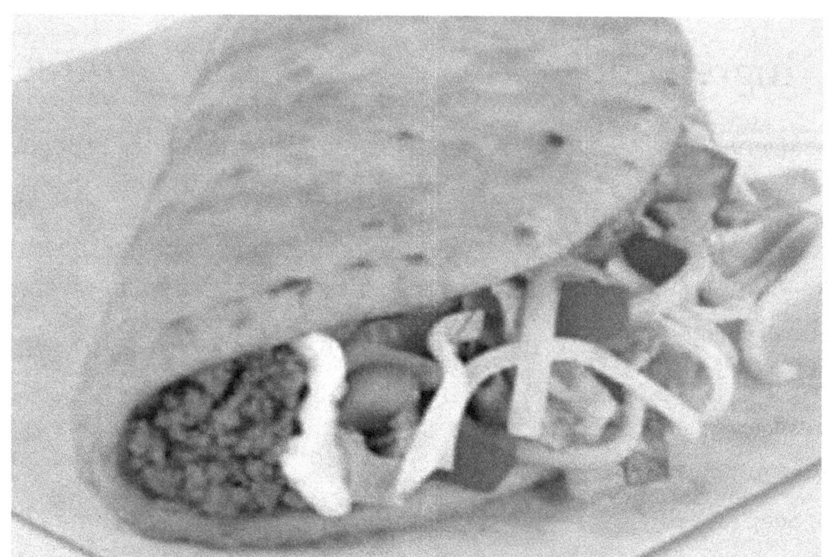

For the Fry Bread:

- ***2 ½ cups all-purpose flour***
- ***1 tablespoon baking powder***
- ***½ teaspoon salt***
- ***1 tablespoon vegetable shortening***
- ***1 cup milk***

For the Filling:

- ***1 tablespoon dried onion flakes***
- ***½ cup water***
- ***1 pound ground beef***
- ***¼ cup flour***
- ***4 teaspoons chili powder***
- ***1 teaspoon paprika***
- ***1 teaspoon ground cumin***
- ***1 teaspoon salt***
- ***½ teaspoon red pepper flakes***

Other Ingredients:

- ***Oil for frying***
- ***Sour cream, for serving***
- ***Lettuce, for serving***
- ***Grated cheese, for serving***
- ***Chopped tomatoes, for serving***

Nutrition

Calories: 80 Fat: 4g Carbs: 20g Sugars: 2g Protein: 15g

Directions

1. Prepare the dough. Combine the flour, baking powder, and salt. Mix the milk and shortening. Do not overwork the dough. Set aside the dough and cover it while you prepare the filling.
2. Mix the onion flakes with the water and set them aside to hydrate.
3. In a skillet, brown the meat and break it into small pieces as it cooks. Drain any excess fat.
4. Sprinkle the flour over the beef. Mix it and let it cook for a minute or two.
5. Add the onion bits and water. Stir in the spices and mix well. Turn the burner to a minimum and cover the skillet.
6. Turn the fried dough out onto a lightly floured surface and divide it into 8 equal pieces. Roll the dough into circles one by one. They should be 8–10 inches across and about a ¼-inch thick. If you want to fold the chalupa, use the rolling pin to press a flat space across the middle of the circle.
7. Heat the oil. Get a small ball of dough (the size of a pea) and drop it in the oil. If the ball immediately floats to the surface, the oil is hot enough.
8. One at a time, lower the dough circles into the oil. Use the tongs to press the dough under the oil, and cook on both sides until golden.
9. For folded chalupas, shape them while they're still hot.
10. Add a portion of the meat filling and layer on the desired toppings.

Preparation Time: 15' *Cooking Time: 4-8'* *Serves: 6-8*

63. Chipotle's Slow Cooked Beef Barbacoa

Ingredients

- *½2 onions, diced*
- *3 tablespoons olive oil*
- *8 garlic cloves, minced*
- *1 tablespoon taco seasoning*
- *½ tablespoon oregano*
- *1 (7-ounce) can of chipotle in adobo sauce*
- *1 cup chicken broth*
- *1 cup water*
- *2 bay leaves*
- *2 tablespoons apple cider vinegar*
- *3 pounds beef roast*

Directions

1. Add all ingredients except the beef in a blender or food processor.
2. Pulse until the spice mixture is well blended.
3. Add a halt of the spice mixture to the bottom of a slow cooker.
4. Place beef in the slow cooker and top with the remaining spice mixture.
5. Slow cook for 8 hours on low or 4 hours on high.
6. Remove the beef from the cooker and shred.
7. If desired, for a saucier barbacoa beef, return shredded beef back to the slow cooker and mix with sauce. Cook for another additional 10–15 minutes on low heat.

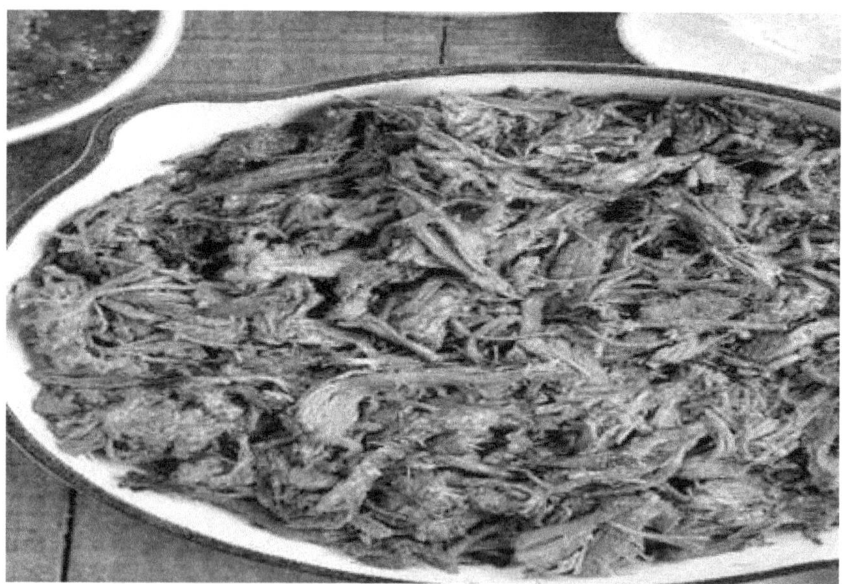

Nutrition

Calories: 178 Fat: 24g Carbs: 123g Sugars: 15g Protein: 27g

Preparation Time: 20' *Cooking Time: 15'* *Serves: 12*

64. Taco Bell's Enchiritos

Ingredients

Seasoning:

- *¼ cup all-purpose flour*
- *1 tablespoon chili powder*
- *1 teaspoon salt*
- *½ teaspoon dried onion flakes*
- *½ teaspoon paprika*
- *¼ teaspoon onion powder*
- *1 dash garlic powder*

Tortillas filling:

- *1 pound lean ground beef*
- *½ cup water*
- *1 (16-ounce) can refried beans*
- *12 small flour tortillas*
- *½ cup onion, diced*
- *1(16-ounce) can red chili sauce*
- *2 cups cheddar cheese, shredded*
- *Some green onions, for serving*
- *Some sour cream, for serving*

Directions

1. Combine all of the seasoning ingredients.
2. Coat the beef in the seasoning using your hands. Make sure that the beef fully absorbs the flavor from the spices.
3. Brown the seasoned beef in the water over medium heat, for 8 to 10 minutes. Stir the beef occasionally to remove lumps.
4. While the beef is browning, microwave the beans on high for 2 minutes.
5. Cover the tortillas in a wet towel and microwave for 1 minute.
6. When the beef is done, assemble the tortillas
7. Place some beans in the middle of the tortilla;
8. Place some beef on top, add some onion;
9. Roll up the tortilla by bringing both ends together in the center;
10. Place the tortilla in a microwave-safe casserole; and
11. Spread the chili sauce and cheddar cheese on top of the tortilla.
12. Heat the entire dish in the microwave for 2-3 minutes. The dish is done when the cheese melts.

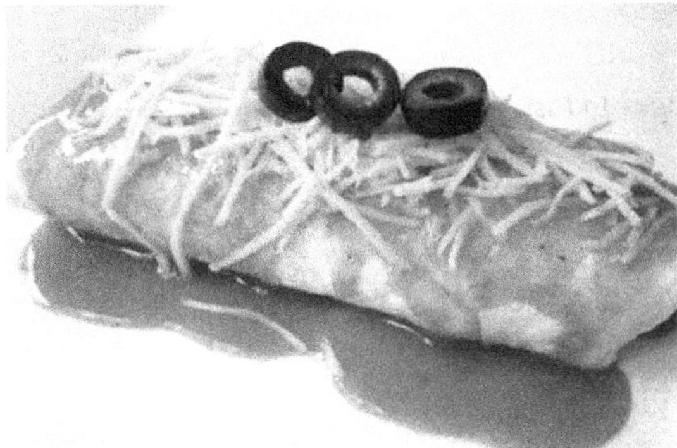

Nutrition

Calories: 119 Fat: 20g Carbs: 76g Sugars: 12g Protein: 10g

Preparation Time: 30' *Cooking Time: 15'* *Serves: 10*

65. Taco Bell's Double Decker Tacos

Ingredients

- ***Taco:***
- ***1 pound ground beef***
- ***2 tablespoons taco seasoning mix, divided***
- ***1 (16-ounces) can refried beans***
- ***2/3 Cup water***
- ***12 crisp taco shells***
- ***Sour cream for serving***
- ***Guacamole:***
- ***2 avocados***
- ***2 tablespoons diced onions***
- ***1 fresh lime, juiced***
- ***Salt and black pepper to taste***
- ***Assembling:***
- ***12 soft flour tortillas, about 7-inch diameter***
- ***2 cups shredded cheddar cheese***
- ***1 cup shredded lettuce***
- ***1 large tomato, chopped***
- ***¼ red onion, chopped***
- ***½ cup sour cream***
- ***Salt and black pepper to taste***

Directions

1. Preheat the oven to 350°F.
2. Cook the beef for 10 to 15 minutes over medium heat, sprinkling it with ¾ ounce of the taco seasoning. When the beef is brown and crumbly, remove it from the heat and set aside.
3. Season the refried beans with the remaining taco seasoning mix by placing the beans, water, and seasoning in a small pot and mixing and mashing everything together. Mash the beans and bring the mixture to a simmer. Heat the taco shells in the oven for 3 to 5 minutes.
4. While the taco shells are being heated, make the guacamole by mashing all the guacamole ingredients together.
5. To assemble the tacos, start by covering one side of each flour tortilla with 2 tablespoons of the bean mixture and wrapping the flour tortilla around a taco shell. Then place the following by layers inside the taco shell

- 2 tablespoons beef
- 2 tablespoons cheese
- Shredded lettuce
- Chopped tomato and onion
- Serve with sour cream on the side.

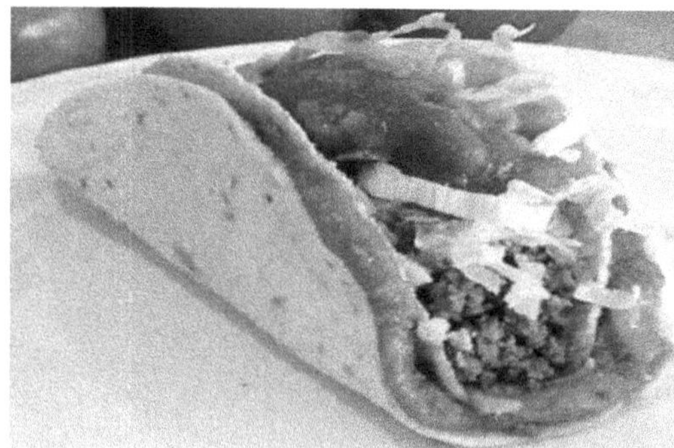

Nutrition

Calories: 184 Fat: 4g Carbs: 57g Sugars: 9g Protein: 12g

Chapter 4
Seafood

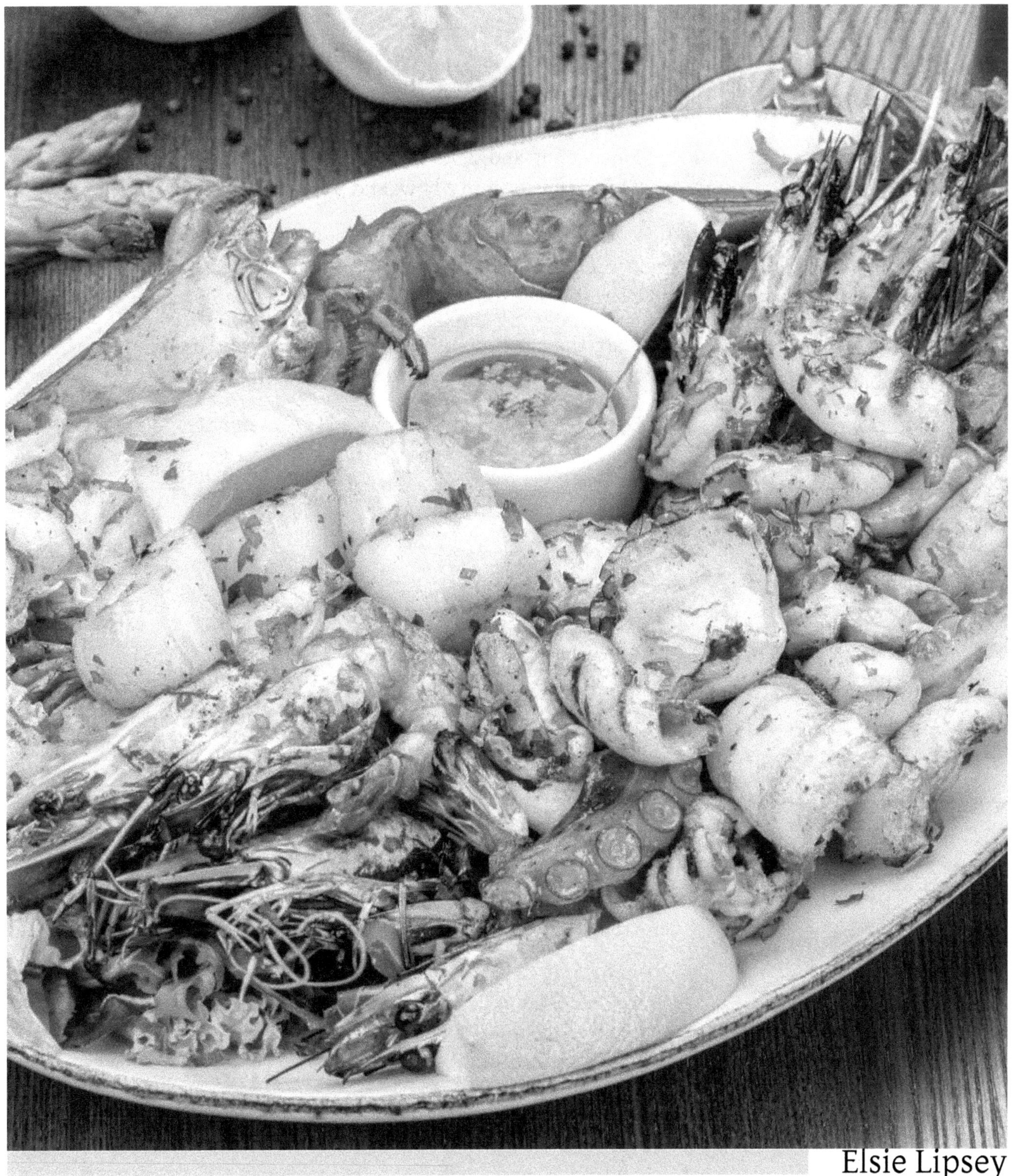

Preparation Time: 10' *Cooking Time: 20'* *Serves: 6*

66. Red Lobster's Crab-Stuffed Mushrooms

Ingredients

- *1 lb. white mushrooms*
- *¼ cup celery*
- *2 tablespoon onion*
- *2 tablespoon red bell pepper*
- *5 lb. crab claw meat*
- *½ cup shredded cheddar cheese*
- *2 cups crushed oyster crackers*
- *.¼ teaspoons Salt & freshly cracked black pepper*
- *½ teaspoons Old Bay Seasoning*
- *¼ teaspoons garlic powder*
- *1 egg*
- *6 slices white cheddar cheese*

Directions

1. Warm the oven at 400° Fahrenheit.
2. Finely chop and sauté the onions, celery, and peppers for two minutes. Transfer it in a bowl and put in the fridge.
3. Rinse the mushrooms and remove the stems (discard half of them). Combine them with the veggies, chopped stems (if desired), rest of the fixings, except for the cheese slices.
4. Place the mushrooms into baking dishes. Put one teaspoon of the mixture into each cup and sprinkle with cheese to bake.
5. Bake them until lightly browned (12–15 minutes).

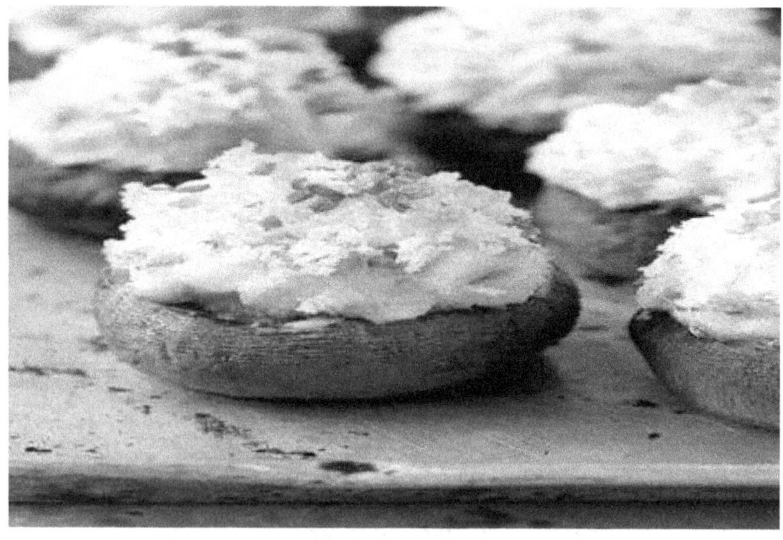

Nutrition

Calories: 115 Fat: 14g Carbs: 78g Sugars: 9g Protein: 8g

Preparation Time: 30' *Cooking Time: 1 hour* *Serves: 4-6*

67. Red Lobster's Shrimp Quiche

Ingredients

- ***1-9 inch Pre-baked pie crust***
- ***4 ounces Petite Alaskan shrimp***
- ***½cup grated Gruyere cheese***
- ***2 Whisked eggs***
- ***1 cup light sour cream***
- ***1 tablespoon green onions/chives***
- ***Black pepper and salt***

Directions

1. Devein, cook, and peel the shrimp.
2. Warm the oven to 350° Fahrenheit.
3. Sprinkle the shrimp over the pie crust, adding the grated cheese.
4. Finely chop the chives or onions. Combine the eggs, pepper, salt, sour cream, and green onions.
5. Pour the mixture into the pie crust.
6. Bake for 25 to 30 minutes.
7. Serve warm or chilled.

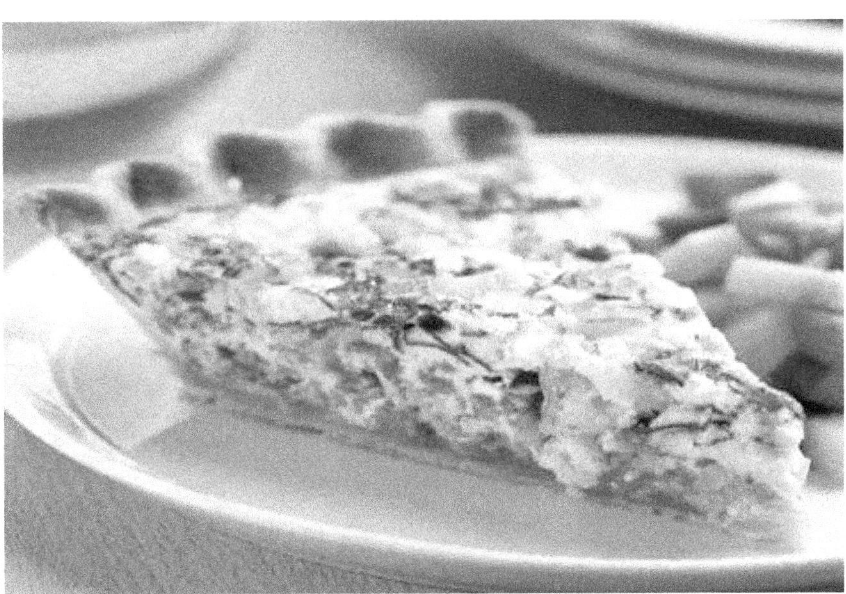

Nutrition

Calories: 112 Fat: 17 Carbs: 50g Sugars: 5g Protein: 7g

Preparation Time: 15' *Cooking Time: 30'* *Serves: 6*

68. Red Lobster's Clam (& Potato) Chowder

Ingredients

- ***2 (6.5) ounces cans minced clams***
- ***2 strips crispy bacon***
- ***1 medium onion***
- ***2 tablespoon all-purpose flour***
- ***4 medium sized potatoes***
- ***1 water***
- ***¼ dried savory***
- ***½ salt***
- ***¼ black pepper***
- ***½ dried thyme***
- ***2 cups milk***
- ***2 tablespoon freshly minced parsley***

Directions

1. Drain the clams, reserving the juice.

2. Fry the bacon in a skillet using the medium temperature setting. Stir it occasionally until it's done and crispy. Place the cooked bacon on a layer of parchment paper or paper towels. Break it apart into bits.

3. Chop and add the onion to the drippings. Simmer and stir them until tender or for four to six minutes. Mix in the flour, thoroughly stirring until it's blended. Slowly stir in water and the reserved clam juice. Continue cooking while stirring until it's bubbly.

4. Peel, slice, and add potatoes and seasonings, bringing it to a boil, stirring often. Lower the temperature setting and continue cooking, covered with a lid on the pot until the potatoes are tender—occasionally stirring (20 to 25 min.)

5. Pour in the milk, parsley, and clams to heat thoroughly. Top with bacon and serve.

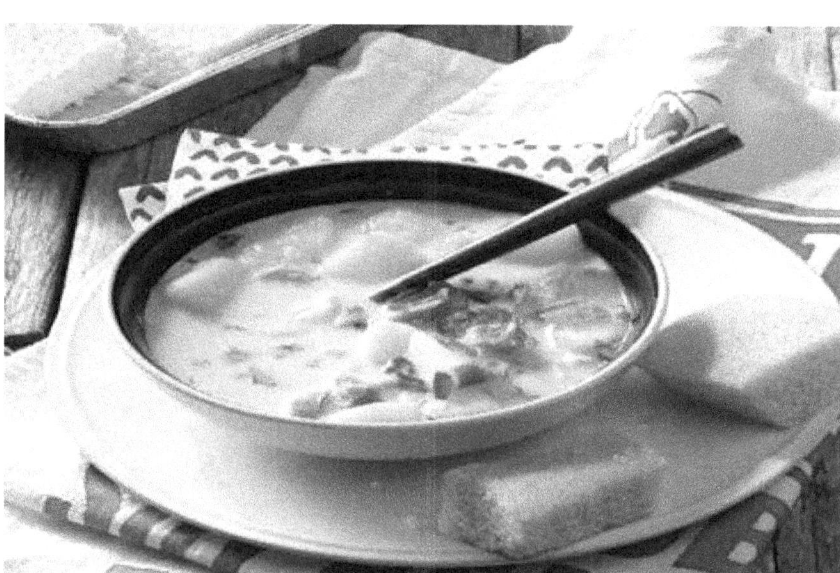

Nutrition

Calories: 178 Fat: 24g Carbs: 123g Sugars: 15g Protein: 27g

Preparation Time: 10' *Cooking Time: 15'* *Serves: 4*

69. Red Lobster's Crab Alfredo

Ingredients

- ***Kosher salt***
- ***3 tablespoon butter***
- ***12 ounces fettuccine or linguine***
- ***3 garlic cloves***
- ***3 tablespoon a-purpose flour***
- ***1 cup chicken broth***
- ***1 cup heavy cream***
- ***1 tablespoon Old Bay***
- ***1 ½ cups freshly grated parmesan***
- ***Black pepper***
- ***2 tablespoonf parsley***
- ***1 lb. lump crab meat***
- ***½ lemon juice***

Directions

1. Prepare a soup pot of salted water and add the noodles and cook until they're al dente. Toss them into a colander to drain and toss back into the pot.
2. Add the butter to a frying pan using the medium heat setting.
3. Mince and add the garlic to sauté for about a minute. Sift and mix in the flour lightly browned.
4. Put the heavy cream and chicken broth into the pot and cook it slowly until it's thickened.
5. Add the parmesan, Old Bay, salt, and pepper, and let melt for about two minutes. Fold in the parsley and crabmeat, tossing until coated. Lastly, add the linguine and stir it well.
6. Garnish with chopped parsley, parmesan, Old Bay, and a squeeze of lemon juice.

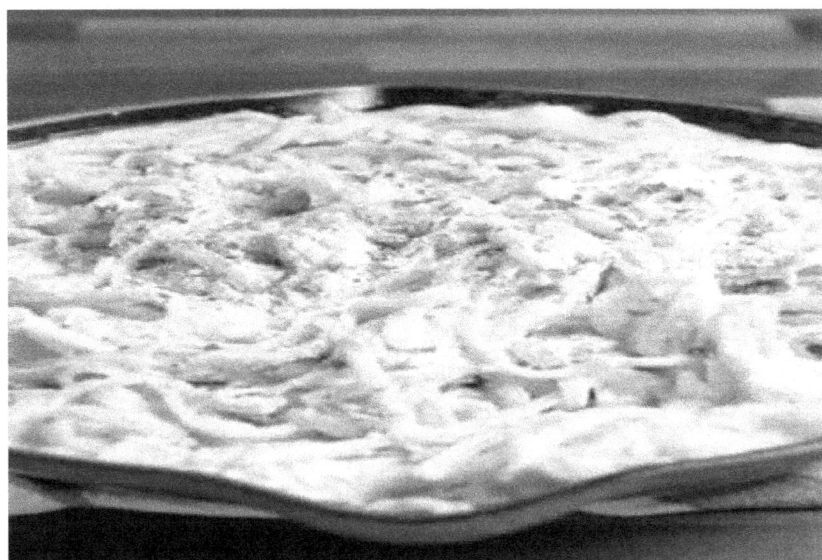

Nutrition

Calories: 119 Fat: 20g Carbs: 76g Sugars: 12g Protein: 10g

Preparation Time: 10' *Cooking Time: 15'* *Serves: 4*

70. Red Lobster's Easy Garlic Shrimp Scampi

Ingredients

- ***1 lb. Jumbo shrimp***
- ***1 teaspoons McCormick's Montreal Chicken Seasoning***
- ***Black pepper & salt***
- ***1 teaspoons olive oil***
- ***3 garlic clove***
- ***3 tablespoon butter, microwaved for 15 seconds to soften***
- ***1/ cup lemon juice***
- ***1 cup low-sugar dry white wine***

Optional: 1 teaspoons Red pepper flakes

- ***¼ cup freshly grated parmesan cheese***
- ***1 teaspoons Italian seasoning***

For the Garnish: Chopped parsley

Directions

1. Peel and devein the shrimp. Give it a good shake of salt, pepper, and chicken seasoning to your liking.
2. Add the oil and warm a skillet using the med-high temperature setting.
3. Toss the shrimp into the pan for three to four minutes. Once it turns pink, set it aside for now.
4. Mince and toss in the garlic to sauté until it is fragrant (1-2 min.)
5. Add and simmer the lemon juice, wine, Italian Seasoning, and pepper flakes (1-2 min). Set to low for two more minutes.
6. Add the butter to the skillet and toss the shrimp back into the pan. Simmer for one to two minutes, and serve using parsley and parmesan cheese.

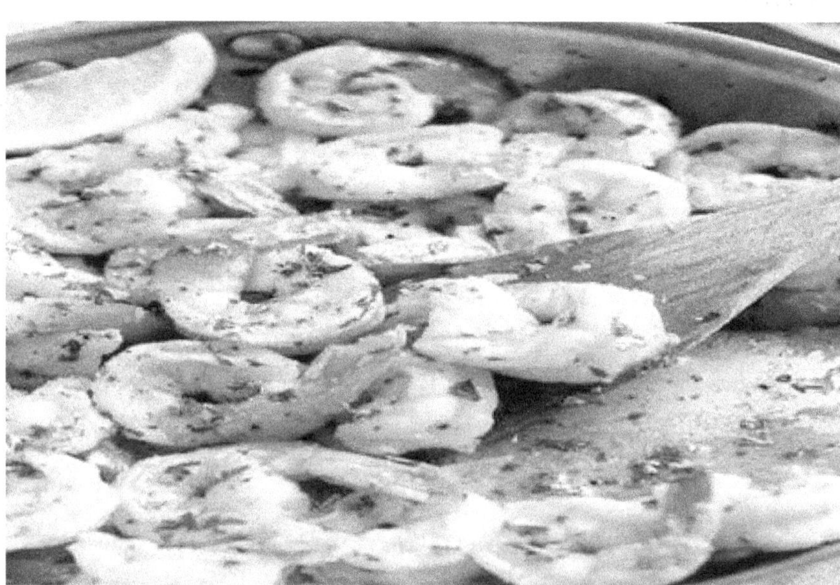

Nutrition

Calories: 184 Fat: 4g Carbs: 57g Sugars: 9g Protein: 12g

Preparation Time: 2 h *Cooking Time: 0* *Serves: 4-6*

71. Red Lobster's Shrimp Gazpacho

Ingredients

- ***20 ounces V-8 vegetable/tomato/ bloody mary mix***
- ***1 tablespoon olive oil***
- ***½ teaspoons worcestershire sauce***
- ***2 tablespoon red wine vinegar***
- ***1 teaspoons fresh cilantro & parsley***
- ***¼ teaspoons tabasco sauce***
- ***1 tablespoonl juice***
- ***1 cup fresh tomatoes***
- ***½ cup Seeded cucumber***
- ***¼ cup Celery***
- ***¼ cup green onions***
- ***¼ cup bell pepper***
- ***Salt and black pepper***
- ***1 cup freshly cooked shrimp***

To serve: 1 lime

Directions

1. Devein and cook the shrimp. Pop it in the fridge to chill.

2. Prep the veggies. Chop the cilantro and parsley. Slice the onions and into ¼-inch pieces. Dice the bell pepper, cucumber, tomatoes, and celery into ¼-inch chunks.

3. Combine all of the fixings (omit the shrimp). Chill it for two hours.

4. Portion into serving dishes and top with two tablespoons of shrimp and a wedge of lime.

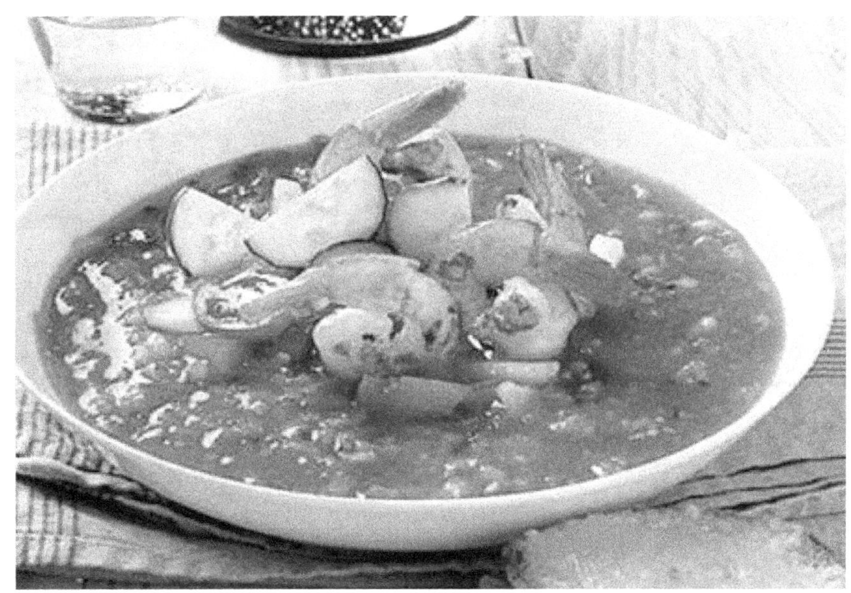

Nutrition

Calories: 147 Fat: 17g Carbs: 87g Sugars: 15g Protein: 14g

Preparation Time: 5' *Cooking Time: 15'* *Serves: 8*

72. Red Lobster's Shrimp Kabobs

Ingredients

- ***1 lb. Uncooked shrimp***
- ***3 tablespoon olive oil***
- ***3 cloves crushed garlic***
- ***½ cup dry bread crumbs***
- ***½ teaspoons seafood seasoning***
- ***Seafood cocktail sauce***
- ***Also Needed: Metal or wooden skewers***

Directions

1. In a shallow mixing container, mix the oil and garlic. Wait for 30 minutes for the flavors to blend.
2. In another mixing container, combine the breadcrumbs and seafood seasoning.
3. Dredge the shrimp through the oil mixture, then coat it using the crumb mixture.
4. Thread the shrimp onto the skewers.
5. Grill the kabobs with the top on the cooker, using medium heat for two to three minutes or until the shrimp turns light pink.
6. Serve with seafood sauce.

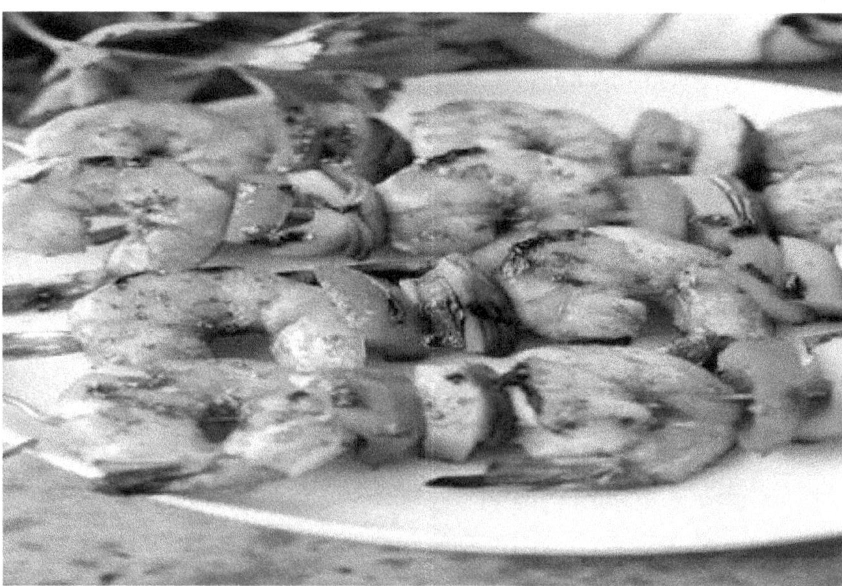

Nutrition

Calories: 158 Fat: 10g Carbs: 71g Sugars: 10g Protein: 16g

Preparation Time: 15' *Cooking Time: 1 hour* *Serves: 6-8*

73. Red Lobster's Shrimp Slaw

Ingredients

- ***3 cups green/white cabbage***
- ***1 cup celery***
- ***1 ½ spinach***
- ***8 ounces Petite Alaskan shrimp***

The Dressing:

- ***½ teaspoons fresh ginger***
- ***½ teaspoons freshly cracked black pepper***
- ***1 teaspoons salt***
- ***¼ cup white wine vinegar***
- ***2 tablespoon honey***
- ***½ cup Mayonnaise***

Directions

1. Shred the cabbage and spinach. Thinly slice the celery. Grate the ginger. Devein, cook, and peel the shrimp.
2. Toss the fixings in a large salad container.
3. Prepare the dressing and spritz the salad thoroughly. Save leftover dressing for a side dish.
4. Chill it for at least an hour.

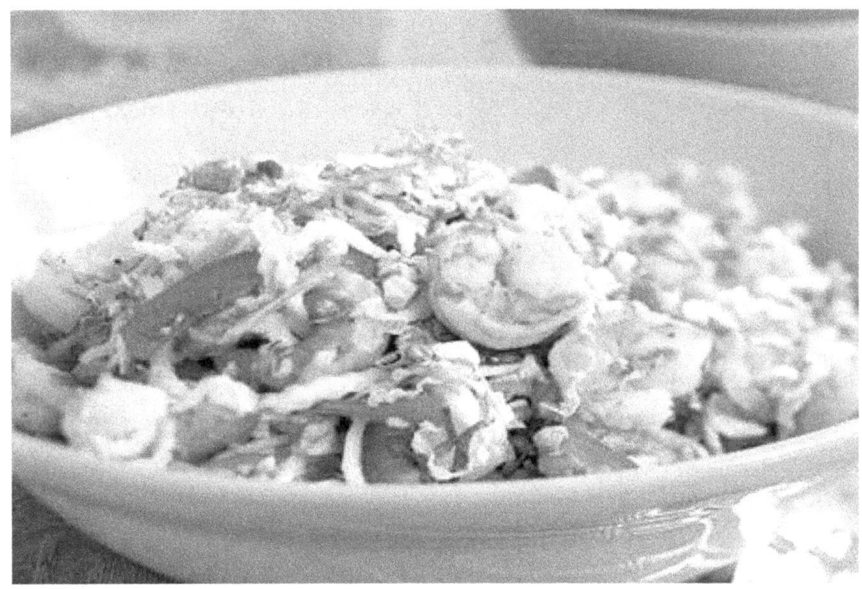

Nutrition

Calories: 136 Fat: 8g Carbs: 56g Sugars: 7g Protein: 13g

Preparation Time: 5' *Cooking Time: 10'* *Serves: 4*

74. Red Lobster's Ginger - Soy Salmon

Ingredients

- *3 tablespoon honey*
- *1 teaspoons dijon-style mustard*
- *¼ cup soy sauce*
- *¼ teaspoons sriracha hot chili sauce/another hot sauce*
- *½ teaspoons grated ginger*
- *2 teaspoons canola oil*
- *4-6 ounces salmon fillets*
- *Black pepper & Kosher salt*
- *Optional l– The Garnish: Sliced scallions*

Directions

1. Set the oven at 400° Fahrenheit
2. Whisk the honey, soy sauce, ginger, mustard, and Sriracha.
3. Warm the oil in an oven-safe skillet using the med-high temperature setting.
4. Dust the salmon with pepper and salt before adding to the skillet.
5. Once the pan is hot, arrange the salmon in the pan and cook for two to three minutes (unmoved to form a crusty layer).
6. At that point, turn them over and place them into the heated oven. Bake them for five to six minutes, leaving the middle slightly pink. Remove and place on the platter to serve.
7. Pour the drippings from the skillet and warm the pan on the stove using the medium-high temperature setting.
8. Dump the soy sauce mixture into the pan and simmer for two to three minutes until thickened.
9. Pour the glaze over the salmon. Top it off with scallions as desired.

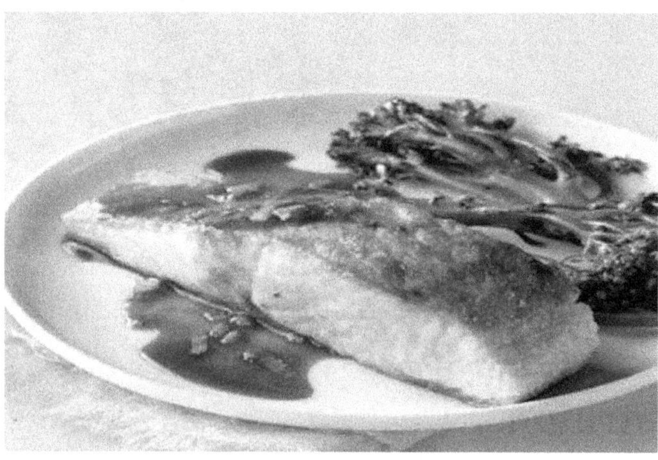

Nutrition

Calories: 242.8 Fat: 6.6g Carbs: 38.4g Sugars: 3g Protein: 8.4g

Chapter 5
Poultry

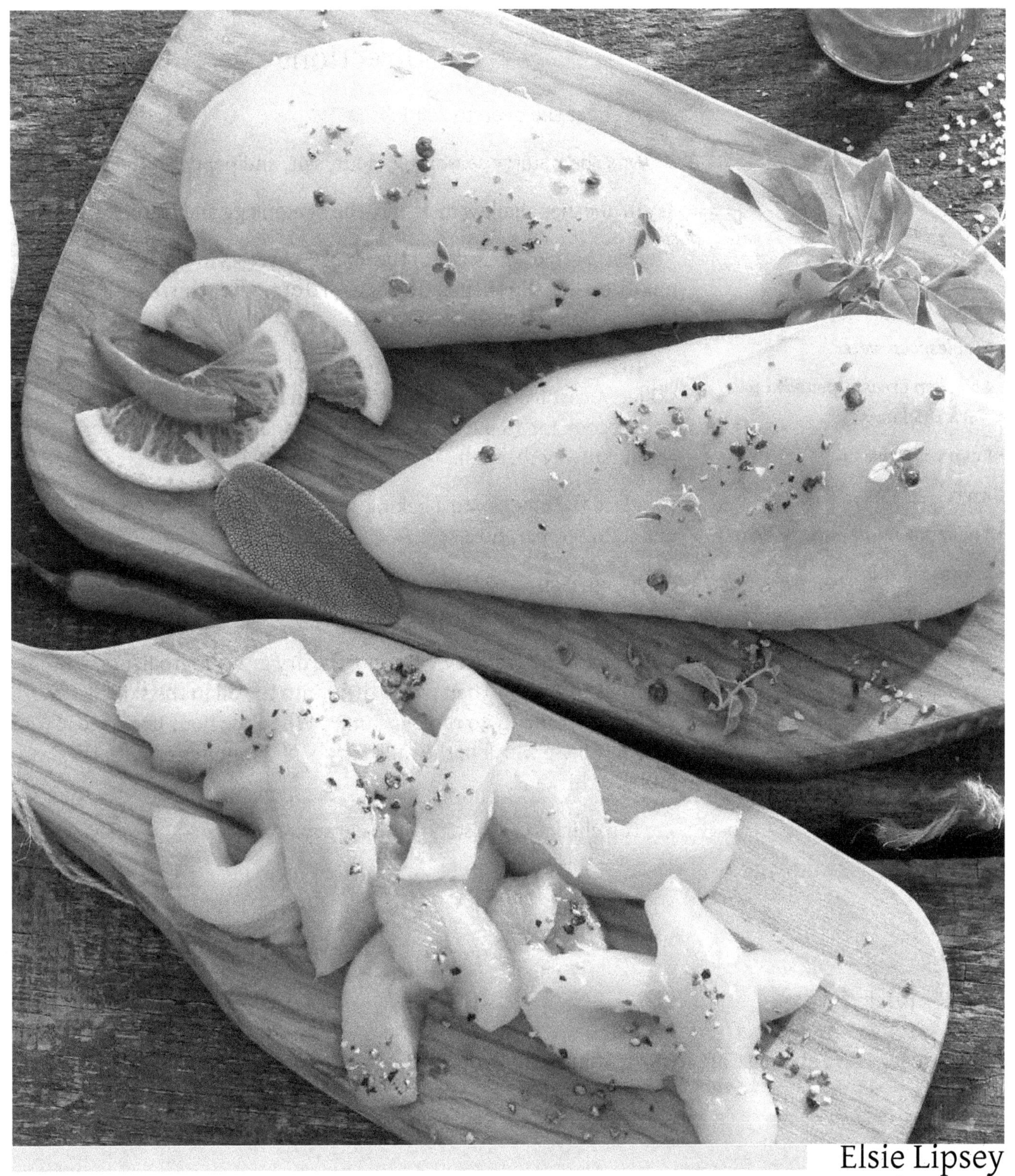

Preparation Time: 15' *Cooking Time: 30'* *Serves: 4*

75. Cracker Barrel's Chicken Fried Chicken

Ingredients

Chicken

- ***½ cup all-purpose flour***
- ***1 teaspoon poultry seasoning***
- ***½ teaspoon salt***
- ***½ teaspoon pepper***
- ***1 egg, slightly beaten***
- ***1 tablespoon water***
- ***4 chicken breasts, pounded to a ½-inch thickness***
- ***1 cup vegetable oil***

Gravy:

- ***2 tablespoons all-purpose flour***
- ***¼ teaspoon salt***
- ***¼ teaspoon pepper***
- ***1¼ cups milk***

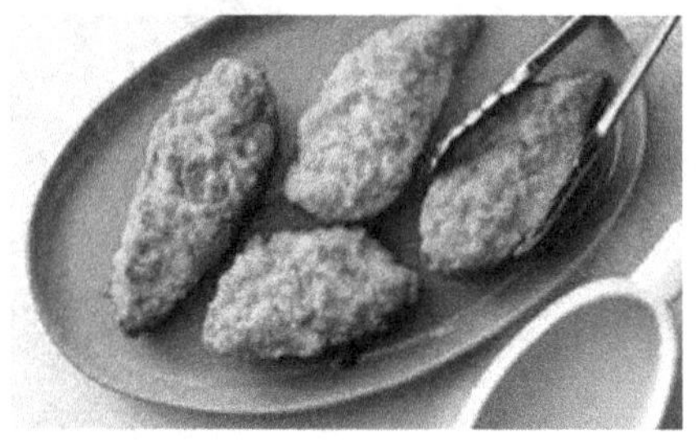

Directions

1. Preheat the oven to 200°F.
2. Mix the poultry seasoning, flour, salt, and pepper.
3. In another shallow dish, mix the beaten egg and water.
4. Coat both of the sides of the chicken breasts in the flour mixture, then dip them in the egg mixture. After this, coat it back into the flour mixture.
5. Heat the vegetable oil over medium-high heat in a large deep skillet. A cast iron is a good choice if you have one. Put the chicken and cook for 15 minutes, or until fully cooked, turning over about halfway through.
6. Place the chicken to a baking sheet and place in the oven to maintain temperature.
7. Remove all but 2 tablespoons of oil from the skillet you cooked the chicken in.
8. Prepare the gravy by whisking the dry gravy ingredients together in a bowl. Then whisk them into the oil in the skillet, stirring thoroughly to remove lumps. When the flour begins to brown, slowly whisk in the milk for about 2 minutes or until the mixture thickens.
9. Top chicken with some of the gravy.

Nutrition

Calories: 242.8 Fat: 6.6g Carbs: 38.4g Sugars: 3g Protein: 8.4g

Preparation Time: 10' *Cooking Time: 45'* *Serves: 4*

76.Cracker Barrel's Broccoli Cheddar Chicken

Ingredients

- ***1-9 inch Pre-baked pie crust***
- ***4 ounces Petite Alaskan shrimp***
- ***½cup grated Gruyere cheese***
- ***2 Whisked eggs***
- ***1 cup light sour cream***
- ***1 tablespoon green onions/chives***
- ***Black pepper and salt***

Directions

1. Preheat the oven to 350°F.
2. Whisk the milk and cheddar cheese soup together in a mixing bowl.
3. Prepare a baking dish by greasing the sides, then lay the chicken in the bottom and season with the salt and pepper.
4. Put the soup mixture on the chicken, then top with the crackers, broccoli, and shredded cheese. Bake for 45 minutes.

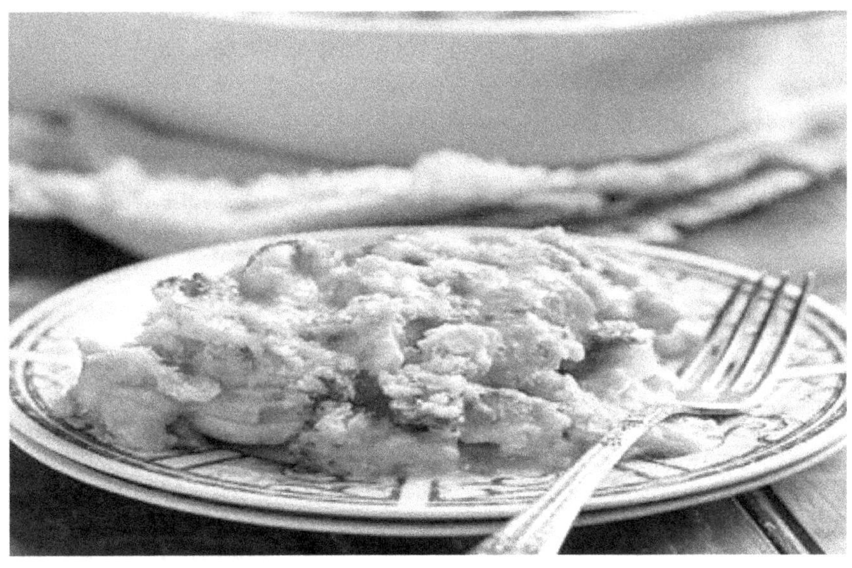

Nutrition

Calories: 150 Fat: 4.2g Carbs: 40g Sugars: 1g Protein: 9g

Preparation Time: 10' *Cooking Time: 30'* *Serves: 4-5*

77. Cracker Barrel's Grilled Chicken Tenderloin

Ingredients

- ***4–5 boneless and skinless chicken breasts, cut into strips, or 12 chicken tenderloins, tendons removed***
- ***1 cup Italian dressing***
- ***2 teaspoons lime juice***
- ***4 teaspoons honey***

Directions

1. Mix together the honey, dressing, and lime juice in a plastic bag. Seal and shake to combine.
2. Place the chicken in the bag. Seal and shake again, then transfer to the refrigerator for at least 1 hour.
3. When ready to prepare, transfer the chicken and the marinade to a large nonstick skillet.
4. Let it boil and allow it to simmer until the liquid has cooked down to a glaze.

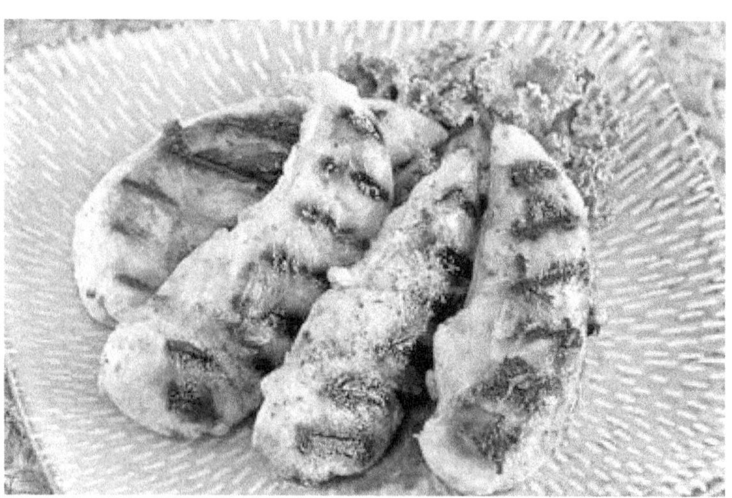

Nutrition

Calories: 100 Fat: 3g Carbs: 21g Sugars: 10g Protein: 5g

Preparation Time: 10' *Cooking Time: 1 h 10'* *Serves: 4*

78. Cracker Barrel's Chicken Casserole

Ingredients

Crust:

- ***1 cup yellow cornmeal***
- ***1/3 Cup all-purpose flour***
- ***1½ teaspoons baking powder***
- ***1 tablespoon sugar***
- ***½ teaspoon salt***
- ***½ teaspoon baking soda***
- ***2 tablespoons vegetable oil***
- ***¾ cup buttermilk***
- ***1 egg***

Filling:

- ***2½ cups bite-sized cooked chicken breast***
- ***¼ cup chopped yellow onion***
- ***½ cup sliced celery***
- ***1 teaspoon salt***
- ***¼ teaspoon ground pepper***
- ***1 can condensed cream (chicken soup)***
- ***1¾ cups chicken broth***
- ***2 tablespoons butter***
- ***½ cup melted butter***

Directions

1. Preheat the oven to 375°F. Combine all of the crust ingredients until smooth.

2. Dump this mixture into a buttered or greased 8×8-inch baking dish. Bake it for 20 minutes, then remove from oven and allow to cool. Reduce oven temperature to 350°F.

3. Crumble the cooled cornbread mixture. Add to a bowl along with ½ cup melted butter. Set aside.

4. Make the chicken filling by adding the butter to a large saucepan over medium heat. Let it melt, then add the celery and onions and cook until soft.

5. Add the chicken broth, cream of chicken soup, salt, and pepper. Stir until everything is well combined. Add the cooked chicken breast pieces and stir again. Cook for 5 minutes at a low simmer.

6. Transfer the filling mixture into 4 individual greased baking dishes or a greased casserole dish. Top with the cornbread mixture and transfer to the oven. Bake for 35–40 minutes for a large casserole dish or 25–30 minutes for individual dishes.

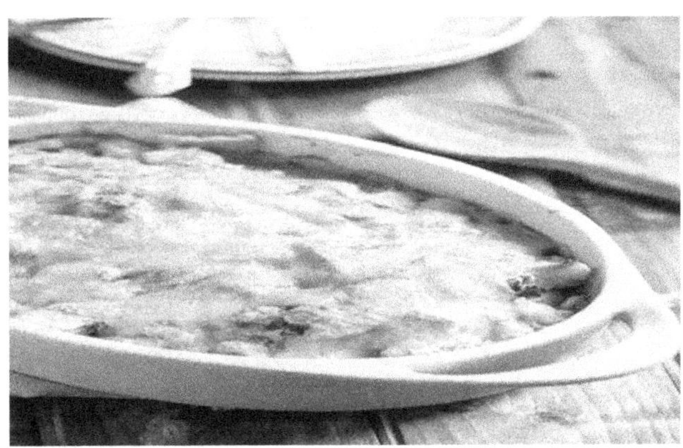

Nutrition

Calories: 178 Fat: 15g Carbs: 50g Sugars: 8g Protein: 9g

Preparation Time: 10' *Cooking Time: 10'* *Serves: 4*

79. Cracker Barrel's Sunday Chicken

Ingredients

- ***Oil for frying***
- ***4 boneless, skinless chicken breasts***
- ***1 cups all-purpose flour***
- ***1 cup bread crumbs***
- ***2 teaspoons salt***
- ***2 teaspoons black pepper***
- ***1 cup buttermilk***
- ***½ cup water***

Directions

1. Add 3–4 inches of oil to a large pot or a deep fryer and preheat to 350°F.
2. Mix the flour, breadcrumbs, salt, and pepper in a shallow dish. To a separate shallow dish, add the buttermilk and water; stir.
3. Pound the chicken breasts to a consistent size. Let it dry paper towel and season with salt and pepper.
4. Dip the seasoned breasts in the flour mixture, then the buttermilk mixture, then back into the flour.
5. Put the breaded chicken to the pan and fry for about 8 minutes. Turn the chicken as necessary so that it cooks evenly on both sides.
6. Remove the chicken to either a wire rack or a plate lined with paper towels to drain.
7. Serve with mashed potatoes or whatever sides you love.

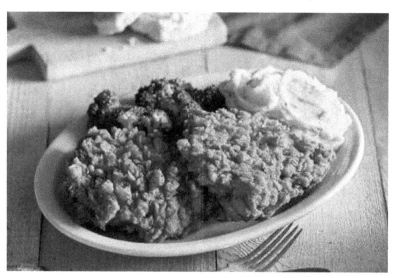

Nutrition

Calories: 150 Fat: 20g Carbs: 50g Sugars: 9g Protein: 15g

Preparation Time: 10' *Cooking Time: 45'* *Serves: 4*

80. Cracker Barrel's Creamy Chicken and Rice

Ingredients

- ***Salt and pepper to taste***
- ***2 cups cooked rice***
- ***1 diced onion***
- ***1 can cream of mushroom soup***
- ***1 packet chicken gravy***
- ***1½ pounds chicken breasts, cut into strips***

Directions

1. Preheat the oven to 350°F.
2. Cook the rice. When it is just about finished, toss in the diced onion so that it cooks too.
3. Spray the baking dish with some nonstick cooking spray.
4. Dump the rice into the prepared baking dish. Layer the chicken strips on top. Pour the cream of mushroom soup on the chicken.
5. Whisk the chicken gravy with 1 cup water, making sure to get all the lumps out. Pour the mixture on top of the casserole.
6. Cover with foil and transfer to the oven and let it bake for 45 minutes or until the chicken is completely cooked.

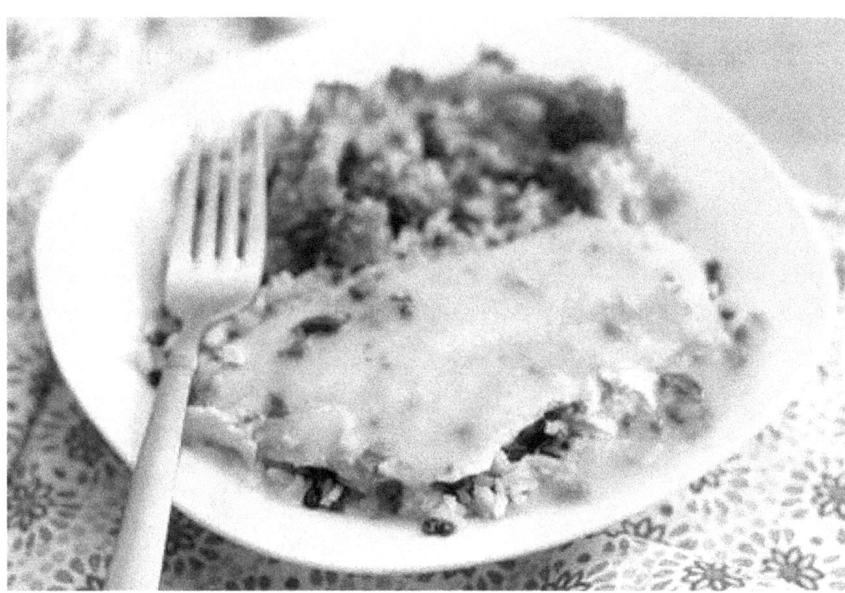

Nutrition

Calories: 160 Fat: 10g Carbs: 50g Sugars: 6g Protein: 12g

Preparation Time: 10' *Cooking Time: 45'* *Serves: 4*

81. Cracker Barrel's Campfire Chicken

Ingredients

- *1 tablespoon paprika*
- *2 teaspoons onion powder*
- *2 teaspoons salt*
- *1 teaspoon garlic powder*
- *1 teaspoon dried rosemary*
- *1 teaspoon black pepper*
- *1 teaspoon dried oregano*
- *1 whole chicken, quartered*
- *2 carrots, cut into thirds*
- *3 red skin potatoes, halved*
- *1 ear of corn, quartered*
- *1 tablespoon olive oil*
- *1 tablespoon butter*
- *5 sprigs fresh thyme*

Directions

1. Preheat the oven to 400°F.
2. Mix the paprika, onion powder, salt, garlic powder, rosemary, pepper, and oregano.
3. Add the chicken quarters and 1 tablespoon of the spice mix to a large plastic freezer bag. Cover and put inside the refrigerator for at least 1 hour.
4. Add the corn, carrots, and potatoes to a large bowl. Drizzle with the olive oil and remaining spice mix. Stir or toss to coat.
5. Preheat a large skillet over high heat. Add some oil, and when it is hot, add the chicken pieces and cook until golden brown.
6. Prepare 4 pieces of aluminum foil and add some carrots, potatoes, corn, and a chicken quarter to each. Top with some butter and thyme.
7. Fold the foil in and make pouches by sealing the edges tightly.
8. Bake for 45 minutes.

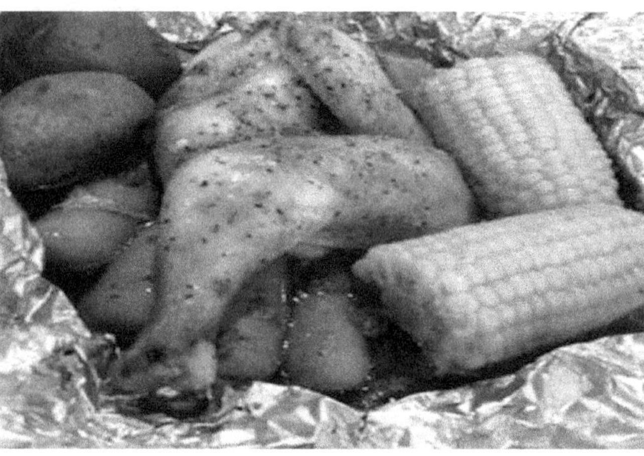

Nutrition

Calories: 140 Fat: 8g Carbs: 30 Sugars: 10g Protein: 25g

Preparation Time: 30' *Cooking Time: 20'* *Serves: 4t*

82. Cracker Barrel's Chicken and Dumplings

Ingredients

- *2 cups flour*
- *½ teaspoon baking powder*
- *1 pinch salt*
- *2 tablespoons butter*
- *1 scant cup buttermilk*
- *2 quarts chicken broth*
- *3 cups cooked chicken*

Directions

1. Mix together in a bowl the salt, flour, and baking powder in a large bowl to make the dumplings. Cut the butter into the flour mixture. Pour in the milk slowly until it forms a dough ball.
2. Cover your countertop with enough flour that the dough will not stick when you roll it out. Roll out the dough relatively thin, then cut into squares to form dumplings.
3. Flour a plate and transfer the dough from the counter to the plate.
4. Bring the chicken broth to a boil in a large saucepan, then drop the dumplings in one by one, stirring continually. The excess flour will thicken the broth. Cook it for 20-25 minutes or until the dumplings are no longer doughy.
5. Add the chicken, stir to combine, and serve.

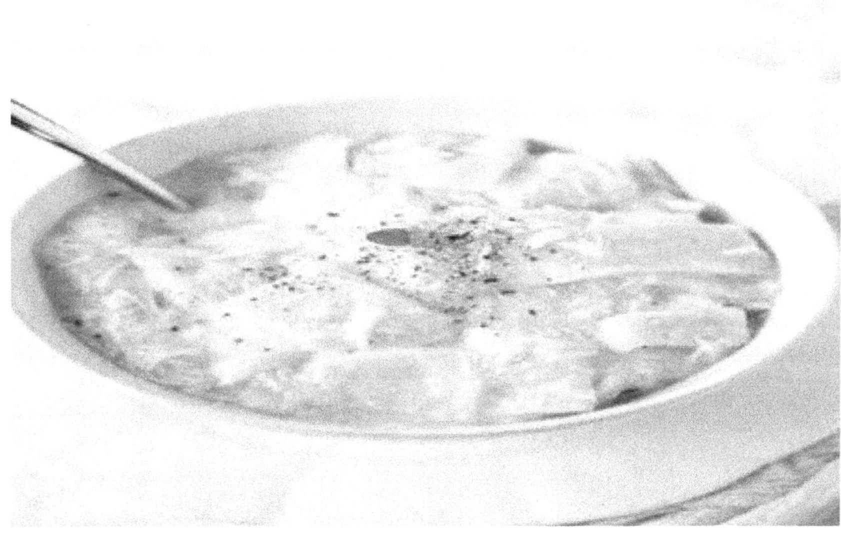

Nutrition

Calories: 115 Fat: 14g Carbs: 78g Sugars: 9g Protein: 8g

Preparation Time: 5' *Cooking Time: 1 h 45'* *Serves: 4-6*

83. Red Lobster's Classic BBQ Chicken

Ingredients

- ***4 pounds chicken***
- ***Salt***
- ***Olive oil***
- ***1 cup barbecue sauce***

Directions

1. Put some olive oil and salt all over the chicken.
2. In the meanwhile, preheat the griddle with high heat.
3. Grill the chicken skin side for 10 minutes.
4. Cover the chicken with foil and grill for 30 minutes in low heat.
5. Put some barbecue sauce all over the chicken.
6. Cook the chicken for another 20 minutes.
7. Baste, cover and cook again for 30 minutes.
8. You will know that the chicken is ready when the internal temperature of the chicken pieces is 165°F and juices run clear.
9. Baste with more barbecue sauce to serve!

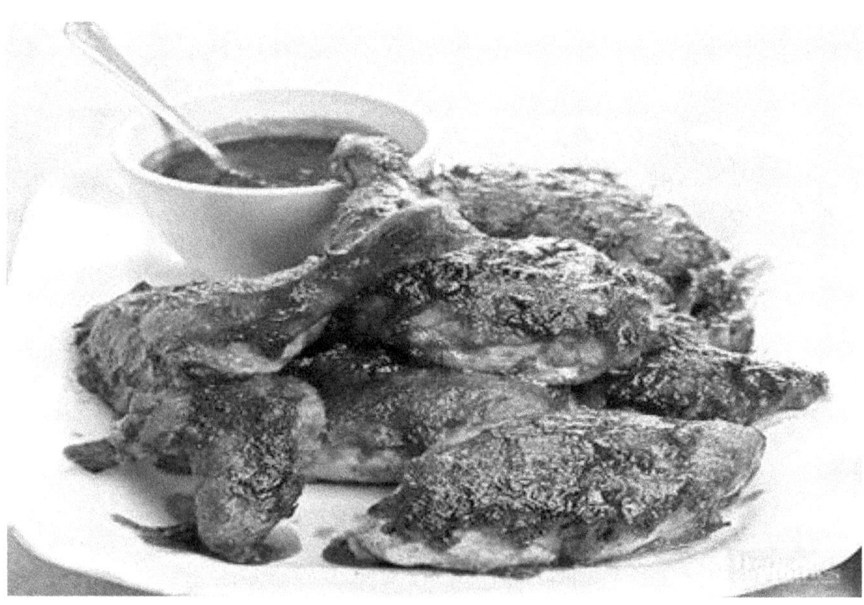

Nutrition

Calories: 539 Fat: 11.6g Carbs: 15.1g Sugar: 0.3g Protein: 87.6g

Preparation Time: 35' *Cooking Time: 15'* *Serves: 4*

84. Chipotle's Grilled Sweet Chili Lime Chicken

Ingredients

- ***½ cup sweet chili sauce***
- ***¼ cup soy sauce***
- ***1 teaspoon marina juice***
- ***1 teaspoon orange juice, fresh squeezed***
- ***1 teaspoon orange marmalade***
- ***2 tablespoons lime juice***
- ***1 tablespoon brown sugar***
- ***1 clove garlic, minced***
- ***4 boneless, skinless chicken breasts***
- ***Sesame seeds, for garnish***

Directions

1. Whisk sweet chili sauce, soy sauce, marina, orange marmalade, lime and orange juice, brown sugar, and the minced garlic together in a small mixing bowl.
2. Set aside ¼ cup the sauce.
3. Coat the chicken in sauce to coat and let it marinate 30 minutes.
4. Preheat your griddle to medium heat.
5. Cook each side of the chicken on the grill for 7 minutes.
6. Baste the cooked chicken with remaining marinade and garnish with sesame seeds to serve with your favorite sides.

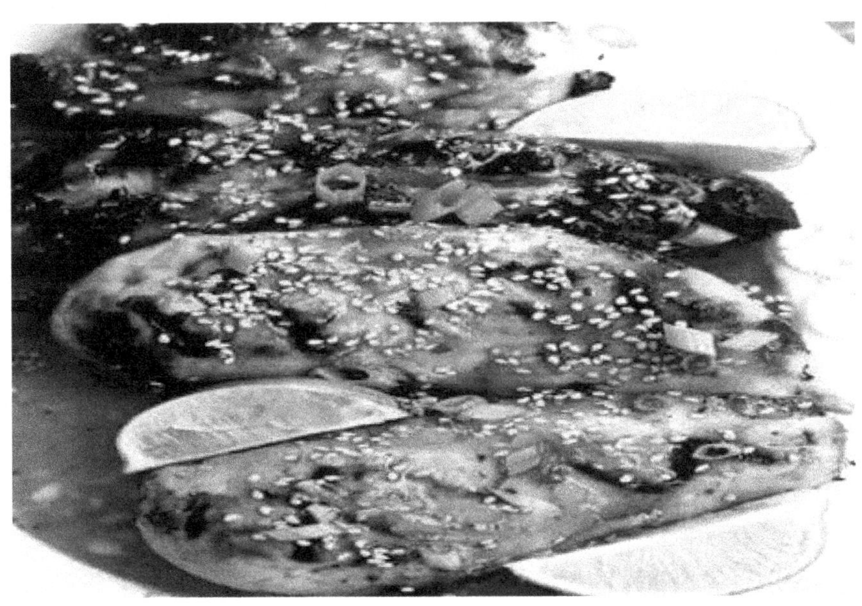

Nutrition

Calories: 380 Sugar: 0.5g Fat: 12g Carbs: 19.7g Protein: 43.8g

Preparation Time: 1-24h *Cooking Time: 20'* *Serves: 4-6*

85. Chipotle's Adobo Chicken

Ingredients

- ***2 lbs. chicken thighs or breasts (boneless, skinless)***

For the marinade:

- ***¼ cup olive oil***
- ***2 chipotle peppers***
- ***1 teaspoon adobo sauce***
- ***1 tablespoon garlic, minced***
- ***1 shallot, finely chopped***
- ***1 ½ tablespoons cumin***
- ***1 tablespoon cilantro, super-finely chopped or dried***
- ***2 teaspoons chili powder***
- ***1 teaspoon dried oregano***
- ***½ teaspoon salt***
- ***Fresh limes, garnish***
- ***Cilantro, garnish***

Directions

1. Preheat grill to medium-high.
2. Blend the marinade ingredients to turn it into paste.
3. Add the chicken and marinade to a sealable plastic bag and massage to coat well.
4. Put in the fridge before grilling.
5. Grill the chicken for 7 minutes, turn and grill and additional 7 minutes; or until good grill marks appear.
6. Continue to grill in low heat until chicken is cooked through and internal temperature reaches 165°F.
7. After that, remove it from the grill and allow to rest 5 to 10 minutes before serving.
8. Squeeze fresh lime and a sprinkle cilantro to serve.

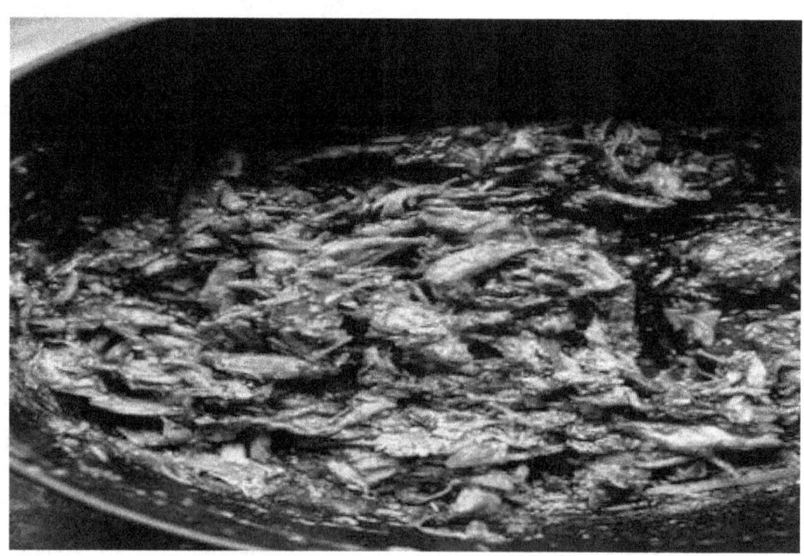

Nutrition

Calories: 561 Sugar: 0.3g Fat: 23.8g Carbs: 18.7g

Preparation Time: 8-24h *Cooking Time: 20'* *Serves: 4*

86. Chipotle'sClassic Grilled Chicken

Ingredients

- ***2 lbs. boneless, skinless chicken thighs***

For the marinade:

- ***¼ cup fresh lime juice***
- ***2 teaspoon lime zest***
- ***¼ cup honey***
- ***2 tablespoons olive oil***
- ***1 tablespoon balsamic vinegar***
- ***½ teaspoon sea salt***
- ***½ teaspoon black pepper***
- ***2 garlic cloves, minced***
- ***¼ teaspoon onion powder***

Directions

1. Mix the ingredients for marinade in a large bowl; reserve 2 tablespoons of the marinade for grilling.
2. Add chicken and marinade to a sealable plastic bag and marinate 8 hours or overnight in the refrigerator.
3. Preheat grill to medium heat and brush lightly with olive oil.
4. Put the chicken on the grill and cook 8 minutes per side.
5. Coat the chicken in the marinade in the last few minutes of cooking until it reaches the internal temperature of 165°F.
6. Place the chicken, tent with foil, and allow resting for 5 minutes.
7. Serve and enjoy!

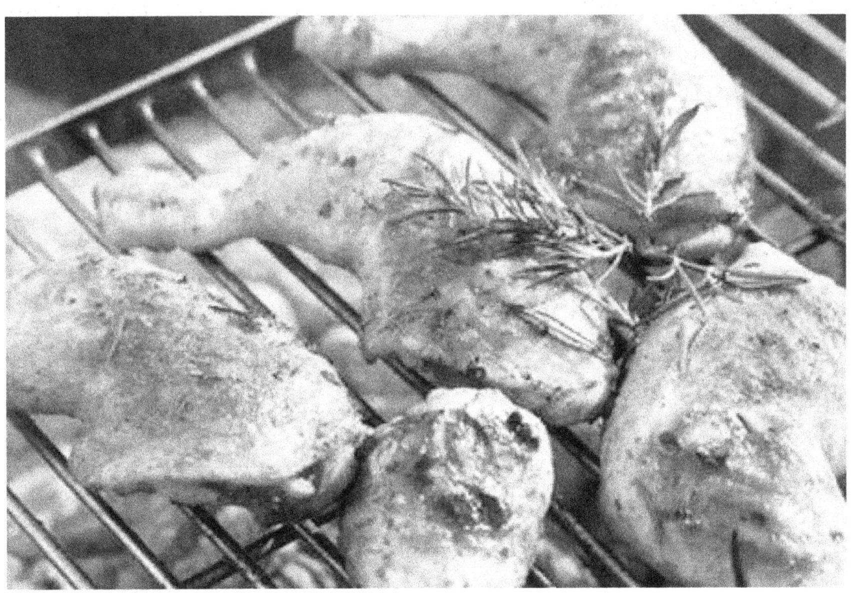

Nutrition

Calories: 381 Sugar: 1.1g Fat: 20.2g Carbs: 4.7g Protein: 44.7g.

Preparation Time: 30'-4h *Cooking Time: 20'* *Serves: 4*

87. Chipotle's Honey Balsamic Marinated Chicken

Ingredients

- ***2 lbs. boneless, skinless chicken thighs***
- ***1 teaspoon olive oil***
- ***½ teaspoon sea salt***
- ***¼ teaspoon black pepper***
- ***½ teaspoon paprika***
- ***¾ teaspoon onion powder***
- ***For the Marinade:***
- ***2 tablespoons honey***
- ***2 tablespoons balsamic vinegar***
- ***2 tablespoons tomato paste***
- ***1 teaspoon garlic, minced***

Directions

1. Add chicken, olive oil, salt, black pepper, paprika, and onion powder to a sealable plastic bag. Seal and toss to coat, covering the chicken with spices and oil; set aside.
2. Whisk together balsamic vinegar, tomato paste, garlic, and honey.
3. Divide the marinade in half. Add one half to the bag of chicken and store the other half in a sealed container in the refrigerator.
4. Put the chicken inside the bag to coat. Refrigerate for 30 minutes to 4 hours.
5. Preheat a grill to medium-high.
6. Place the chicken to the grill and cook 7 minutes per side.
7. During last minute of cooking, brush remaining marinade on top of the chicken thighs. Serve immediately.

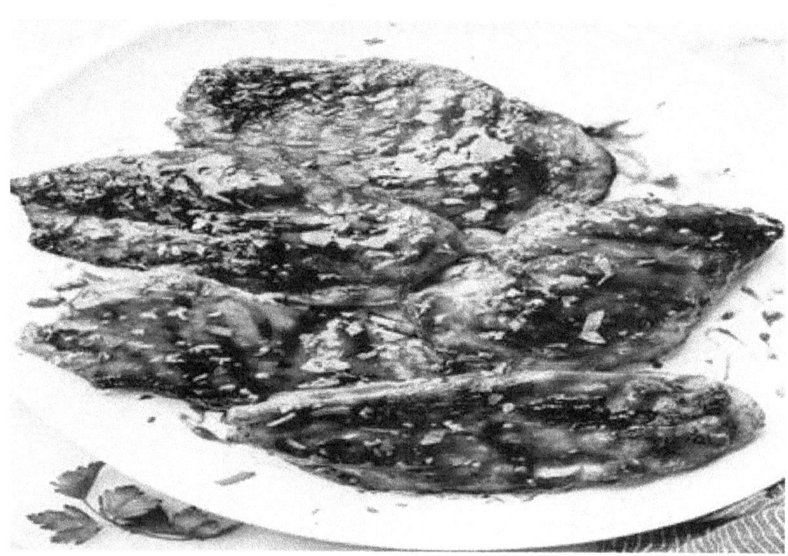

Nutrition

Calories: 485 Sugar: 0.5g Fat: 18.1g Carbs: 11g Protein: 66.1g

Preparation Time: 35' *Cooking Time: 20'* *Serves: 4*

88. Chipotle's California Grilled Chicken

Ingredients

4 boneless, skinless chicken breasts

3/4 cup balsamic vinegar

2 tablespoons extra virgin olive oil

1 tablespoon honey

1 teaspoon oregano

1 teaspoon basil

1 teaspoon garlic powder

For garnish:

Sea salt

Black pepper, fresh ground

4 slices fresh mozzarella cheese

4 slices avocado

4 slices beefsteak tomato

Balsamic glaze, for drizzling

Directions

1. Mix the balsamic vinegar, honey, olive oil, oregano, basil and garlic powder in a large mixing bowl.
2. Add chicken to coat and marinate for 30 minutes in the refrigerator.
3. Preheat grill and cook the chicken for 7 minutes each side.
4. Top each chicken breast with mozzarella, avocado, and tomato and tent with foil on the grill to melt for 2 minutes.
5. Drizzle some of balsamic glaze, and a pinch of sea salt and black pepper.

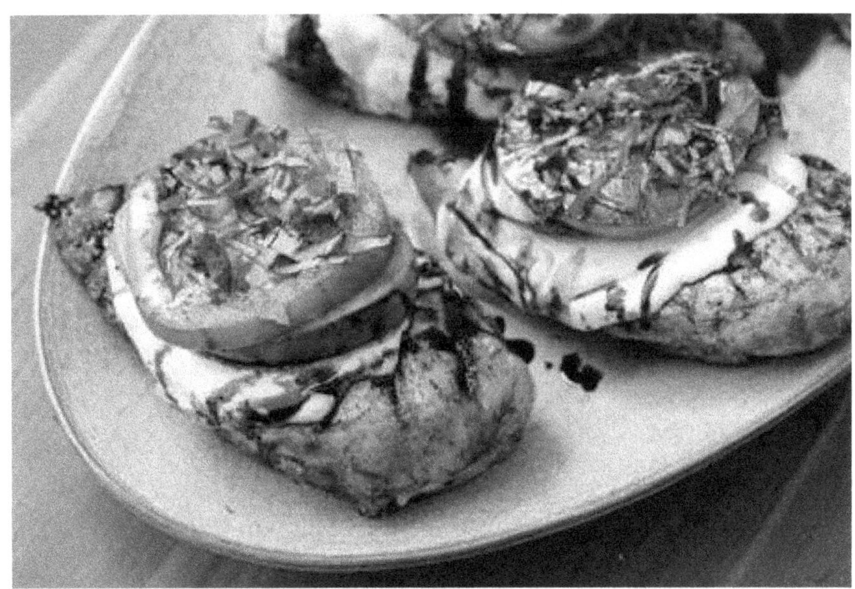

Nutrition

Calories: 883 Sugar: 15.2g Fat: 62.1g Carbs: 29.8g Protein: 55.3g

Preparation Time: 4h 35' *Cooking Time: 4h 50'* *Serves: 6*

89. Chipotle's Salsa Verde Marinated Chicken

Ingredients

6 boneless, skinless chicken breasts

1 tablespoon olive oil

1 teaspoon sea salt

1 teaspoon chili powder

1 teaspoon ground cumin

1 teaspoon garlic powder

For the salsa Verde marinade:

3 teaspoons garlic, minced

1 small onion, chopped

6 tomatillos, husked, rinsed and chopped

1 medium jalapeño pepper, cut in half, seeded

¼ cup fresh cilantro, chopped

½ teaspoon sugar or sugar substitute

Directions

1. Add salsa Verde marinade Ingredients to a food processor and pulse until smooth. Mix sea salt, chili powder, cumin, and garlic powder together in a small mixing bowl.

2. Season the chicken with olive oil and seasoning mix, and lay in glass baking dish. Spread a tablespoon of salsa Verde marinade over each chicken breast to cover; reserve remaining salsa for serving. Refrigerate for 4 hours. Brush some olive oil on the griller and preheat.

3. Add the chicken to the grill and cook 7 minutes per. Serve each with additional salsa Verde and enjoy!

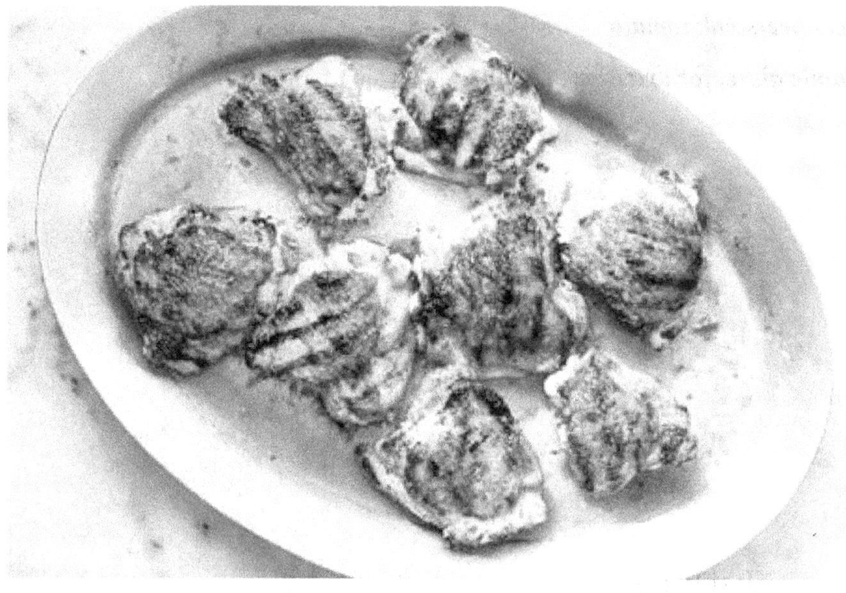

Nutrition

Calories: 321 Sugar: 1.3g Fat: 13.7g Carbs: 4.8g Protein: 43g

Preparation Time: 1h 10' *Cooking Time: 15'* *Serves: 4-5*

90. Chipotle's Hawaiian Chicken Skewers

Ingredients

- ***1 lb. boneless, skinless chicken breast, cut into 1 ½ inch cubes***
- ***3 cups pineapple, cut into 1 ½ inch cubes***
- ***2 large green peppers, cut into 1 ½ inch pieces***
- ***1 large red onion, cut into 1 ½ inch pieces***
- ***2 tablespoons olive oil, to coat veggies***
- ***For the marinade:***
- ***1/3 cup tomato paste***
- ***1/3 cup brown sugar, packed***
- ***1/3 cup soy sauce***
- ***¼ cup pineapple juice***
- ***2 tablespoons olive oil***
- ***1 ½ tablespoon mirin or rice wine vinegar***
- ***4 teaspoons garlic cloves, minced***
- ***1 tablespoon ginger, minced***
- ***½ teaspoon sesame oil***
- ***Pinch of sea salt***
- ***Pinch of ground black pepper***
- ***10 wooden skewers, for assembly***

Directions

1. Combine marinade Ingredients in a mixing bowl until smooth. Reserve a ½ cup the marinade in the refrigerator.

2. Put the chicken and marinade to a sealable plastic bag and refrigerate for 1 hour. Soak 10 wooden skewer sticks in water for 1 hour. Preheat the grill to medium heat.

3. Add red onion, bell pepper and pineapple to a mixing bowl with 2 tablespoons olive oil and toss to coat.

4. Thread red onion, bell pepper, pineapple and chicken onto the skewers until all of the chicken has been used.

5. Place skewers on grill and grab your reserve marinade from the refrigerator; grill for 5 minutes then brush with remaining marinade and rotate.

6. Brush again with marinade and grill about 5 additional minutes or until chicken reads 165°F on a meat thermometer. Serve warm.

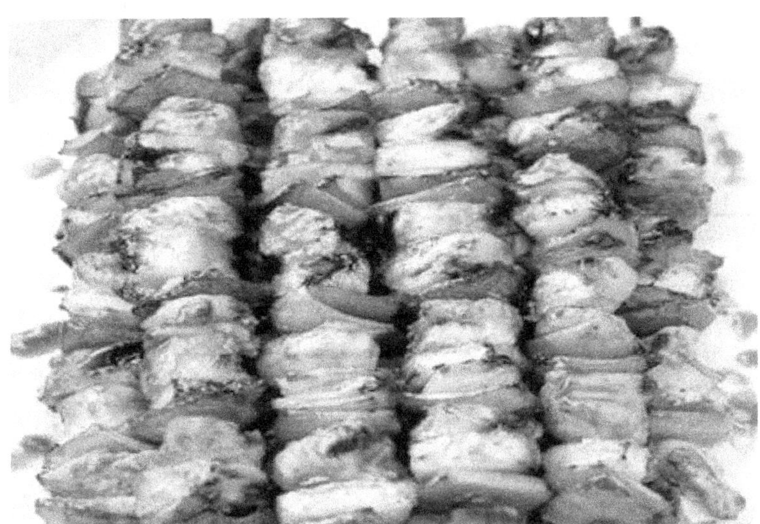

Nutrition

Calories: 311 Sugar: 4.2g Fat: 8.8g Carbs: 38.1g Protein: 22.8g

Preparation Time: 20' *Cooking Time: 25'* *Serves: 4t*

91. Applebee's Three Cheese Penne with Chicken

Ingredients

- ***1 pound chicken breasts, diced***
- ***1/3 cup Italian dressing***
- ***3 cups penne pasta, uncooked***
- ***2 tablespoons butter***
- ***2 cups Alfredo sauce***
- ***8 ounces Italian blend shredded cheese***
- ***4 tomatoes, diced***
- ***1 teaspoon dried basil***
- ***2 cloves garlic, minced***
- ***6 tablespoons olive oil***

Directions

1. Preheat the oven to 350°F. Coat baking dish with cooking spray.

2. Let the chicken be marinated with the Italian dressing for at least 30 minutes.

3. Cook the pasta in pan with water. Drain well and place it in the baking dish.

4. Heat a skillet over medium-high heat. Add the butter, and brown the chicken on all sides.

5. Add the chicken to the pasta, and stir in the alfredo sauce. Top with cheese, and bake for 25 minutes, until the pasta is heated through and the cheese is melted and bubbly.

6. Meanwhile, combine the tomatoes, basil, garlic, and olive oil in a small dish and stir to combine.

7. When the casserole is bubbly, remove it from the oven and serve topped with the tomato mixture.

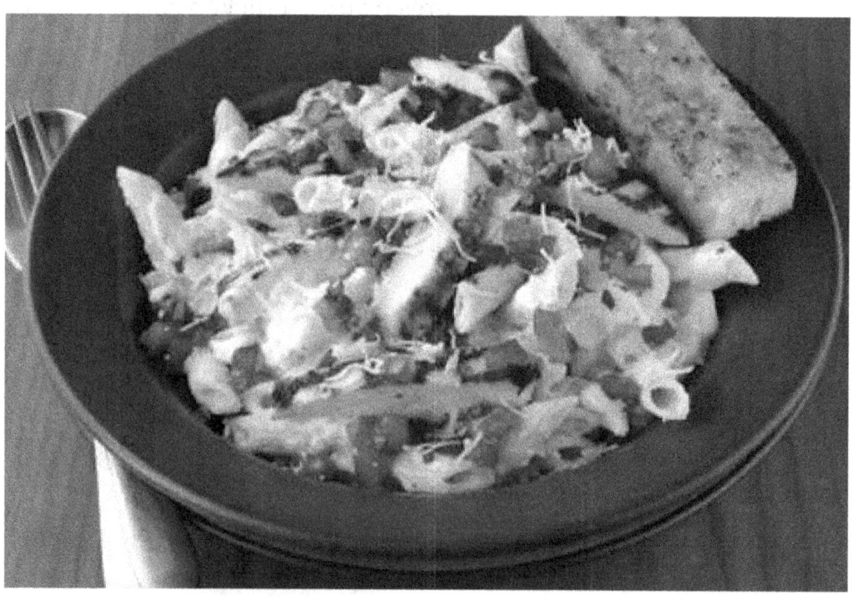

Nutrition

Calories: 242.8 Fat: 6.6g Carbs: 38.4g Sugars: 3g Protein: 8.4g

Preparation Time: 30' *Cooking Time: 50'* *Serves: 4-6*

92. Applebee's Mac and Cheese Honey Pepper Chicken

Ingredients

- *6 slices thick-cut bacon, cooked and chopped*
- *Seasoned flour:*
- *2 cups all-purpose flour*
- *3 tablespoons paprika*
- *1 ½ tablespoons kosher salt*
- *1 ½ tablespoons dry mustard*
- *1 ½ tablespoons garlic powder*
- *1 ½ tablespoons onion powder*
- *1 tablespoon seasoned salt*
- *¾ tablespoon black pepper*
- *½ tablespoon celery seed*
- *½ teaspoon dried ginger*
- *½ teaspoon dried thyme*
- *½ teaspoon dried basil*
- *½ teaspoon dried oregano*
- *Fried chicken:*
- *1 pound chicken tenders*
- *2 cups buttermilk*
- *2–3 cups oil for frying*
- *Honey pepper sauce:*
- *¾ cup honey*
- *¼ cup brown sugar*
- *¼ cup pineapple juice*
- *3 tablespoons apple cider vinegar*
- *3 tablespoons soy sauce*
- *Juice of 1 lemon*
- *1 teaspoon black pepper*
- *¼ teaspoon cayenne pepper (or to taste)*
- *4 cheese sauce and pasta:*
- *¼ cup butter*
- *3 cloves garlic, minced*
- *1 jalapeño pepper, diced*
- *3 tablespoons all-purpose flour*
- *2 cups heavy cream*
- *½ cup Parmesan cheese, grated*
- *¾ cup mozzarella cheese, shredded*
- *½ cup Romano cheese, shredded*
- *½ cup asiago cheese, shredded*
- *½ teaspoon dried basil*
- *Black pepper to taste*
- *Fresh parsley for garnish*
- *1 pound cavatappi pasta, uncooked (or other short cut pasta)*
- *2 tablespoons olive oil, for drizzling*

Nutrition

Calories 150 Fat 4.2g Carbs 40g Sugars 1g Protein 9g

Directions

1. Mix the chicken in a bowl together with the buttermilk. Rotate the chicken in the bowl to make sure each piece is covered.
2. In a large re-sealable bag, combine all the ingredients for the seasoned flour and shake it up.
3. Combine all the ingredients for the honey pepper sauce. Bring it to a boil over medium-high heat, and then reduce the heat to low and let it simmer until the sauce thickens. Remove it from the heat.
4. Remove the chicken from the buttermilk, then place them in the bag with the seasoned flour and shake to coat. Set them on a baking tray while you coat the remaining pieces. Repeat until all the chicken has been coated with the seasoned flour.
5. Put the oil in a skillet in medium heat. Cook the tenders in the hot oil until they are golden brown and cooked through completely. Set aside.
6. After that, cook the pasta in a pot of boiling water until it is al dente. Drain and put some olive oil to keep it from sticking together. Cover.
7. Melt the butter in a medium saucepan over medium to medium-low heat. Add the garlic and diced pepper and sauté until the garlic is fragrant. Add the flour and whisk to combine. Cook till it turns brown.
8. Gradually add in the heavy cream, whisking constantly. Allow it to cook for 5 minutes, whisking the entire time. The cream should thicken and will coat your spoon.
9. Gradually stir in your cheeses until they are completely melted. Stir in the basil and pepper.
10. Mix the pasta to the cheese sauce and combine well to make sure it is all coated.
11. Plate some of the mac and cheese on a serving plate.
12. Coat the chicken tenders in the honey pepper sauce and lay them on top of the mac and cheese.
13. Serve, and enjoy!

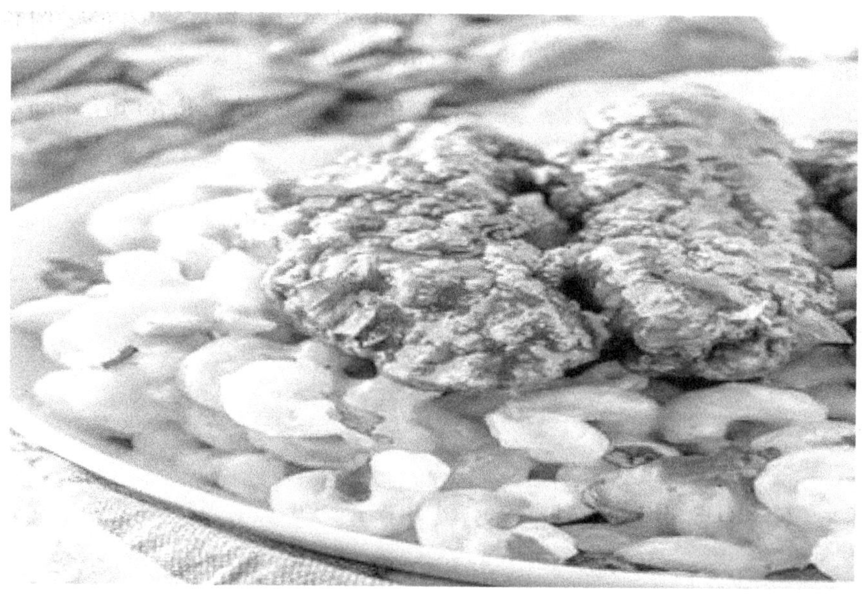

Preparation Time: 20' *Cooking Time: 25'* *Serves: 5*

93. Applebee's Chicken Cavatappi

Ingredients

- *2 boneless skinless chicken breasts*
- *½ cup Italian salad dressing*
- *4 Roma tomatoes, seeded and diced*
- *¼ cup chopped fresh basil*
- *2 tablespoons olive oil*
- *¼ teaspoon kosher salt*
- *¼ teaspoon pepper*
- *1 pound cavatappi pasta*
- *½ cup unsalted butter*
- *4 cloves garlic, crushed*
- *2 cups heavy cream*
- *½ cup mozzarella cheese, shredded*
- *½ cup Parmesan cheese, grated*
- *½ cup Asiago cheese, shredded*
- *4 ounces mascarpone cheese*
- *¼ teaspoon kosher salt*
- *¼ teaspoon pepper*
- *½ teaspoon crushed red pepper flakes*
- *2 ounces prosciutto*

Directions

1. Put the chicken in bags that are re-sealable and pour in the Italian dressing. Seal the bag and let them marinade in the refrigerator for at least 1 hour.

2. In a mixing bowl, combine the tomatoes, basil, olive oil, and salt. Stir to combine, then cover and set to the side.

3. Cook the cavatappi in a pot of boiling water until al dente.

4. After your chicken has marinated, heat a skillet over medium-high heat. Melt a little of the butter and brown the chicken breasts for about 5 minutes on each side or until fully cooked. Slice them into thin slices.

5. Let the butter melt in the saucepan and add the garlic and let it cook until fragrant. Put in the heavy cream and let it simmer. Reduce the heat and add all the cheeses. Put some salt, pepper, and red pepper flakes. Stir constantly until the cheese has melted.

6. Pour the cheese sauce over the cooked pasta, and stir to coat the pasta.

7. Crisp up the prosciutto in a small skillet.

8. Serve by placing some pasta on a plate. Top it with chicken, the tomato mixture, and crispy prosciutto.

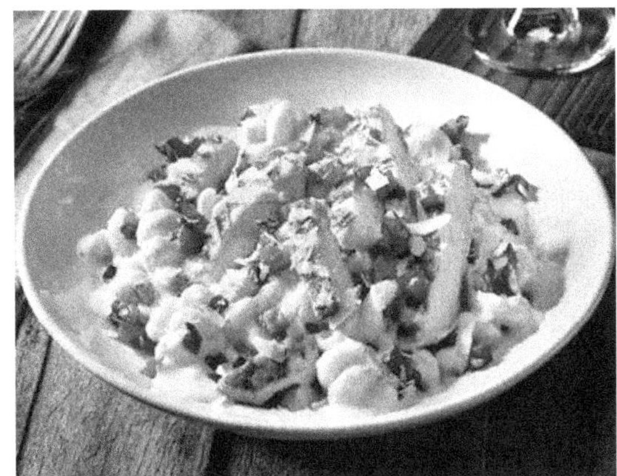

Nutrition

Calories: 100 Fat: 3g Carbs: 21g Sugars: 10g Protein: 5g

Preparation Time: 15' *Cooking Time: 6'* *Serves: 1*

94. Applebee's Chicken Quesadilla

Ingredients

- ***2 (12-inch) flour tortillas***
- ***1 tablespoon butter, melted***
- ***2 tablespoons chipotle pepper sauce (optional)***
- ***4 ounces grilled chicken (spicy seasoning optional)***
- ***¼ cup pepper jack cheese, shredded***
- ***¼ cup tomato, diced***

Optional totppings:

- ***Jalapeño pepper, diced***
- ***Onion, diced***
- ***Cilantro, minced***
- ***Bacon, fried and crumbled***
- ***1 cup lettuce, shredded***

To serve:

- ***Sour cream***
- ***Green onion***
- ***Salsa***

Directions

1. Preheat a large skillet over medium heat.
2. Put some melted butter on one side of the tortilla. Place one tortilla butter side down on your counter or cutting board.
3. Top the tortilla with chipotle sauce, then sprinkle on the grilled chicken. Add the cheese, tomato, and other desired toppings. Cover the other tortilla on top, butter side up, and transfer it to the skillet.
4. Cook for 3 minutes (or until the tortilla starts to crisp up), then flip and cook on the other side, making sure the cheese has melted completely, but not so long that the lettuce (if used) is wilted.
5. Serve the quesadilla with sour cream, green onion, and salsa.

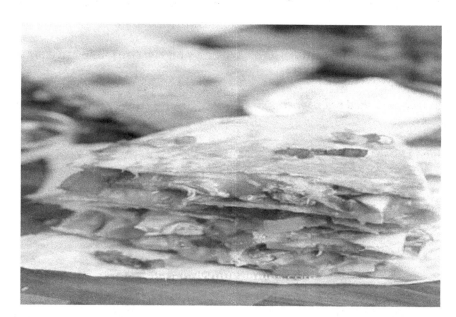

Nutrition

Calories: 178 Fat: 15g Carbs: 50g Sugars: 8g Protein: 9g

Preparation Time: 10’ *Cooking Time: 20’* *Serves: 4*

95. Applebee’s Fiesta Lime Chicken

Ingredients

4 boneless skinless chicken breasts

2 tablespoons olive oil

Salt and pepper to taste

¼ cup ranch dressing

¼ cup Greek yogurt

1 tablespoon lime juice

¼ cup fresh cilantro chopped

1 clove garlic, minced

½ cup Colby cheese, shredded

½ cup Monterey jack cheese, shredded

• For serving:

Mexican Rice

Pico de Gallo

Tortilla strips

Directions

1. Preheat the grill to 400°F.
2. Cover the chicken with olive oil, then season with salt and pepper as desired.
3. Grill the chicken for about 10 minutes on each side, or bake for 20 minutes in the oven.
4. Combine the ranch dressing, yogurt, lime juice, cilantro, and garlic. Stir well.
5. Just before the chicken is done, spread a bit of the dressing mixture over each breast and top with a portion of the cheeses. Continue to cook until the cheese is melted.
6. To serve, plate a scoop of Mexican rice and place a chicken breast on top. Add Pico de Gallo and tortilla strips.

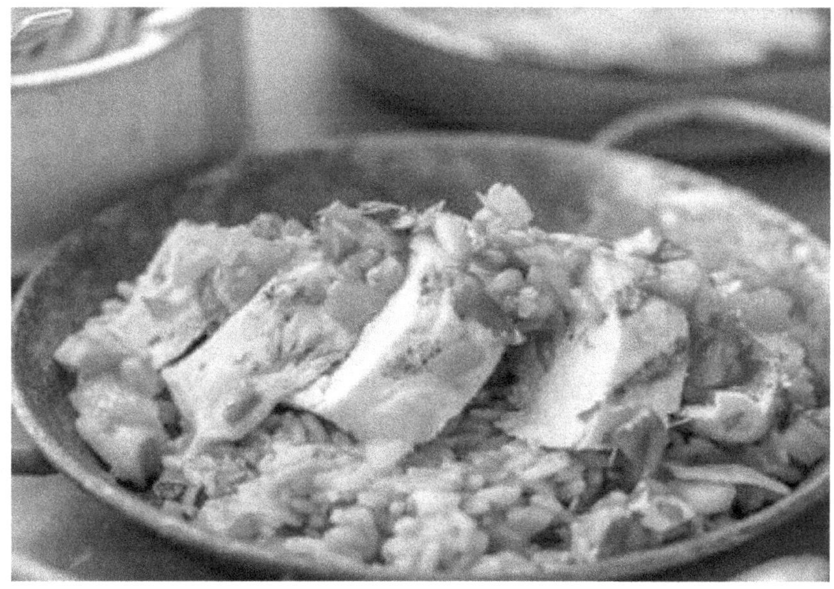

Nutrition

Calories: 150 Fat: 20g Carbs: 50g Sugars: 9g Protein: 15g

Preparation Time: 20' *Cooking Time: 25'* *Serves: 4*

96. Applebee's Margherita Chicken

Ingredients

- ***4 boneless skinless chicken breasts***
- ***Spice rub***
- ***2 tablespoons packed brown sugar***
- ***Juice of 1 lime***
- ***1 tablespoon oil***
- ***2 tablespoons paprika***
- ***1 tablespoon chili powder***
- ***1 tablespoon ground cumin***
- ***1 ½ teaspoons salt***
- ***1 teaspoon pepper***

Glaze:

- ***½ cup ketchup***
- ***¼ cup balsamic vinegar***
- ***1 teaspoon oregano***
- ***¼ cup packed brown sugar***
- ***Cheese topping***
- ***1 cup mozzarella cheese, shredded***
- ***½ cup Parmesan cheese, grated***

Brustchetta:

- ***2 cloves garlic, chopped***
- ***2 teaspoons balsamic vinegar***
- ***½ teaspoon kosher salt***
- ***¼ teaspoon fresh cracked pepper***
- ***2 tablespoons chopped fresh basil***
- ***3 tablespoons olive oil***
- ***6 Roma tomatoes, diced***

Directions

1. Combine all the rub ingredients and spread the mixture over the chicken, using your fingers to massage it into the meat. Cover the chicken with wrap and refrigerate for at least an hour.

2. When the chicken is almost done marinating, make the bruschetta. Combine the garlic, vinegar, salt, pepper and basil in a small bowl. Stir to combine. Add in the olive oil add the tomatoes. Cover with plastic wrap and set aside until you are ready to assemble.

3. In a small bowl, combine the glaze ingredients.

4. After your chicken has marinated preheat the grill and set the oven to broil. Cook the chicken over medium-high heat until the juices run clear and the meat has an internal temperature of 165°F. While the chicken is cooking, occasionally brush glaze over the breasts but watch them carefully so they don't burn.

5. When chicken is done on the grill, place it on a baking tray and top it with both the mozzarella and Parmesan cheeses. Put them under the broiler and cook until the cheese is melty and a bit bubbly.

6. Serve the chicken topped with the bruschetta topping.

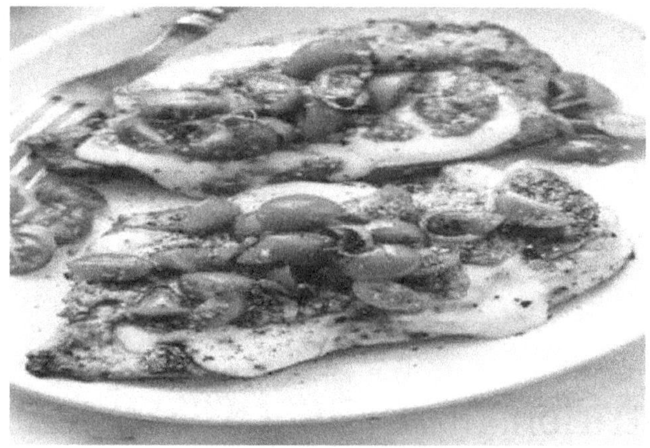

Nutrition

Calories 160 Fat 10g Carbs 50g Sugars 6g Protein 12g Lunch 2

Preparation Time: 15' *Cooking Time: 1'* *Serves: 4*

97. BJ Restaurant's Caprese Piadina

Ingredients

- ***4 Piadina bread, sliced***
- ***2 balls buffalo mozzarella, sliced***
- ***2 large, ripe tomatoes, thinly sliced***
- ***2 cups freshly washed and dried arugula***
- ***2 tablespoons fresh basil pesto***
- ***3 tablespoons extra virgin olive oil***
- ***Salt & pepper***

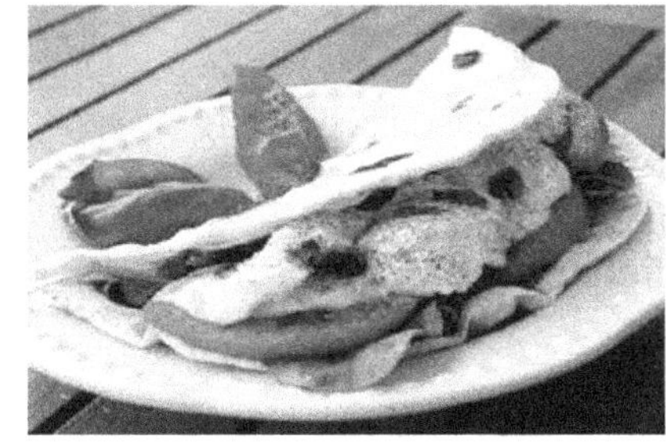

Directions

1. Wash the arugula in a colander and leave it to drain all the excess liquid;
2. Cut the tomatoes into thin slices and keep them aside;
3. Take the buffalo mozzarella and slice the balls into thick slices;
4. Place a suitable skillet on medium heat and grease it with olive oil;
5. Add arugula and sauté for 1 minute on medium heat;
6. Remove from the heat and allow the arugula to cool down;
7. Place the Piadina on the working surface and slice it into 2 halves;
8. Top the lower halves of the Piadina bread slice with basil pesto;
9. Divide the arugula on top of the basil pesto;
10. Top each Piadina slice with a tomato slice and a slice of mozzarella cheese;
11. Sprinkle salt and black pepper over the cheese to adjust the seasoning;
12. Place the top halves of the Piadina slices over the cheese slices;
13. Transfer the Piadina to the serving plates;
14. Serve fresh.

Nutrition

Calories: 242.8 Fat: 6.6g Carbs: 38.4g Sugars: 3g Protein: 8.4g

Preparation Time: 20' *Cooking Time: 15'* *Serves: 4*

98. BJ Restaurant's Spicy Garlic Wings

Ingredients

- *1 cup Frank's Red-Hot Sauce*
- *1/3 cup vegetable oil*
- *2 teaspoons sugar*
- *2 teaspoons garlic powder*
- *½ teaspoon black pepper*
- *½ teaspoon cayenne pepper*
- *1 teaspoon worcestershire sauce*
- *1 tablespoon butter*
- *1 egg yolk*
- *3 teaspoons water*
- *3 teaspoons cornstarch*
- *1 dozen chicken wings*
- *Salt, to taste*
- *Black pepper, to taste*

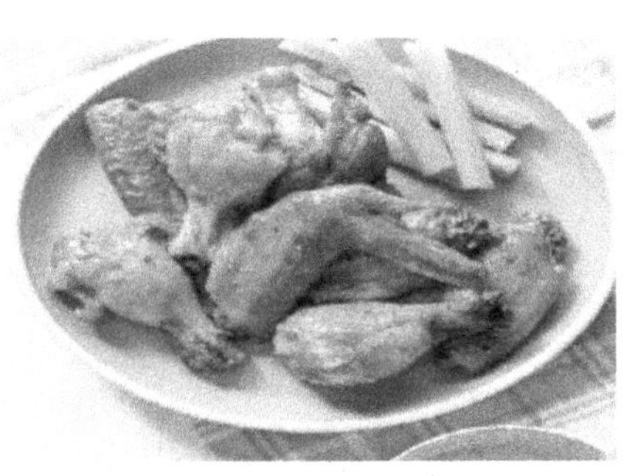

Directions

1. Mix red hot sauce with vegetable oil, sugar, garlic powder, black pepper, cayenne pepper, Worcestershire sauce and butter in a bowl.
2. Pour this hot sauce mixture into a small saucepan.
3. Cook this mixture to a boil then reduce the heat to a simmer.
4. Cook the hot sauce for 5 minutes with occasional stirring.
5. After that, transfer to a bowl to allow it to cool down.
6. Meanwhile, beat egg yolk with cornstarch and water in a suitable bowl.
7. Add this egg yolk mixture into the hot sauce mixture and mix well until well incorporated.
8. Sprinkle pepper and salt on the chicken wings and toss to coat.
9. Set a charcoal grill on medium heat and grease its grilling grates with cooking spray.
10. Place the chicken wings on the grilled grates and grill the wings for 5 minutes.
11. Brush the hot sauce mixture over the wings and flip them.
12. Grill them for 5 minutes and brush again with the hot sauce mixture.
13. Continue grilling the wings until golden brown on both the sides.
14. Cook the wings in batches to avoid overcrowding.
15. Transfer the cooked wings to a bow.
16. Pour the remaining hot sauce over the cooked wings and toss well.
17. Serve warm and fresh

Nutrition

Calories: 150 Fat: 4.2g Carbs: 40g Sugars: 1g Protein: 9g

Preparation Time: 20' *Cooking Time: 10'* *Serves: 4*

99. BJ Restaurant's Chicken Pot Stickers with Dipping Sauce

Ingredients

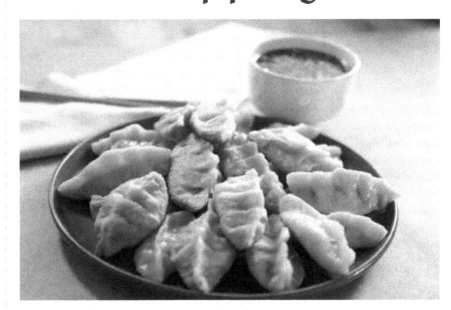

- ***Dough:***
- ***1 cup all-purpose flour***
- ***¼ cup boiling water***
- ***½ cup cold water***
- ***Filling:***
- ***½ lb. ground chicken***
- ***1/6 cup chicken broth***
- ***1 teaspoon sugar***
- ***1 teaspoon soy sauce***
- ***1 teaspoon rice vinegar***
- ***½ teaspoon freshly grated ginger***
- ***1 pinch salt***
- ***1 scallion, finely chopped***
- ***Freshly ground black pepper***
- ***2 teaspoons olive oil***
- ***Dipping Sauce:***
- ***1 tablespoon soy sauce***
- ***½ tablespoon rice vinegar***
- ***1 teaspoon sesame oil***
- ***½ scallion, finely chopped***
- ***A pinch of crushed dried red pepper***

Nutrition

Calories: 100 Fat: 3g Carbs: 21g Sugars: 10g Protein: 5g

Directions

1. First, prepare the dough and take a small bowl.
2. Mix flour and salt in this bowl then slowly pour in hot water.
3. Continue mixing the flour until it forms a coarse meal mixture.
4. Stir in ½ cup cold water then mix until it forms a smooth texture.
5. Knead this smooth flour dough on a floured surface for 10 minutes.
6. Cover this dough for 20 minutes with a damp towel.
7. Meanwhile, prepare the filling for pot stickers.
8. Mix ground chicken with chicken broth, soy sauce, sugar, salt, ginger, vinegar, scallions, and pepper.
9. Mix well until chicken is thoroughly mixed with the spices.
10. Now take the prepared dough and divide it into 12 balls and roll each ball into 4-inches circle.
11. Add 1 tablespoon of chicken filling onto the center of each circle and fold the circle in half.
12. Pinch the edges of the dumplings and seal them together.
13. Place a large pot on medium heat to cook the dumplings and fill it with water.
14. As the water boils, add the dumplings and cook for 4 minutes.
15. Cook the dumplings in batches to avoid overcrowding.
16. Take away the dumplings from the water and drain the excess water.
17. Place a non-stick skillet over medium heat and add olive oil to heat.
18. Sear these dumplings in a skillet for 2 minutes per side.
19. Prepare the dipping sauce by mixing soy sauce, sesame oil, red pepper, scallion, and vinegar in a small bowl.
20. Serve the seared dumplings with the dipping sauce.

Chapter 6
Beef

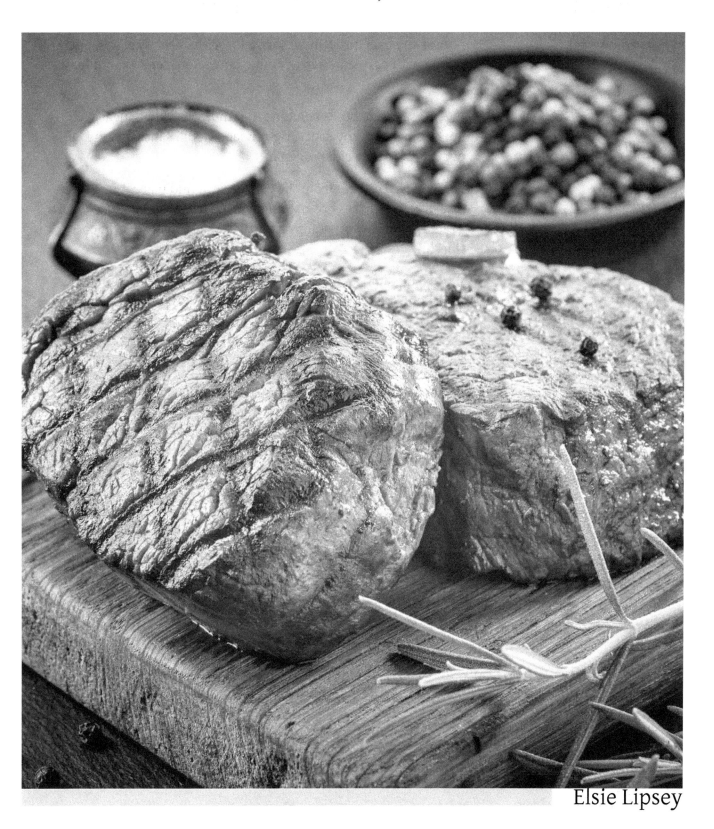

Preparation Time: 20' *Cooking Time: 15'* *Serves: 4*

100. Panda Express's Beijing Beef

Ingredients

- *1 pound flank steak*
- *1 cup canola oil*
- *4 cloves garlic, minced*
- *1 yellow onion*
- *1 red bell pepper*
- *2 tablespoons + 1 teaspoon cornstarch, divided*
- *¼ teaspoon salt*
- *3 egg whites, beaten*
- *½ cup water*
- *¼ cup sugar*
- *3 tablespoons ketchup*
- *6 tablespoons hoisin sauce*
- *1 tablespoon soy sauce*
- *2 teaspoons oyster sauce*
- *4 teaspoons sweet chili sauce*
- *1 teaspoon crushed red peppers*
- *2 tablespoons apple cider vinegar*

Directions

1. Cut the beef into ¼-inch slices. Place the beef, egg, salt, and 1 teaspoon of cornstarch in a mixing bowl. Refrigerate for at least an hour.

2. In a separate bowl, combine together the water, sugar, ketchup, hoisin sauce, soy sauce, oyster sauce, chili sauce, crushed red pepper and apple cider vinegar.

3. Remove the beef from the refrigerator and place it in a separate dish. Discard the remaining marinade. Sprinkle the beef with 2 tablespoons of cornstarch and stir. Shake off any excess cornstarch.

4. In a medium saucepan, heat the oil over medium-high heat. When hot, fry the beef in batches, about 2–3 minutes. Remove from oil and set on a paper-towel-lined plate to drain.

5. To a large skillet, add 2 tablespoons of the same oil you fried the beef in. Heat over medium-high heat. Add the onion and pepper and let it cook for about 3 minutes.

6. Add the garlic and cook about 30 seconds more, then remove from the skillet and add to the plate with the beef.

7. Pour the sauce you prepared to the skillet and cook over high heat until it thickens. Add the beef and vegetables, stirring to coat.

Nutrition

Calories: 160 Fat: 10g Carbs: 50g Sugars: 6g Protein: 12g

Preparation Time: 30' *Cooking Time: 15'* *Serves: 4*

101. Panda Express's Copycat Beef and Broccoli

Ingredients

- *2 tablespoons cornstarch, divided*
- *3 tablespoons Chinese rice wine, divided*
- *1 pound flank steak, cut thinly against the grain*
- *1 pound broccoli florets*
- *2 tablespoons oyster sauce*
- *2 tablespoons water*
- *1 tablespoon brown sugar*
- *1 tablespoon soy sauce*
- *1 tablespoon cornstarch*
- *2 tablespoons canola oil*
- *¼ teaspoon sesame oil*
- *1 teaspoon ginger, finely chopped*
- *2 cloves garlic, finely chopped*
- *2 teaspoons sesame seeds*

Directions

1. In a plastic bag, put 1 tablespoon cornstarch and 2 tablespoons Chinese rice wine. Place beef inside and seal tightly. Massage bag to fully coat beef. Marinate for at least 20 minutes.

2. Rinse broccoli and place in a nonreactive bowl. Place a wet paper towel on top, then microwave for 2 minutes. Set aside.

3. Stir oyster sauce, water, 1 tablespoon Chinese rice wine, brown sugar, soy sauce, and remaining cornstarch in a bowl until well mixed. Set aside.

4. Heat wok over high heat. You want the wok to be very hot. Then, heat canola and sesame oil in wok and wait to become hot.

5. Working in batches, add steak and cook over high heat for 1 minute. Flip, and cook other side for another 1 minute. Transfer to a plate.

6. To the same wok, add garlic and ginger. Sauté for about 10 to 15 seconds then return beef to wok. Toss in heated broccoli. Slightly stir prepared sauce to make sure cornstarch is not settled on the bottom, then add to wok. Toss everything in the sauce to combine. Continue cooking until sauce becomes thick.

7. Garnish with sesame seeds. Serve.

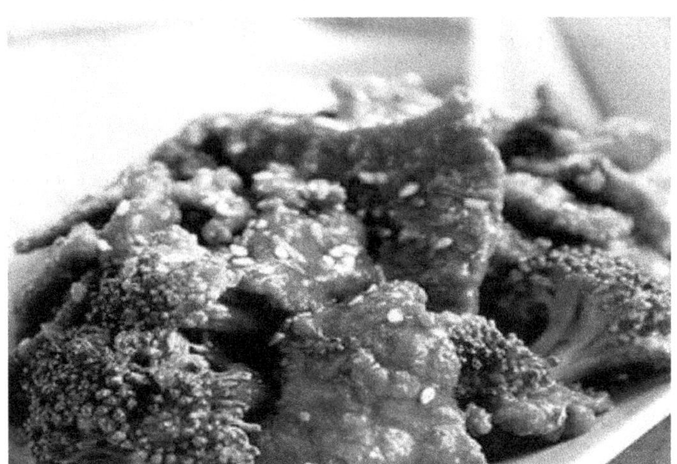

Nutrition

Calories: 140 Fat: 8g Carbs: 30 Sugars: 10g Protein: 25g

Preparation Time: 20' *Cooking Time: 10'* *Serves: 4-6*

102. PF Chang's Beef A La Sichuan

Ingredients

Stir-fry

- ***1 pound flank steak or sirloin, sliced thin***
- ***4 medium celery ribs***
- ***2 medium carrots***
- ***1 green onion***
- ***¼ cup peanut oil or canola oil***
- ***¼ cup cornstarch***
- ***½ teaspoon red pepper flakes***
- ***1½ teaspoons sesame oil***

Sauce:

- ***3 tablespoons soy sauce***
- ***2 tablespoons hoisin sauce***
- ***1 tablespoon garlic and red chili paste***
- ***½ teaspoon Chinese hot mustard***
- ***1 teaspoon rice wine vinegar***
- ***½ teaspoon chili oil***
- ***2 teaspoons brown sugar***
- ***1 teaspoon garlic, minced***
- ***½ teaspoon fresh ginger, minced***
- ***½ teaspoon red pepper flakes***

Directions

1. Mix all of the ingredients for the sauce in a mixing bowl. Set aside.
2. Slice the carrots and celery as thinly as possible and set aside.
3. Sprinkle the beef with the cornstarch in a bowl. Make sure every piece is coated. Allow to sit for 10 minutes.
4. Put oil in a skillet or work over medium-high heat and cook the beef until crispy, about 4–5 minutes. When done, remove beef from the oil to a paper-towel-lined plate to drain.
5. Discard any oil remaining in the skillet.
6. Put some of the sesame oil to the same skillet and heat over high heat. Add the celery, stir and cook for about 1 minute. Add the crushed red pepper and stir. Add the carrots, cooking and stirring for another 30 seconds.
7. Add the beef and green onions and stir, then pour the sauce into the skillet and bring to a boil. Let it cook for a minute, then serve over rice. v

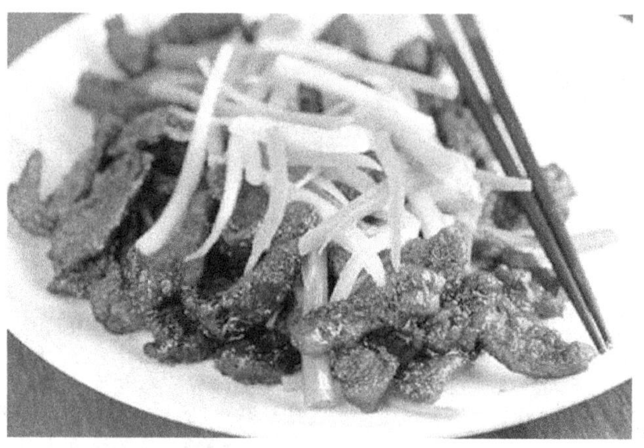

Nutrition

Calories: 112 Fat: 17 Carbs: 50g Sugars: 5g Protein: 7g

Preparation Time: 45' *Cooking Time: 15'* *Serves: 4*

103. P.F. Chang's Beef and Broccoli

Ingredients

- *1/3 cup oyster sauce*
- *2 teaspoons toasted sesame oil*
- *1/3 cup sherry*
- *1 teaspoon soy sauce*
- *1 teaspoon white sugar*
- *1 teaspoon corn starch*
- *Beef and Broccoli*
- *¾ pound beef round steak, cut into 1/8-inch thick strips*
- *3 tablespoons vegetable oil*
- *1 thin slice of fresh ginger root*
- *1 clove garlic, peeled and smashed*
- *1 pound broccoli*

Directions

1. Combine together the ingredients for the marinade and marinate the beef in the mixture for 30 minutes.
2. Sauté the garlic and ginger for a minute in a pan with oil.
3. After that, remove the ginger and garlic from the pan and add the broccoli and cook it until tender. Transfer it to a bowl.
4. In the same pan, cook the beef and the marinade for about 5 minutes.
5. Pour the broccoli back in and keep cooking for another 3 minutes.
6. Place it in a bowl of plate.

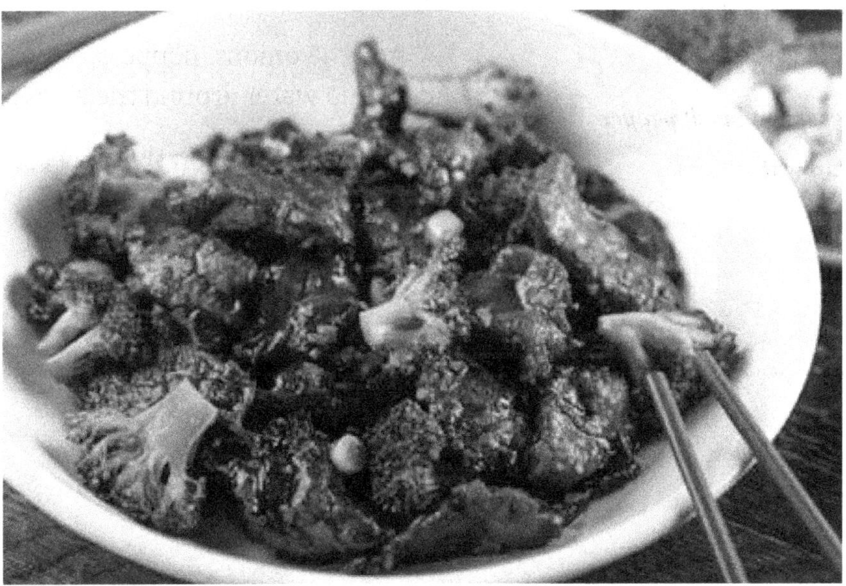

Nutrition

Calories: 80 Fat: 4g Carbs: 20g Sugars: 2g Protein: 15g

Preparation Time: 15' *Cooking Time: 3 h* *Serves: 4*

104. PF Chang's Pepper Steak

Ingredients

- ***1 ½ pounds beef sirloin***
- ***Garlic powder to taste***
- ***2 ½ tablespoons vegetable oil***
- ***1 cube or 1 teaspoon beef bouillon***
- ***¼ cup hot water***
- ***½ tablespoon cornstarch***
- ***□ cup onion, roughly chopped***
- ***1 green bell pepper, roughly chopped***
- ***1 red bell pepper, roughly chopped***
- ***2 ½ tablespoons soy sauce***
- ***1 teaspoon white sugar***
- ***½ teaspoon salt***
- ***½ teaspoon black pepper***
- ***½ cup water***

Directions

1. Cut the beef into pieces approximately 1½ inches long and 1 inch wide.
2. Sprinkle the garlic powder over the beef and give it a quick stir.
3. Dissolve the bouillon in the hot water. Stir until the bouillon has completely dissolved, then stir in the cornstarch until that is completely mixed in as well.
4. Put the oil to heat in a skillet or wok over medium-high heat. When hot, add the beef and vegetables. Cook just long enough to brown the beef, then transfer to a crock pot.
5. Stir the bouillon mixture a bit, then pour it over the beef in the slow cooker.
6. Add the onions, peppers, soy sauce, sugar, salt, and pepper. Add ½ cup water around the sides of the cooker.
7. Place the cover on the slow cooker and cook for about 3 hours on high or 6 hours on low.
8. Serve with rice.

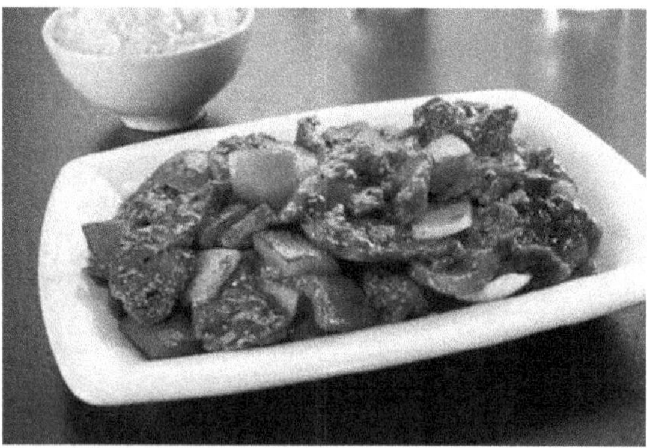

Nutrition

Calories: 178 Fat: 24g Carbs: 123g Sugars: 15g Protein: 27g

Chapter 7 Vegetables

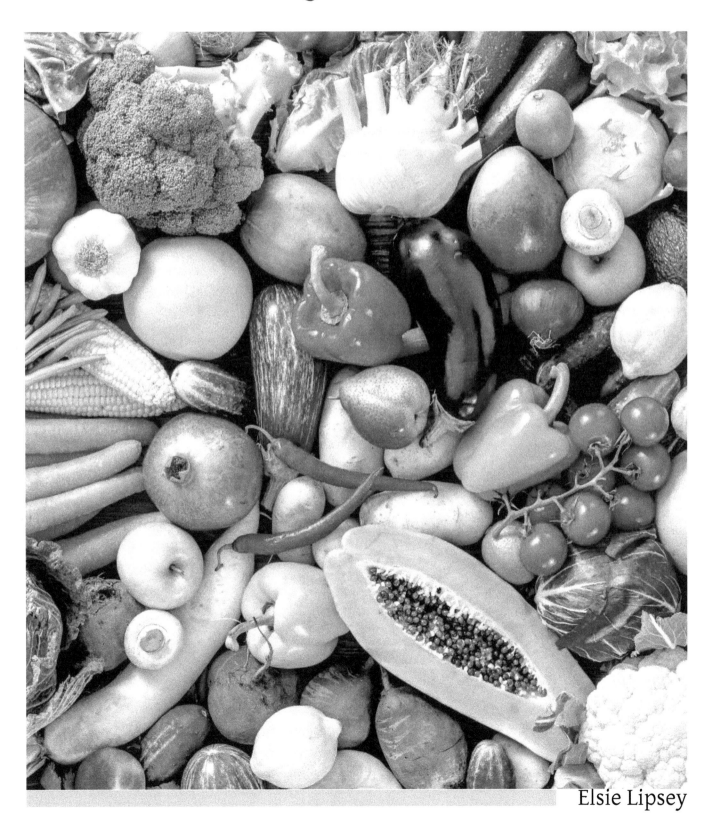

Preparation Time: 10' *Cooking Time: 45'* *Serves: 6*

105. Olive Garden's Stuffed Mushrooms

Ingredients

- ***Stuffed Mushrooms***
- ***12 fresh mushrooms, washed, de-stemmed, and dried***
- ***1 teaspoon flat-leaf parsley, minced***
- ***¼ teaspoon dry oregano***
- ***¼ cup + 1 tablespoon butter, divid-ed; melted, cooled***
- ***¼ cup mozzarella cheese, finely grated***
- ***Some fresh parsley for garnish***

Stuffing:

- ***1 can (6 ounces) clams, drained, finely minced; save ¼ cup juice***
- ***1 green onion, finely minced***
- ***1 egg, beaten***
- ***½ teaspoon garlic, minced***
- ***1/8 teaspoon garlic salt***
- ***½ cup Italian breadcrumbs***
- ***1 tablespoon red bell pepper, finely diced***
- ***2 tablespoons parmesan cheese, finely grated***
- ***1 tablespoon Romano cheese, finely grated***
- ***2 tablespoons mozzarella cheese, finely grated***

Directions

1. Grease a small baking pan and preheat the oven to 350°F.
2. Thoroughly mix all the stuffing ingredients EXCEPT the clam juice and the cheeses.
3. When everything is blended, add in the clam juice and mix again. Next, add in the cheeses and continue mixing.
4. Stuff each of the mushrooms with about 1½ teaspoons of the mixture.
5. Pour 1 tablespoon of the butter into the baking pan and ar-range the mushrooms on the pan.
6. Mix ¼ cup the melted butter with the oregano and the parsley. Pour the butter mixture over the mushrooms.
7. Cover the pan and bake for 35–40 minutes.
8. Uncover the mushrooms and sprinkle the remaining mozza-rella cheese over the top and bake until the cheese melts.
9. Transfer to a serving plate. Garnish with parsley, if desired.

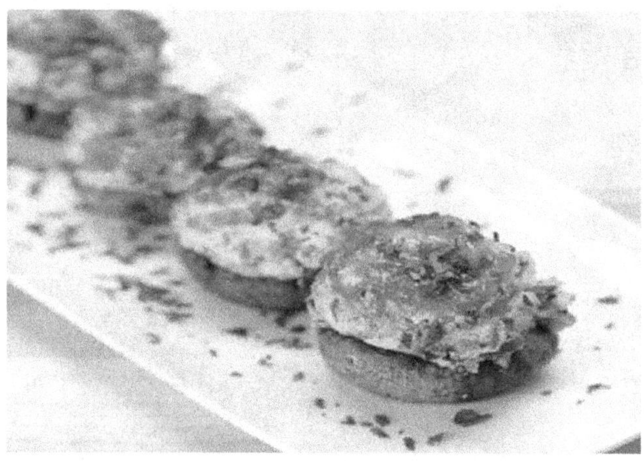

Nutrition

Calories: 293.1 Total Fat: 20.3g Carbs: 13.6g Protein: 14.7g Sodium: 618.8mg

Preparation Time: 10' *Cooking Time: 10'* *Serves: 4*

106. P.F. Chang's Spicy Green Beans

Ingredients

- ***1 pound green beans, rinsed and trimmed***
- ***2 tablespoons fresh ginger, grated***
- ***2 tablespoons garlic, minced***
- ***2 tablespoons cooking oil***
- ***¼ cup water***

Sauce:

- ***2 tablespoons soy sauce***
- ***1 tablespoon rice vinegar***
- ***2 teaspoons sugar***
- ***2 tablespoons Szechuan peppercorn***

Directions

1. Mix all of the ingredients for sauce and bring some water to a boil and add the green beans. Cook for 3-5 minutes, or until crispy.
2. Sauté the garlic and ginger in the oil. When the mixture becomes aromatic, add in the green beans and cook for 2 to 3 minutes, or until soft
3. Add in the sauce and continue stirring the beans.
4. Serve with rice.

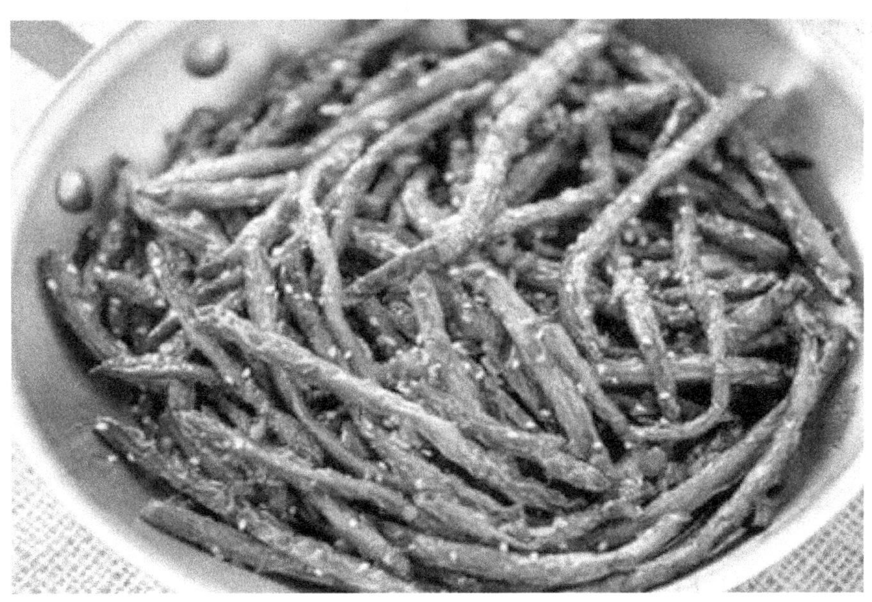

Nutrition

Calories: 117.4 Total Fat: 7.1g Carbs: 12.4g Protein: 3.3g Sodium: 511.1mg

Preparation Time: 5' *Cooking Time: 25'* *Serves: 6*

107. Chili's Black Bean

Ingredients

- ***2 cans (15.5 ounces each) black beans***
- ***½ teaspoon sugar***
- ***1 teaspoon ground cumin***
- ***1 teaspoon chili powder***
- ***½ teaspoon garlic powder***
- ***2 tablespoon red onion, diced finely***
- ***½ teaspoon fresh cilantro, minced (optional)***
- ***½ cup water***
- ***Salt and black pepper to taste***
- ***Pico de Gallo and or sour cream for garnish (optional)***

Directions

1. Combine the beans, sugar, cumin, chili powder, garlic, onion, cilantro (if using), and water in a saucepan and mix well.
2. Over medium-low heat, let the bean mixture simmer for about 20-25 minutes. Season with salt and pepper to taste.
3. Remove the beans from heat and transfer to serving bowls.
4. Garnish with Pico de Gallo and/or a dollop of sour cream, if desired.

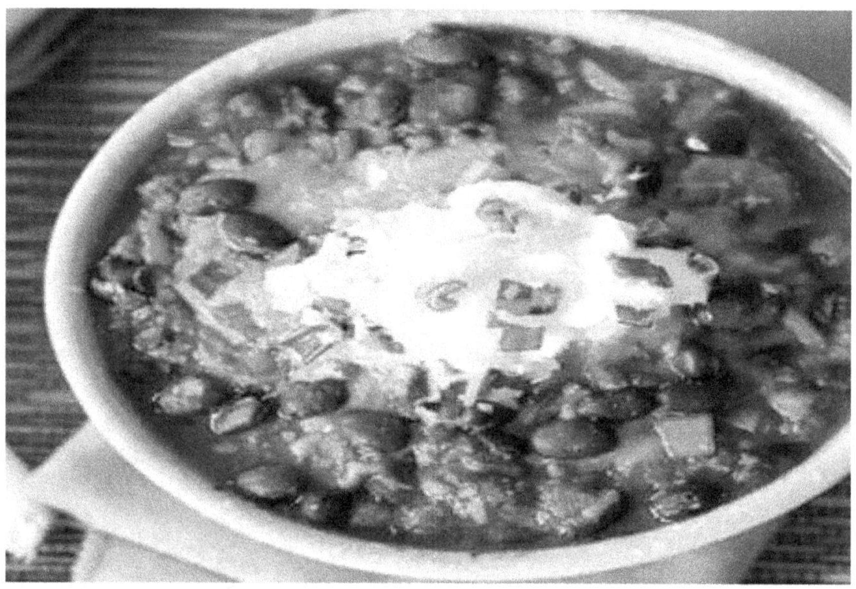

Nutrition

Calories: 143.8 Total Fat: 0.7g Carbs: 25g Protein: 9.5.2g Sodium: 5.5mg

Preparation Time: 10' *Cooking Time: 30'* *Serves: 6*

108. In "N" Out's Animal Style Fries

Ingredients

32 ounces frozen French fries

2 cups cheddar cheese, shredded

1 large onion, diced

2 tablespoons raw sugar

2 tablespoons olive oil

1 ½ cups mayonnaise

¾ cup ketchup

¼ cup sweet relish

1 ½ teaspoon white sugar

1 ½ teaspoon apple cider vinegar

½ teaspoon salt

½ teaspoon black pepper

Directions

1. 1. Let the oven be preheated at 350°F and place the oven grill in the middle position.

2. 2. Put the fries on a large baking sheet and bake in the oven according to package directions.

3. 3. Put the olive oil in a non-stick skillet over medium heat. Add the onions and sauté for about 2 minutes until fragrant and soft.

4. 4. Add raw sugar and continue cooking until the onions caramelize. Remove from heat and set aside.

5. 5. Add the mayonnaise, ketchup, relish, white sugar, salt, and black pepper to a bowl and mix until well combined. Set aside.

6. 6. Once the fries are cooked, remove from heat and set the oven to broil.

7. 7. Sprinkle with the cheddar cheese over the fries and place under the broiler until the cheese melts, about 2-3 minutes.

8. 8. Add the cheese fries to serving bowls or plates. Add some caramelized onions on top and smother with mayonnaise sauce. Serve immediately.

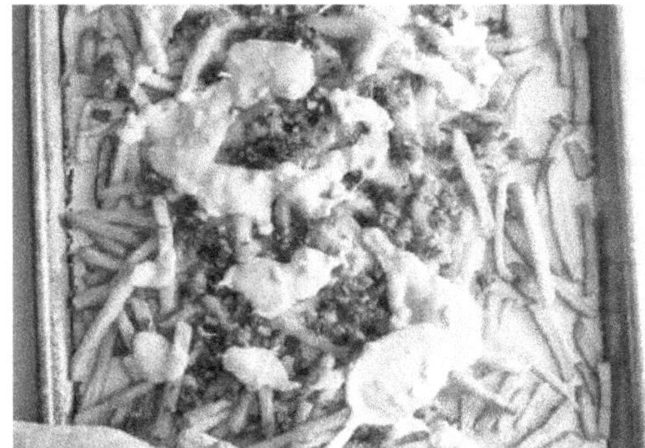

Nutrition

Calories 75Total Fat 42 g Carbs 54 g Protein 19 g Sodium 1105 mg

Preparation Time: 15' *Cooking Time: 0'* *Serves: 10*

109. KFC's Coleslaw

Ingredients

- ***8 cups cabbage, finely diced***
- ***¼ cup carrot, finely diced***
- ***2 tablespoons onions, minced***
- ***1/3 cup granulated sugar***
- ***½ teaspoon salt***
- ***1/8 Teaspoon pepper***
- ***¼ cup milk***
- ***½ cup mayonnaise***
- ***¼ cup buttermilk***
- ***1½ tablespoons white vinegar***
- ***2½ tablespoons lemon juice***

Directions

1. Combine the cabbage, carrot, and onions in a bowl.
2. Place the rest of the ingredients in a blender or food processor and blend until smooth. Pour the sauce over the cabbage mixture.
3. Put inside the refrigerator for several hours before serving.

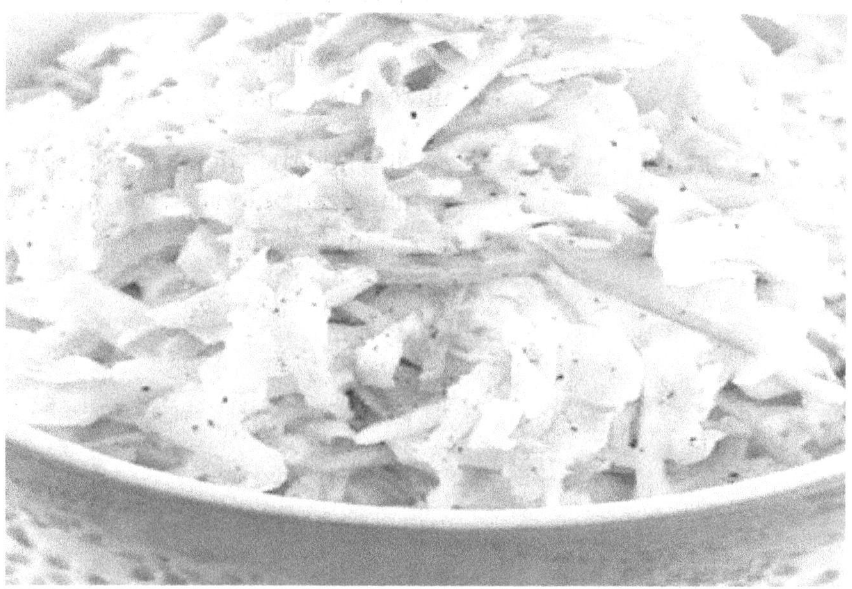

Nutrition

Calories 49.6 Total Fat 0.3 g Carbs 11.3 g Protein 1.2 g Sodium 138.3 mg

Preparation Time: 5' *Cooking Time: 45'* *Serves: 6*

110. Cracker Barrel's Baby Carrot

Ingredients

- *1 teaspoon bacon grease, melted*
- *2 pounds fresh baby carrots*
- *Some water*
- *1 teaspoon salt*
- *¼ cup brown sugar*
- *¼ cup butter, melted*
- *¼ cup honey*

Directions

1. Heat the bacon grease in a pot. Place the carrots in the grease and sauté for 10 seconds. Cover the carrots with water and add the salt.

2. Bring the entire mixture to a boil over medium heat, then reduce the heat to low and allow it to simmer for another 30 to 45 minutes. By this time, the carrots should be half cooked.

3. Remove half the water from the pot and add the rest of the ingredients.

4. Keep cooking until the carrots become tender. Transfer to a bowl and serve.

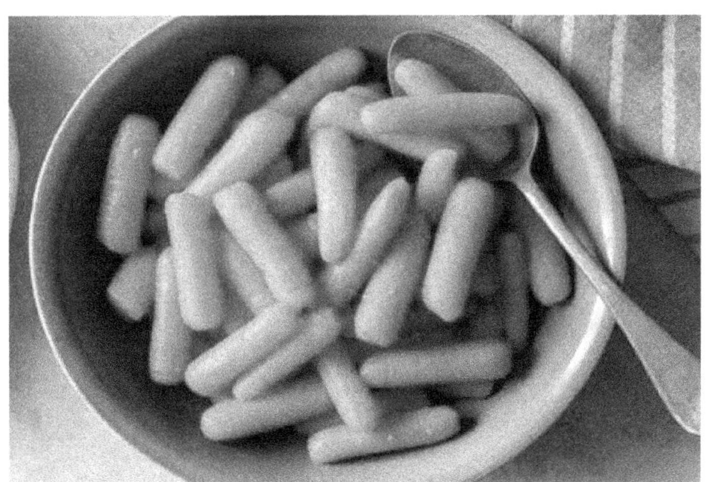

Nutrition

Calories: 205 Total Fat: 8.6g Carbs: 33.1g Protein: 1.1g Sodium: 577.4mg

Chapter 8
Tasty Pasta

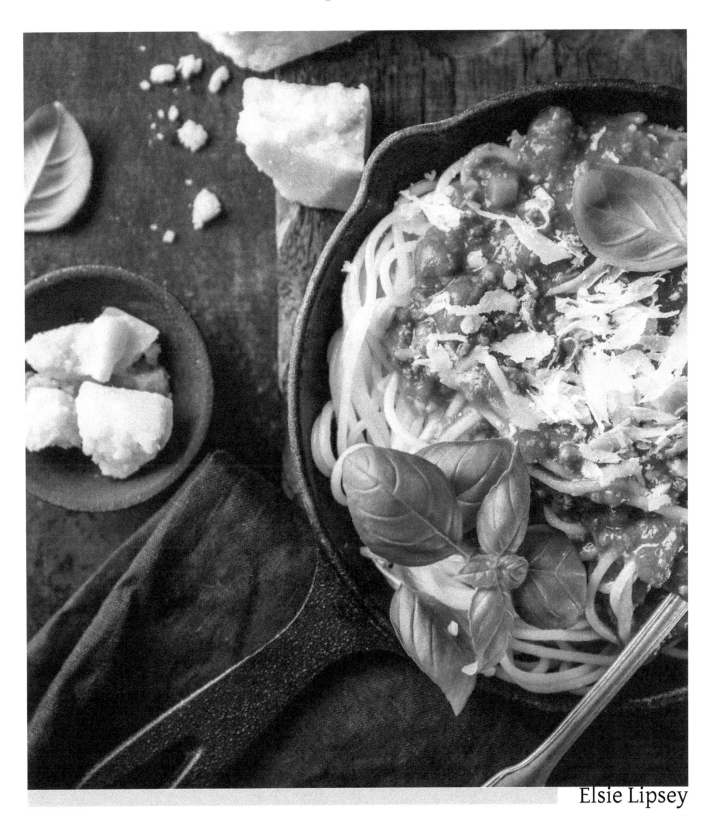

Preparation Time: 15' *Cooking Time: 20'* *Serves: 4*

111. Mediterranean's Garlic, Oil and Hot Pepper Spaghetti

Ingredients

- ***13 ounces whole wheat spaghetti***
- ***6 tablespoon olives***
- ***1 hot pepper***
- ***1 garlic clove***
- ***Salt***
- ***Parmesan***

Directions

1. Mince the garlic and the hot pepper. Cook the spaghetti in salted boiling water.
2. Put some of the olive oil in a pan and add the garlic and hot pepper. Cook for some minutes.
3. Once the spaghetti are cooked, drain it and pour it in the pan together with the garlic and hot pepper.
4. Season with some parmesan.

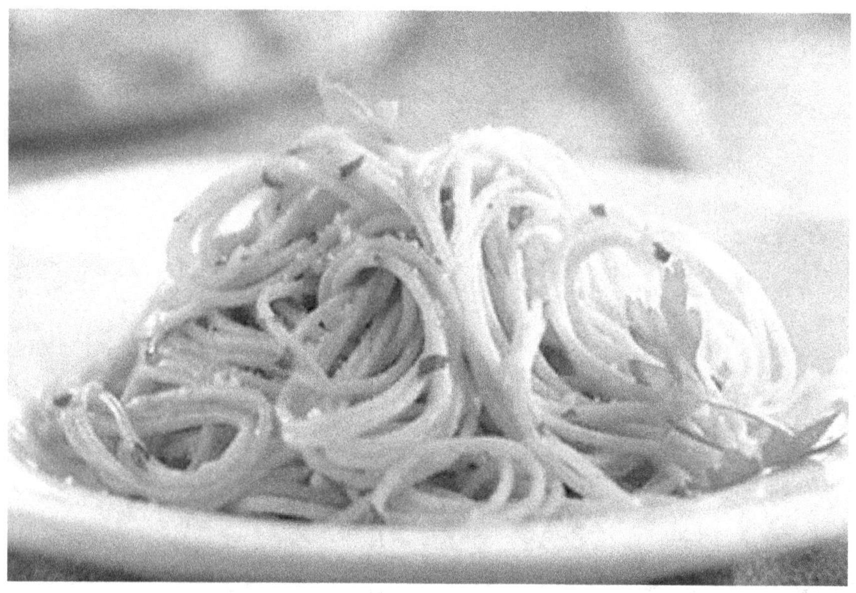

Nutrition

Calories: 152 Protein: 20g Carbohydrate: 32g Fat: 5g

Preparation Time: 15' *Cooking Time: 40'* *Serves: 4*

112. Mediterranean's Carbonara Spaghetti

Ingredients

- ***10 ounces spaghetti***
- ***6 yolks***
- ***5 ounces pork cheek***
- ***Pepper***
- ***2 ounces roman pecorino***
- ***Salt***

Directions

1. Cut the pork cheek in □ inches strips. In a pan, cook the pork cheek over medium heat for 10 minutes.
2. Meanwhile, cook the spaghetti in salted boiling water.
3. In a bowl beat the yolks, add most of the roman pecorino and some pepper. Mix everything.
4. When the spaghetti pasta is cooked, drain it and pour it in the pork cheek pan with the heat off.
5. Add the bowl compound and stir fast; the yolks must not cook.
6. Serve the spaghetti seasoned with some more cheese.

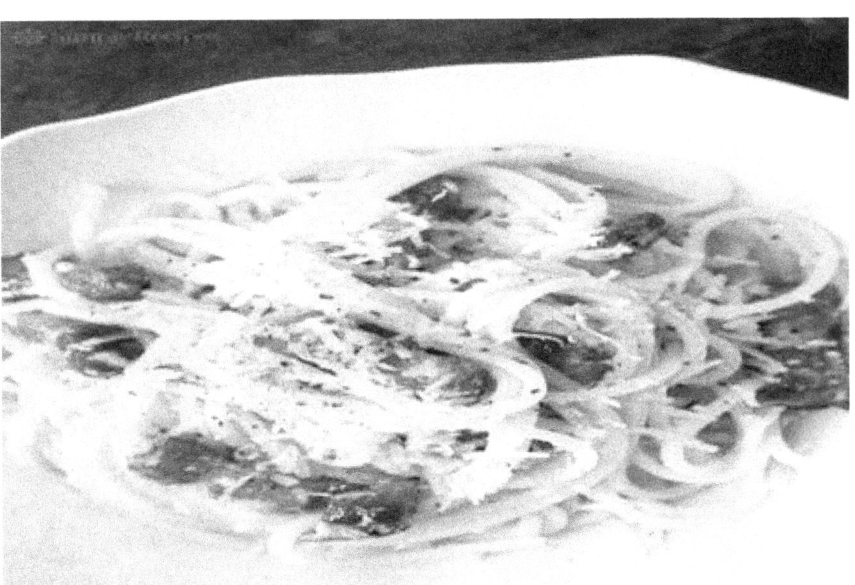

Nutrition

Calories: 186 Protein: 22g Carbohydrate: 38g Fat: 8g

Preparation Time: 15' *Cooking Time: 30'* *Serves: 4*

113. Mediterranean's Bolognese Spaghetti

Ingredients

- ***13 ounces whole wheat spaghetti***
- ***26 ounces minced meat***
- ***1 onion***
- ***½ celery***
- ***1 carrot***
- ***14 ounces tomato sauce***
- ***1 cup white dry wine***
- ***Salt and pepper***
- ***Olive oil***

Directions

1. Mince the vegetables and heat some oil in a deep pan.
2. Cook the vegetables in the pan for some minutes, add the meat and break it. Add the white wine and let evaporate.
3. Add salt, pepper and tomato sauce. Cook for 2 hours over low heat.

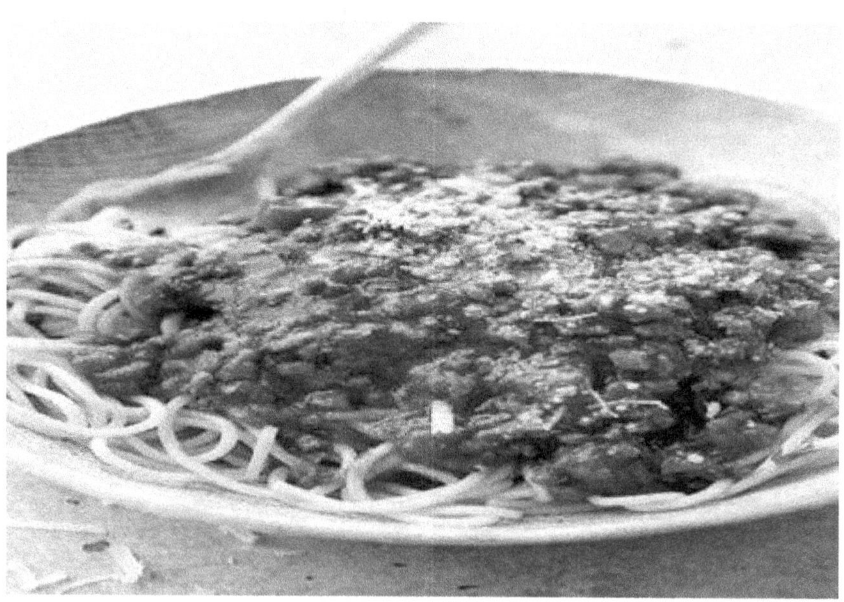

Nutrition

Calories: 136 Protein: 17g Carbohydrate: 18g Fat: 5g

Preparation Time: 15' *Cooking Time: 30'* *Serves: 4*

114. Mediterranean's Gricia Spaghetti

Ingredients

- ***13 ounces whole wheat spaghetti***
- ***5 ounces pork cheek***
- ***2 ounces roman pecorino***
- ***Salt***

Directions

1. Cut the pork cheek in □ inches strips.
2. In a pan, cook the pork cheek over medium heat for 10 minutes.
3. Meanwhile, cook the spaghetti in salted boiling water.
4. When the spaghetti pasta is cooked, drain it and pour it in the pork cheek pan. Add the roman pecorino and mix everything.

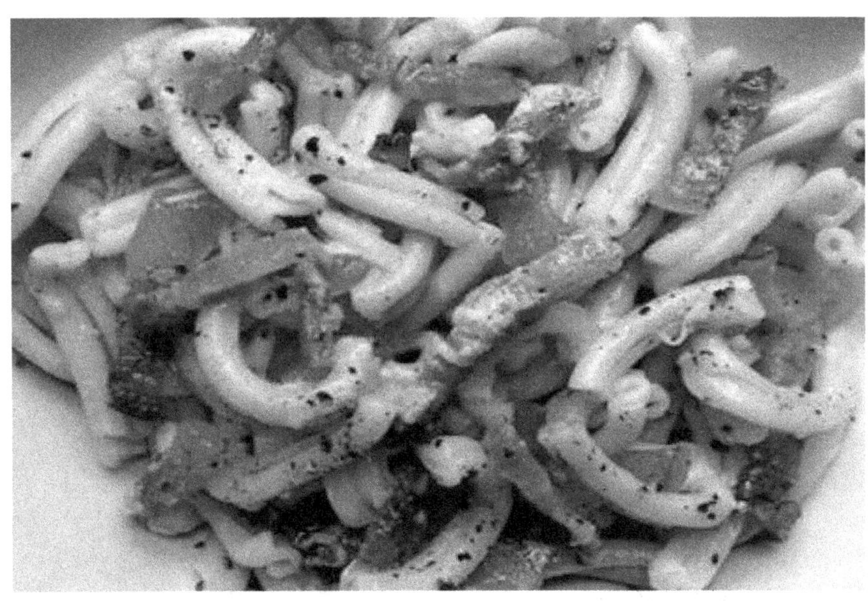

Nutrition

Calories: 110 Protein: 10g Carbohydrate: 28g Fat: 7g

Preparation Time: 10’ *Cooking Time: 30’* *Serves: 4*

115. Mediterranean’s Italian Pasta

Ingredients

- *3 anchovies*
- *9 ounces mozzarella cheese*
- *13 ounces whole-wheat pasta*
- *2 tablespoon olives*
- *3 tomatoes*
- *3 tablespoon olive oil*
- *Pepper*
- *Salt*

Directions

1. Cook the pasta in boiling water.
2. Meanwhile chop the tomatoes, the mozzarella, and the anchovies.
3. Once the pasta is cooked, use some cold water to cool it.
4. Season with the chop ingredients, add the olive oil, some salt, pepper, and basil.

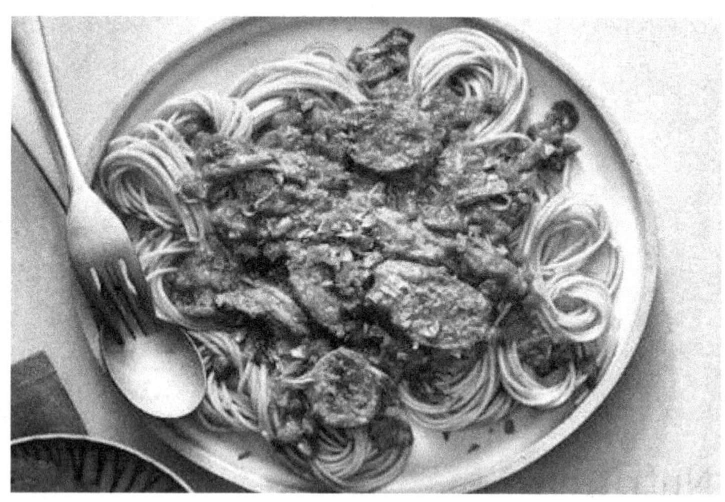

Nutrition

Calories: 100 Protein: 8g Carbohydrate: 18g Fat: 6g

Preparation Time: 15' *Cooking Time: 25'* *Serves: 4*

116. Mediterranean's Zucchini Carbonara Pasta

Ingredients

- ***13 ounces whole-wheat pasta***
- ***2 eggs***
- ***2 tablespoon olive oil***
- ***2 zucchini***
- ***1 garlic clove***
- ***2 tablespoon milk***
- ***Salt***
- ***Parmesan***

Directions

1. Cut the zucchinis into small pieces. Put olive oil in a pan to let it heat and add the garlic clove. After a few minutes add the zucchinis and cook for 10 minutes.
2. Cook the pasta in boiling water, meanwhile beat the eggs together with the milk in a big bowl. Add the parmesan and some salt.
3. If the pasta is cooked already, drain it and add it into the pan. Pour the pan content into the bowl and mix everything.

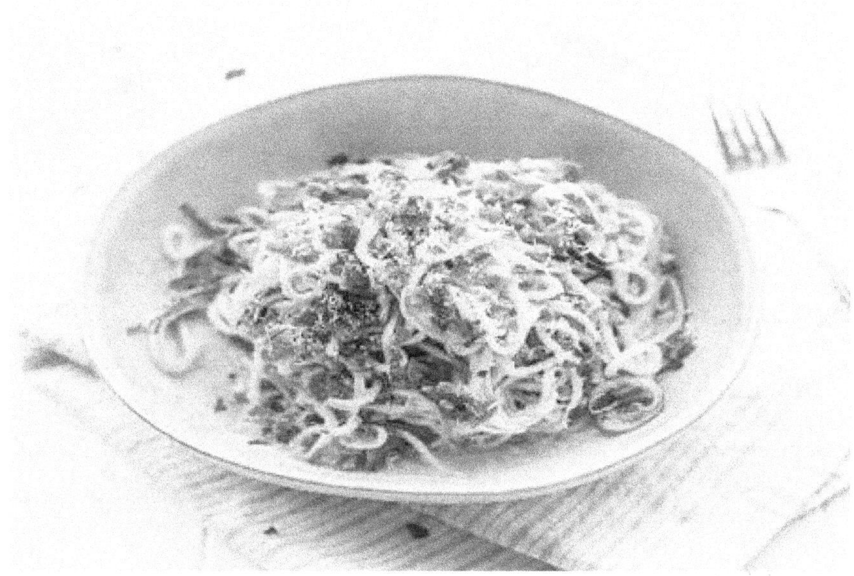

Nutrition

Calories: 105 Protein: 10g Carbohydrate: 23g Fat: 9g

Preparation Time: 15' *Cooking Time: 10'* *Serves: 4*

117. Mediterranean's Fresh Pasta with Turnip Greens

Ingredients

- ***18 ounces fresh pasta (orecchiette)***
- ***30 ounces turnip greens***
- ***2 garlic cloves***
- ***6 tablespoon olive oil***
- ***Parmesan***
- ***Salt***

Directions

1. Wash and cook the turnip greens in boiling water for a few minutes.
2. Keep the water, mince the garlic, and put in a pan with the oil. Cook together with the turnip greens, add some salt.
3. Cook the pasta in the turnip greens water, drain the pasta and mix it in the pan together with the turnip greens, add some parmesan.

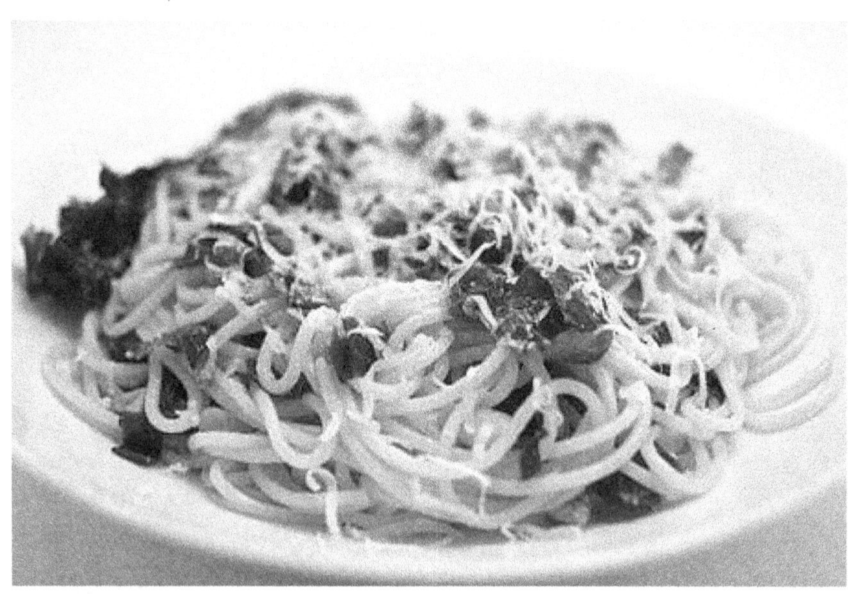

Nutrition

Calories 115 Protein 11g Carbohydrate 22g Fat 5g

Preparation Time: 15' *Cooking Time: 25'* *Serves: 4*

118. Mediterranean's Tomatoes and Mozzarella Pasta

Ingredients

- ***13 ounces of whole-wheat pasta***
- ***20 cherry tomatoes***
- ***1 onion***
- ***3 tablespoon olive oil***
- ***7 ounces mozzarella cheese***
- ***Basil***
- ***Salt***

Directions

1. Boil some water to cook the pasta, cut the tomatoes in half and mince the onion.
2. Heat the oil in a pan and sauté the onion, add the tomatoes and the basil and cook for 7-8 minutes. Turn the heat off.
3. Place the pasta in the pan with boiling water and salt to cook and cut the mozzarella into cubes.
4. When the pasta is already cooked mix it into the pan together with the tomatoes, cook for a few minutes while adding the mozzarella.

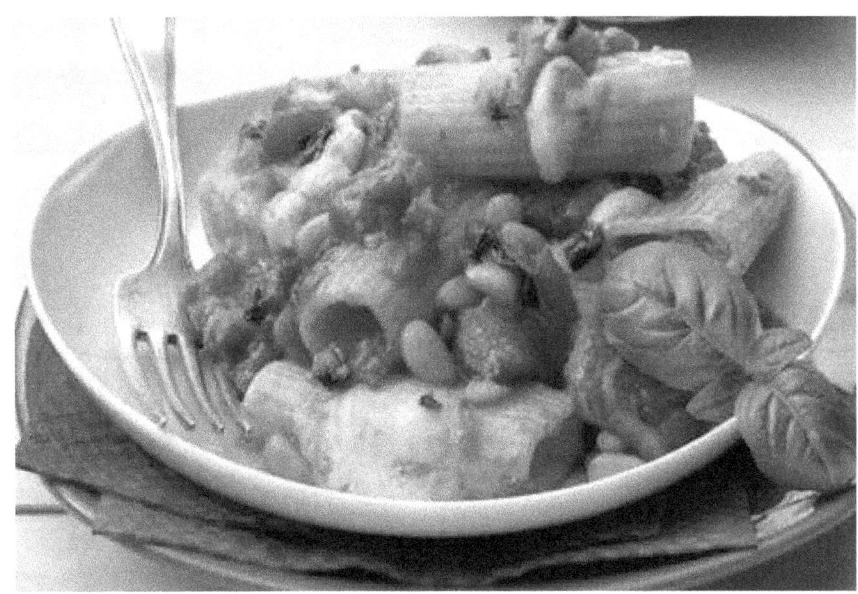

Nutrition

Calories: 105 Protein: 10g Carbohydrate: 23g Fat: 9g

Preparation Time: 10' *Cooking Time: 25'* *Serves: 4*

119. Mediterranean's Smoked Salmon Pasta

Ingredients

- ***18 ounces fresh pasta (fettuccini)***
- ***4 ounces smoked salmon***
- ***½ cup cooking cream***
- ***3 tablespoon olive oil***
- ***Salt***

Directions

1. Cut the salmon into strips and cook it with the olive oil in a pan.
2. After 2 minutes add the cooking cream and cook for 5 minutes.
3. Cook the pasta in boiling water with a pinch of salt, drain it, and add it into the pan with the salmon. Cook for a few minutes.

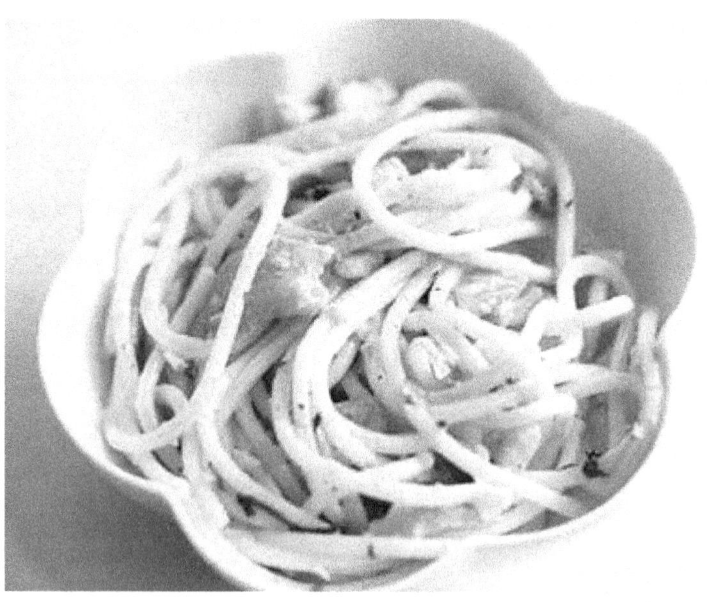

Nutrition

Calories: 110 Protein: 9g Carbohydrate: 20g Fat: 11g

Preparation Time: 10' *Cooking Time: 20'* *Serves: 4*

120. Mediterranean's Mushroom and Yogurt Pasta

Ingredients

- ***13 ounces whole-wheat pasta (fettuccini)***
- ***14 ounces of mixed mushrooms***
- ***1 onion***
- ***1 garlic clove***
- ***4 Tablespoon white yogurt***
- ***5 Tablespoon olive oil***
- ***Salt***

Directions

1. Cut the onion, wash the mushrooms, and cut them. Boil some water to cook the pasta.
2. Heat a large pan in medium and add the olive oil, the garlic clove, and the minced onion then add the mushrooms and cook for 10 minutes.
3. Once the pasta is cooked drain it and add it into the pan, add the yogurt, and mix.

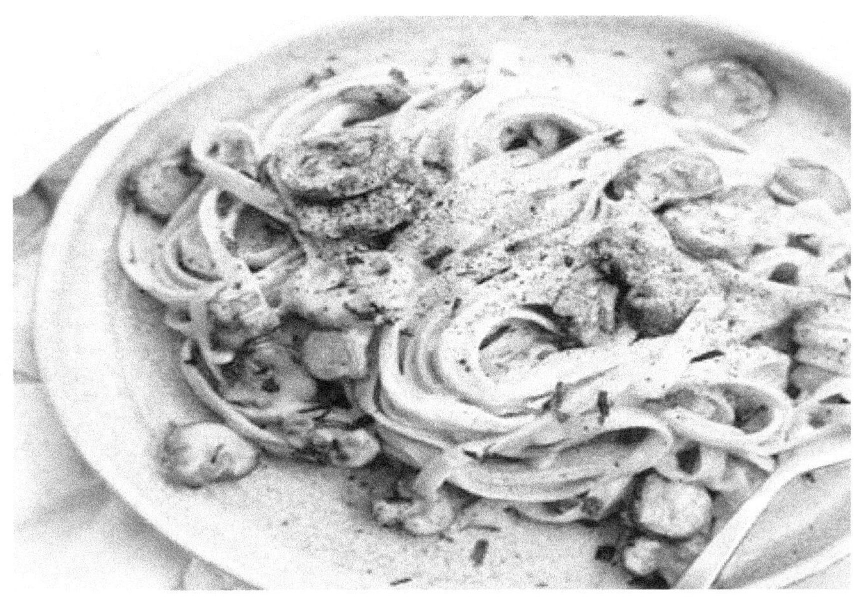

Nutrition

Calories: 105 Protein: 10g Carbohydrate: 23g Fat: 9g

Preparation Time: 15' *Cooking Time: 20'* *Serves: 4*

121. Mediterranean's Treviso Fettuccine

Ingredients

- ***8 ounces dry egg fettucine***
- ***2 red chicory***
- ***1 shallot***
- ***1 cup white wine***
- ***4 Tablespoon olive oil***
- ***Salt***
- ***Pepper***
- ***Parmesan***

Directions

1. Wash and cut the chicory into strips, mince the shallot.
2. Put the shallot in a pan with some oil, add the chicory and cook for some minutes.
3. Pour the wine, salt, and pepper and cook for 5 minutes.
4. Cook the fettuccine in boiling water, drain them, and pour them into the pan together with the chicory.
5. Season with some parmesan.

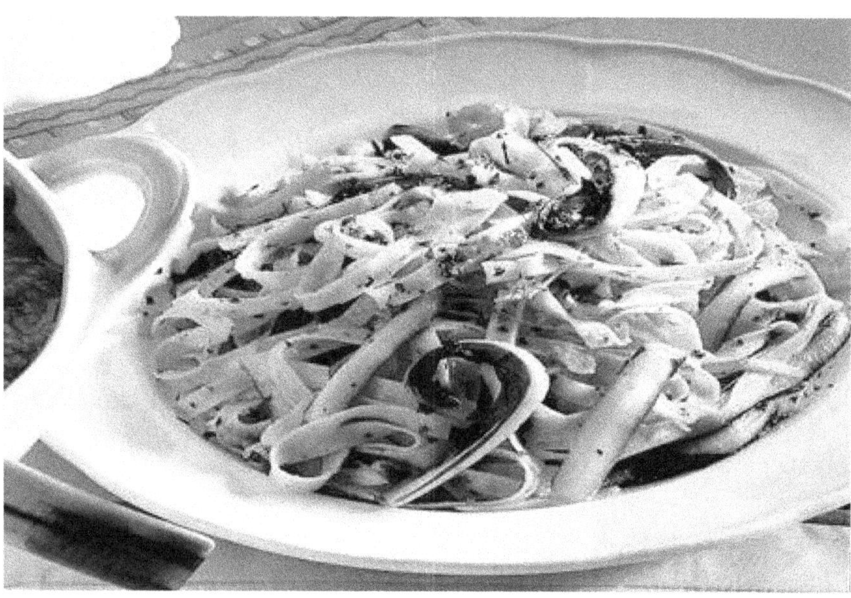

Nutrition

Calories 101 Protein 8g Carbohydrate 13g Fat 5g

Preparation Time: 10' *Cooking Time: 25'* *Serves: 2*

122. Mediterranean's Pesto Pasta

Ingredients

- ***13 ounces whole wheat pasta***
- ***1 garlic clove***
- ***1 bunch of basil***
- ***1 cup olive oil***
- ***2 ounces of pine nuts***
- ***Salt***
- ***Parmesan***

Directions

1. In a mixer, mix the basil, the garlic, some parmesan, the oil, the pine nuts, and some salt.
2. In a pan, let water boil and put the pasta to cook. Drain it afterward.
3. Combine and mix the pesto sauce in the pasta and cook for 1 minute.

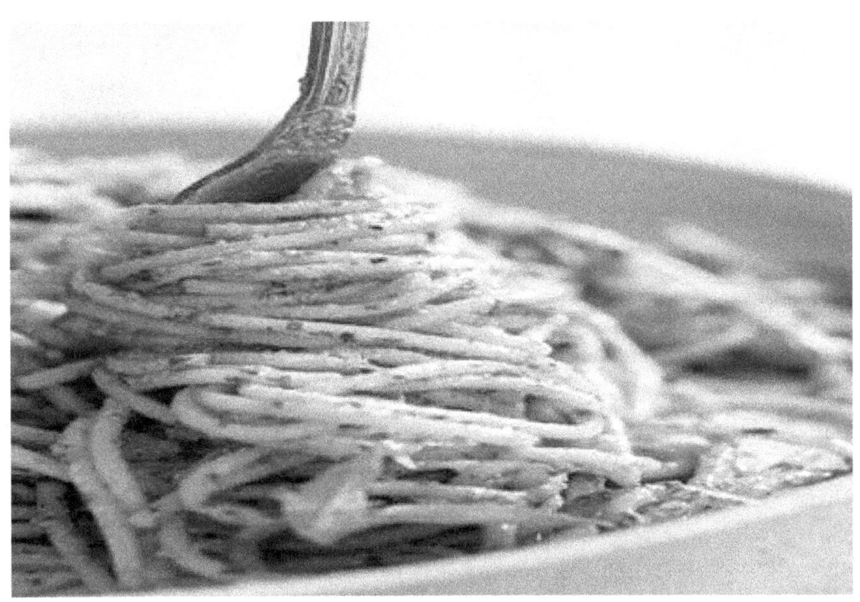

Nutrition

Calories: 105 Protein: 10g Carbohydrate: 23g Fat: 9g

Preparation Time: 15' *Cooking Time: 20'* *Serves: 2*

123. Mediterranean's Vegetarian Pasta

Ingredients

- ***13 ounces of pasta***
- ***1 eggplant***
- ***2 zucchini***
- ***1 red pepper***
- ***1 yellow pepper***
- ***Olive oil***
- ***1 onion***
- ***Salt***

Directions

1. Cut the vegetables into slices. Heat some oil in the pan.
2. Cook the vegetables in the pan, add some water, and wait 20 minutes.
3. Meanwhile, cook the pasta into some boiling water.
4. After that, drain the pasta and pour it in the vegetable pan.

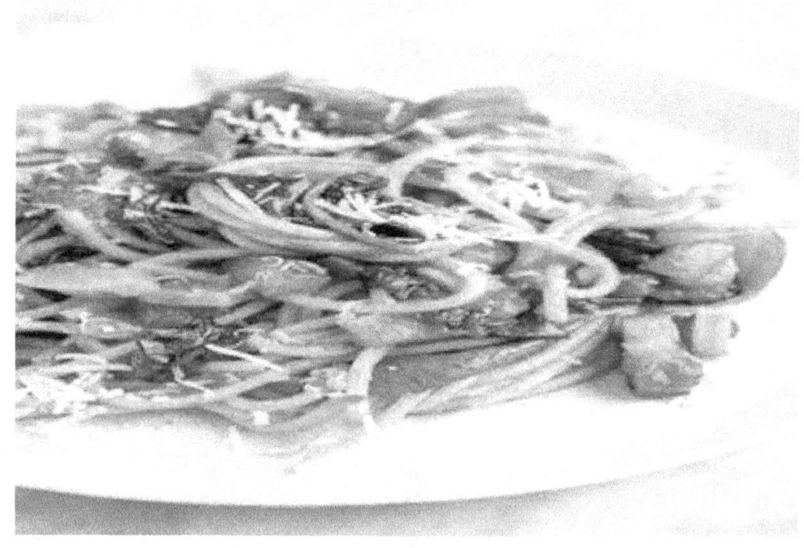

Nutrition

Calories: 103 Protein: 8.9g Carbohydrate: 19g Fat: 9g

Preparation Time: 10' *Cooking Time: 20'* *Serves: 2*

124. Mediterranean's Amatriciana Pasta

Ingredients

- ***13 ounces whole wheat spaghetti***
- ***6 ounces pork cheek***
- ***1 chili pepper***
- ***14 ounces tomato sauce***
- ***3 ounces roman pecorino***
- ***Salt***
- ***3 Tablespoon olive oil***

Directions

1. Cut the pork cheek in inches strips. Pour the olive oil in the pan and add the chili pepper, add the pork cheek and cook for 8 minutes in low heat.
2. Meanwhile, cook the pasta in salted boiling water. Add the tomato sauce in the pork cheek pan and cook for 10 minutes.
3. Once the pasta is cooked, drain it and add it into the sauce. Add the roman pecorino.

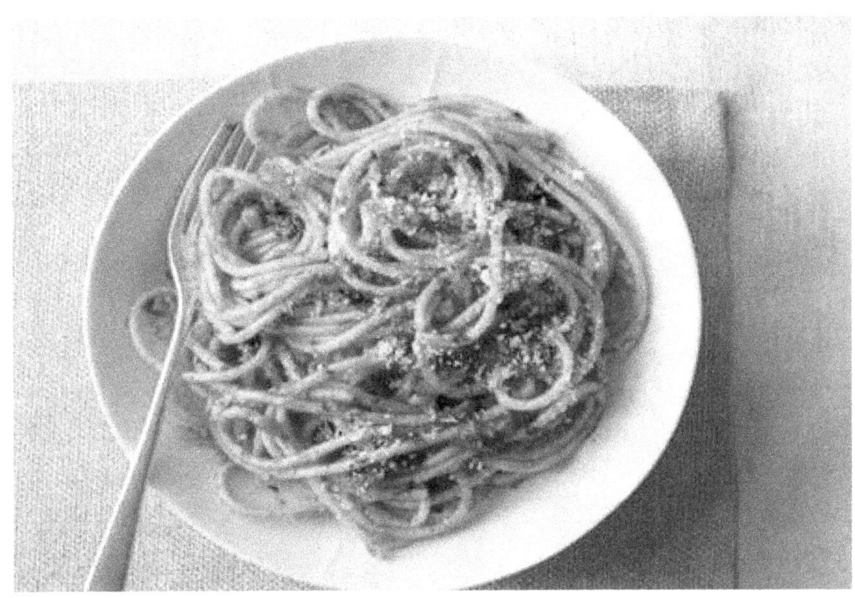

Nutrition

Calories: 105 Protein: 10g Carbohydrate: 23g Fat: 9g

Chapter 9
Soup

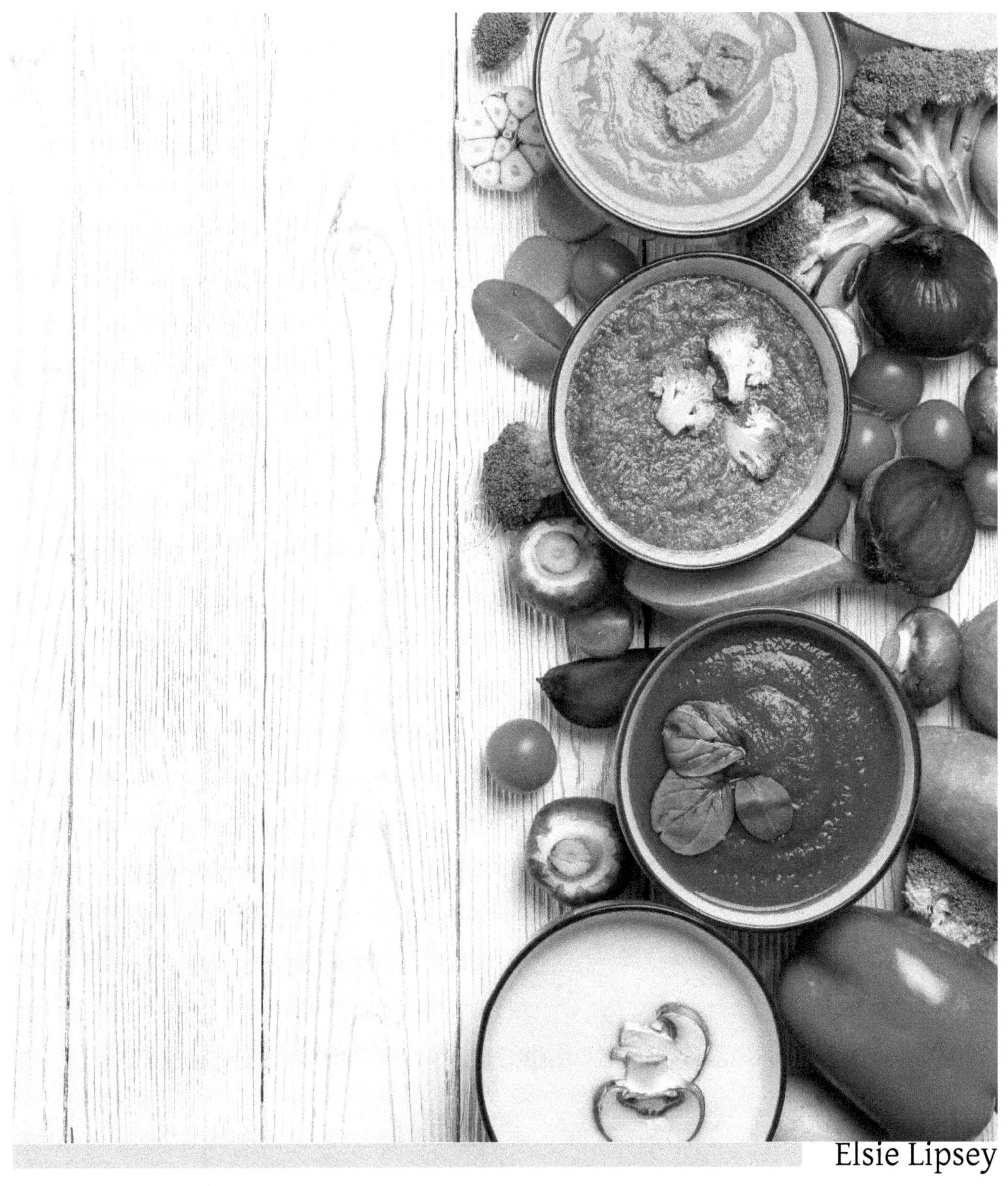

Preparation Time: 25' *Cooking Time: 1 hour* *Serves: 6*

125. Olive Garden's Creamy Zuppa Toscana

Ingredients

- ***1 pound Italian sausage, ground***
- ***1¼ teaspoon red pepper flakes, ground***
- ***4 bacon slices, cut into ½-inch pieces***
- ***1 large onion, diced***
- ***1 tablespoon minced garlic***
- ***5 (13¾-ounce) cans chicken broth***
- ***6 potatoes, finely chopped***
- ***1 cup heavy cream***
- ***2 cups fresh spinach leaves***

Directions

1. Cook the sausage and red pepper flakes on medium-high heat for at least 10 minutes or until brown. Drain. Transfer to a bowl and set aside.

2. In the same pot, cook bacon on medium heat for 10 minutes or until crunchy. Drain drippings until only a few tablespoons are left at the bottom of the pot. Mix the in onions and garlic with the bacon.

3. Add chicken broth into the pot and adjust heat to high. Bring to a boil. Add potatoes and boil for 20 minutes. Adjust heat to medium and mix in the cream and cooked sausage to reheat.

4. Stir in spinach and serve.

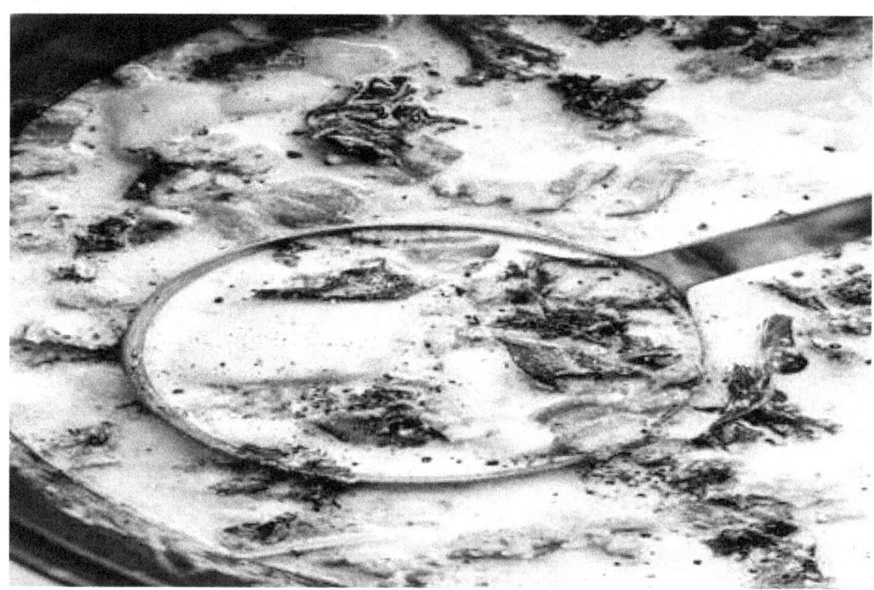

Nutrition

Calories: 554 Total Fat: 33g Carbs: 46g Protein: 20g Sodium: 2386mg

Preparation Time: 15' *Cooking Time: 50'* *Serves: 8*

126. Panera's Broccoli Cheddar Soup

Ingredients

- ***1 tablespoon butter***
- ***½ onion, diced***
- ***¼ cup melted butter***
- ***¼ cup flour***
- ***2 cups milk***
- ***2 cups chicken stock***
- ***1½ cup broccoli florets, diced***
- ***1 cup carrots, cut into thin strips***
- ***1 stalk celery, sliced***
- ***2½ cups Cheddar cheese, grated***
- ***Salt and pepper, to taste***

Directions

1. Let 1 tablespoon of butter melt in a skillet and cook onion over medium heat for 5 minutes or until caramelized. Set aside.
2. In a saucepan, mix melted butter and flour, then cook on medium-low heat. Add 1 or 2 tablespoons milk to the flour to prevent from burning. Cook for at least 3 minutes or until smooth.
3. While stirring, gently pour the rest of the milk in with the flour. Mix in chicken stock. Let it simmer for 20 minutes. Toss in broccoli, carrots, cooked onion, and celery. Cook until vegetables turn soft.
4. Mix in cheese and stir until the cheese is completely melted. Season with salt and pepper, to taste.
5. Transfer into individual bowls. Serve.

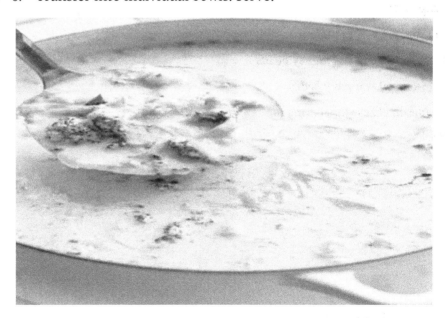

Nutrition

Calories: 304 Total Fat: 23g Carbs: 11g Protein: 14g Sodium: 624mg

Preparation Time: 10' *Cooking Time: 20'* *Serves: 8*

127. Olive Garden's Pasta e Fagioli

Ingredients

- *1 cup ditalini pasta*
- *2 tablespoons olive oil, divided*
- *1 pound Italian sausage*
- *3 garlic cloves, finely chopped*
- *1 onion, chopped*
- *3 carrots, peeled and chopped*
- *2 stalks celery, chopped*
- *3 cups chicken broth*
- *1 16-ounce can tomato sauce*
- *1 15-ounce can diced tomatoes*
- *1 teaspoon dried basil*
- *1 teaspoon dried oregano*
- *¾ teaspoon dried thyme*
- *1 cup water*
- *Salt and pepper, to taste*
- *1 (15-ounce) can red kidney beans*
- *1 (15-ounce) can navy beans*
- *Parmesan cheese for serving (optional)*

Directions

1. Cook pasta in water that is boiling. Drain and set aside.
2. Pour a tablespoon oil to a pot and heat. Sauté sausage in the pot for at least 3 minutes or until brown over medium heat. Drain and set aside.
3. Pour oil in the same pot over medium-low heat. Add garlic, onion, carrots, and celery. Mix from time to time while cooking for at least 3 minutes or until vegetables soften.
4. Pour in broth, tomato sauce, tomatoes, basil, oregano, thyme, cooked sausage, and water. Add salt and pepper, to taste. Once boiling, adjust heat to low and let simmer for another 10 minutes or until all vegetables are soft.
5. Mix in cooked pasta and beans to reheat.
6. Put some parmesan cheese on top if desired and serve.

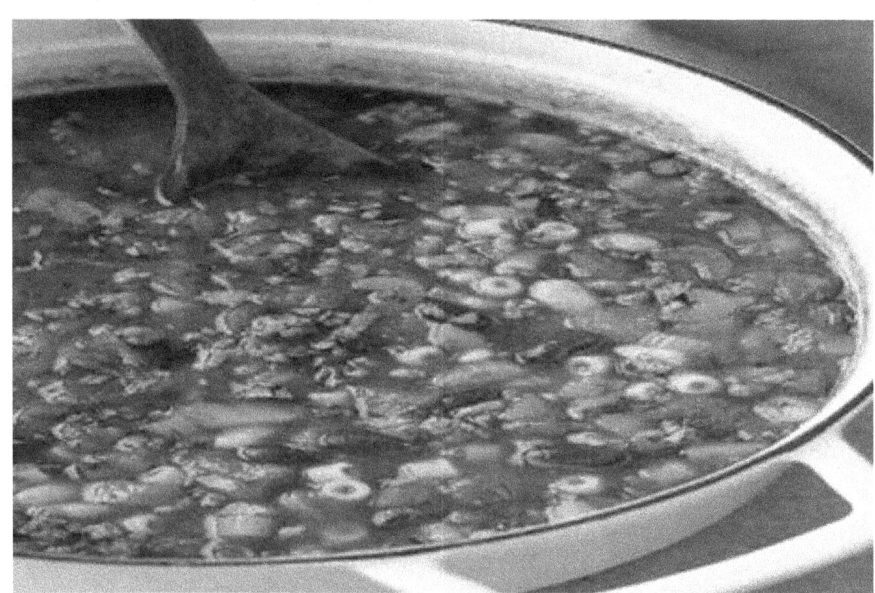

Nutrition

Calories: 340 Total Fat: 10g Carbs: 44g Protein: 22g Sodium: 889mg

Preparation Time: 10' *Cooking Time: 45'* *Serves: 8*

128. Carrabba'sMinestrone Soup

Ingredients

- ***2 teaspoons olive oil***
- ***1 large stalk celery, finely chopped***
- ***2 large carrots, cut thinly***
- ***½ small onion, finely chopped***
- ***4 garlic cloves, finely chopped***
- ***Salt and pepper, to taste***
- ***½ cup green beans, cut into 1-inch pieces***
- ***4 cups cabbage, finely chopped***
- ***1 small summer squash, roughly chopped***
- ***1 small zucchini, roughly chopped***
- ***1 tablespoon fresh parsley, finely chopped***
- ***½ tablespoon dried basil***
- ***1 (14-ounce) can white kidney beans***
- ***1 (14-ounce) can garbanzo beans***
- ***4 cups vegetable broth***
- ***4 cups water***
- ***2 bay leaves***
- ***1 (14-ounce) can diced tomatoes***
- ***2 tablespoons Parmesan cheese, grated***
- ***1½ cups red potatoes, diced***

Directions

1. Put oil in a large pan on medium heat. Cook celery, carrots, onion, and garlic with salt and pepper for at least 5 minutes or until vegetables are tender.
2. Toss in green beans, cabbage, zucchini, squash, parsley, and basil. Cook for another 5 minutes.
3. Grind half of the white kidney and garbanzo beans in a blender.
4. Add to the pan the stock, water, bay leaves, tomatoes, ground and unground beans, parmesan rind, and potatoes. Let it simmer until potatoes are tender.
5. Serve.

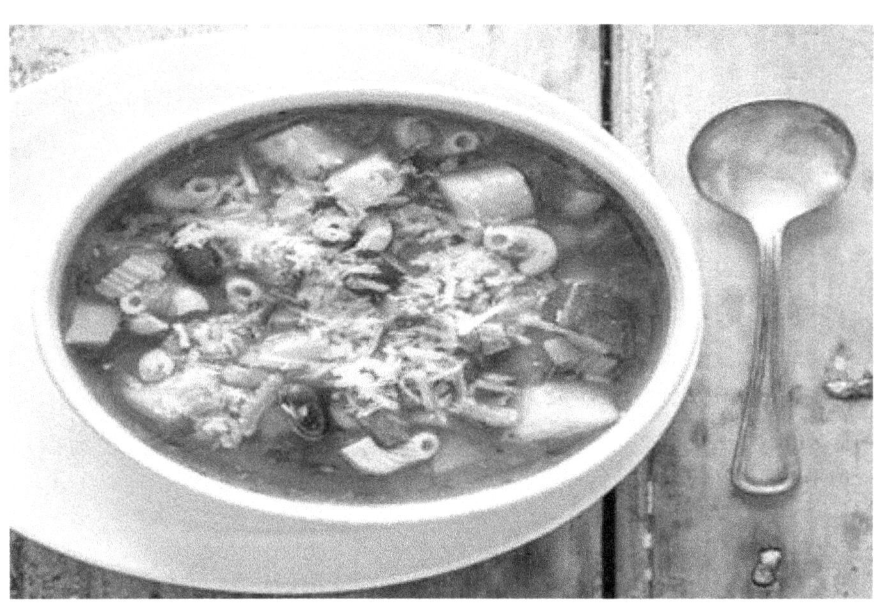

Nutrition

Calories 370 Total Fat: 9g Carbs: 51g Protein: 23g Sodium: 590mg

Preparation Time: 10' *Cooking Time: 20'* *Serves: 8*

129. Applebees's Tomato Basil Soup

Ingredients

- *3 tablespoons olive oil*
- *1 small garlic clove, finely chopped*
- *1 (10 ¾-ounce) can condensed tomato soup*
- *¼ cup bottled marinara sauce*
- *5 ounces water*
- *1 teaspoon fresh oregano, diced*
- *½ teaspoon ground black pepper*
- *1 tablespoon fresh basil, diced*
- *6 Italian-style seasoned croutons*
- *2 tablespoons Parmesan cheese, shredded*

Directions

1. Put oil in a medium sized pan over medium heat. Add garlic and stir fry for 2 to 3 minutes or until garlic is soft and aromatic.
2. Pour tomato soup and marinara sauce into pan and stir. Add water gradually. Toss in oregano and pepper. Once simmering, reduce heat to low. Cook for 15 minutes until all the flavors are combined. Add basil and stir.
3. Transfer to bowls. Add croutons on top and sprinkle with Parmesan cheese.
4. Serve.

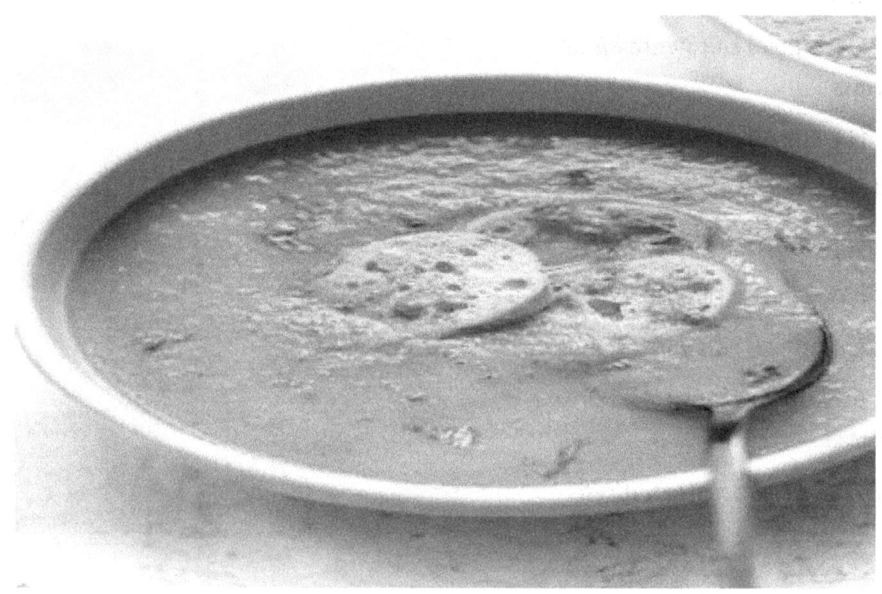

Nutrition

Calories 350 Total fat 26g Carbs 28g Sugar 14g Protein 6g

Preparation Time: 10' *Cooking Time: 1 hour* *Serves: 12*

130. Panera's Lemon Chicken Orzo Soup

Ingredients

- *Water, for boiling*
- *Salt, to taste*
- *8 ounces orzo pasta*
- *1 teaspoon olive oil*
- *3 carrots, diced*
- *3 ribs celery, diced*
- *1 onion, diced*
- *2 cloves garlic, finely chopped*
- *½ teaspoon dried thyme*
- *½ teaspoon dried oregano*
- *Salt, to taste*
- *Pepper, to taste*
- *1 bay leaf*
- *3 (32-ounce) cartons chicken broth*
- *½ cup fresh lemon juice*
- *1 lemon, zested*
- *8 ounces cooked chicken breast, diced*
- *1 (8-ounce) package baby spinach leaves*
- *1 lemon, sliced*
- *¼ cup Parmesan cheese, shredded*

Directions

1. Pour water and add a pinch of salt to a pot and bring to a boil and put the orzo and cook until pasta is al dente. Remove from heat and drain.
2. Put olive oil in medium heat. Add carrots, celery, and onion. Sauté for about 5 to 7 minutes until vegetables become tender and onion is translucent. Stir in garlic. Cook for another minute or until aromatic. Toss in the thyme, oregano, salt, black pepper, and bay leaf. Add chicken broth. Bring to a boil.
3. Bring heat to medium-low. Let it simmer for 10 minutes.
4. Add orzo and lemon zest. Pour in lemon juice and the chicken. Cook everything for about 3 minutes until both the chicken and orzo are heated thoroughly. Toss in spinach and cook for about 2 to 3 minutes. The soup is ready once the spinach wilts into the broth and the orzo is soft.
5. Transfer into bowls and serve with lemon slices and Parmesan cheese.

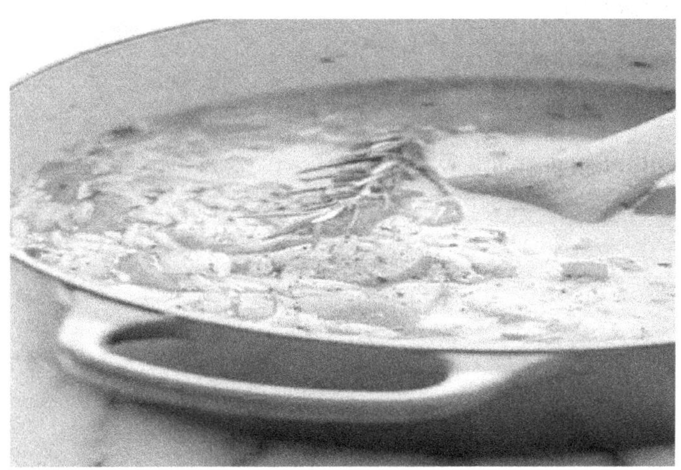

Nutrition

Calories: 167 Total Fat: 4g Carbs: 22g Sugar: 4g Protein 12g Sodium 187 mg

Preparation Time: 30' *Cooking Time: 30'* *Serves: 6*

131. Olive Garden's Chicken and Gnocchi Soup

Ingredients

- *¼ cup butter*
- *1 tablespoon extra-virgin olive oil*
- *1 large zucchini, chopped*
- *2 stalks celery, chopped*
- *1 yellow onion, chopped*
- *½ red bell pepper, chopped*
- *2 carrots, grated*
- *4 garlic cloves, finely chopped*
- *¼ cup all-purpose flour*
- *3 cups chicken broth*
- *3 cups half-and-half*
- *2 cups rotisserie chicken meat, shredded*
- *1 (16-ounce) package small gnocchi*
- *2 cups fresh spinach, chopped*
- *Salt and pepper, to taste*
- *½ teaspoon ground thyme*
- *¼ teaspoon nutmeg, grated*

Directions

1. Heat butter together with olive oil on medium heat. Add zucchini, celery, onion, red bell pepper, carrots, and garlic. Sauté for about 8 to 10 minutes until tender, then mix in flour to coat vegetables. Cook for another 2 minutes.
2. Pour chicken broth in pot and stir for 5 minutes until ingredients are combined and soup is smooth and has thickened. Then, stir in half-and-half and cook for another 5 minutes until soup is a bit thicker. Slowly stir in chicken, gnocchi, and spinach. Sprinkle in salt, pepper, thyme, and nutmeg.
3. Serve.

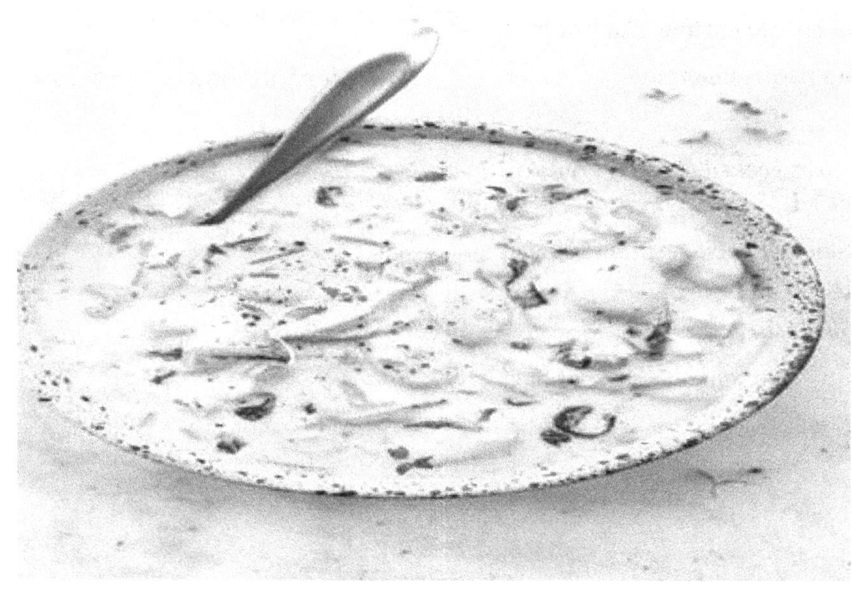

Nutrition

Calories: 416 Total Fat: 24g Carbs: 35g Sugar: 8g Fibers: 3g Protein: 17g

Preparation Time: 5' *Cooking Time: 1h 10'* *Serves: 4*

132. Denny's Broccoli Cheese Soup

Ingredients

- ***1/8 teaspoon of white pepper***
- ***¼ teaspoon of salt***
- ***4 cups chopped broccoli florets***
- ***2 ¼ cups chicken broth***
- ***3 cups shredded mild cheddar cheese***
- ***1 ½ cups whole milk***
- ***¼ cup all-purpose flour***
- ***¼ cup butter***

Directions

1. Let the butter melt in medium heat then add the flour and cook for about 1 minute, while stirring constantly.

2. Prepare a roux by whisking some milk in the saucepan, adding some cheese to it, and stirring until the cheese has melted.

3. Add the remaining ingredients, stir them all together and continue cooking until the soup boils. Let it simmer in low heat for 60 minutes while stirring often. Make sure the broccoli is tender before serving.

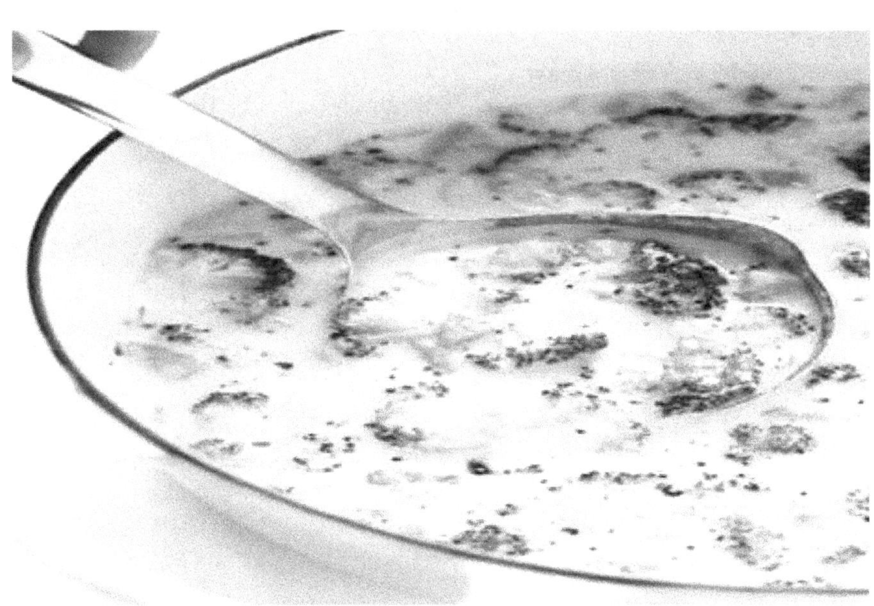

Nutrition

Calories: 324 Fat: 23g Carbs: 26g Protein: 31g

Preparation Time: 5' *Cooking Time: 1h 10'* *Serves: 8*

133. Hard Rock Café's Homemade Chicken Noodle Soup

Ingredients

- *3 cups wide egg noodles, dry*
- *1 teaspoon minced fresh parsley*
- *1 teaspoon freshly ground black pepper*
- *1 teaspoon salt*
- *4 cups water*
- *4 cups chicken broth*
- *½ cup diced celery*
- *2 medium carrots, peeled and diced*
- *1 cup diced onion*
- *1 tablespoon butter*
- *2 tablespoons vegetable oil*
- *1 pound skinless chicken thigh fillets*
- *1 pound skinless chicken breast fillets*
- *Garnish*
- *Minced fresh parsley*

Directions

1. Pour vegetable oil in a pot over medium heat. Sauté the chicken breasts and thighs for about 10 to 15 minutes, or until the chicken gets slightly brown on both sides, and they are cooked through. Take the chicken out of the pot, and place them on a cutting board.

2. After that, add the butter to the pot, then the celery, carrot, and onion. Sauté the veggies for about 10 minutes, while stirring constantly, until the carrots start to soften.

3. Slice the chicken into cubes, then add them into the large pot alongside the chicken broth, water, veggies, salt, pepper, and a teaspoon of parsley. Boil them all together, and when the soup reaches a boiling point, lower the heat and let it simmer for 10 more minutes. Combine the noodles to the soup, and continue to simmer for 15 more minutes, until the noodles are soft.

4. Serve the soup in a bowl with sprinkled minced fresh parsley on top.

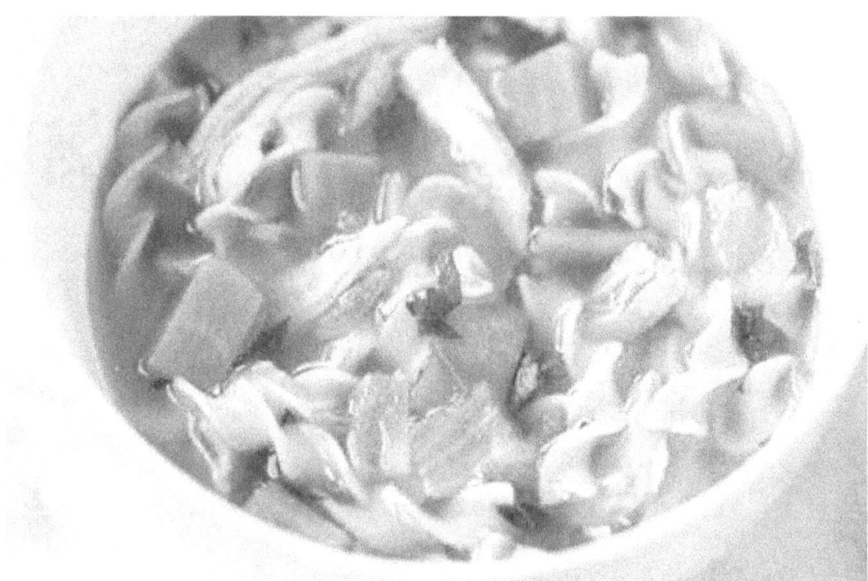

Nutrition

Calories: 302 Fat: 21g Carbs: 18g Protein: 30g

Preparation Time: 6' *Cooking Time: 1h 40'* *Serves: 6*

134. Mimi's Cafe French Market Onion Soup

Ingredients

- ***6 tablespoons shredded Parmesan cheese***
- ***6 slices mozzarella cheese***
- ***6 slices Swiss cheese***
- ***6 to 12 slices French bread***
- ***3 tablespoons Kraft grated Parmesan cheese***
- ***¼ teaspoon garlic powder***
- ***1 teaspoon salt***
- ***3 (14-ounce) cans beef broth***
- ***3 medium white onions, sliced***
- ***¼ cup butter***

Directions

1. Melt some butter in pot and sauté the onions in it for about 15 to 20 minutes, until they become transparent (when they begin to brown).

2. Pour in the beef broth, and add the garlic powder and salt to the existing onions. Boil the mixture and let it simmer uncovered for about 1 hour. Add grated Parmesan cheese within the last 10 minutes of cooking the soup.

3. When the soup has finished cooking, prepare the oven by preheating it to 350ºF in order to toast the baguette slices for 10 to 12 minutes, or until they start to turn brown. When done, take them out and set the oven to broil.

4. To prepare a serving of soup, take 1 cup soup and pour it into an oven-safe bowl. Place one or two slices toasted baguette on top to float and a slice of Swiss cheese on top of the bread slice. Add a slice of mozzarella and sprinkle 1 tablespoon of shredded Parmesan cheese over top.

5. Put the bowl of soup on a baking sheet and broil in the oven until the cheese starts to turn brown.

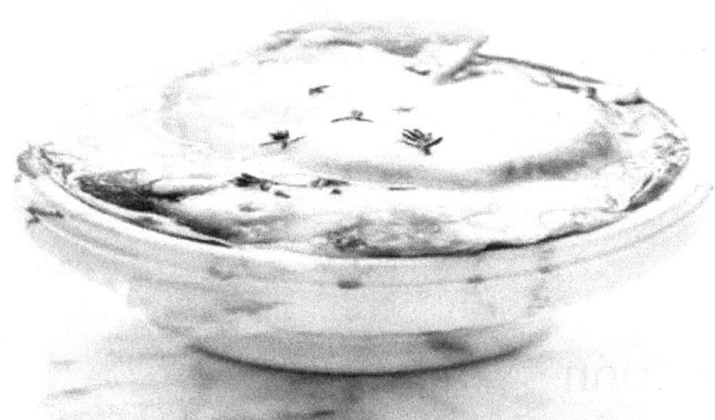

Nutrition

Calories: 292 Fat: 18g Carbs: 20g Protein: 27g

Preparation Time: 7' *Cooking Time: 45'* *Serves: 8*

135. Olive Garden's Minestrone Soup

Ingredients

- *½ cup seashell pasta*
- *4 cups fresh baby spinach*
- *3 cups hot water*
- *2 bay leaves*
- *¼ teaspoon dried basil*
- *½ teaspoon ground black pepper*
- *1 ½ teaspoons salt*
- *1 ½ teaspoons dried oregano*
- *2 tablespoons minced fresh parsley*
- *½ cup shredded carrot*
- *1 (14-ounce) can diced tomatoes*
- *2 (15-ounce) cans red kidney beans, drained*
- *4 cups vegetable broth*
- *4 teaspoons minced garlic*
- *¼ cup minced celery*
- *½ cup frozen cut Italian green beans*
- *½ cup chopped zucchini*
- *1 cup minced white onion*
- *3 tablespoons olive oil*

Directions

1. Pour the olive oil in a large saucepan over medium heat. Sauté the green beans, zucchini, onion, garlic, and celery for about 5 minutes, or until the onion starts to turn translucent.

2. Mix the broth in the pot, add the drained beans, carrots, spices, tomatoes, bay leaves, and hot water, and boil them all together. When the soup reaches the boiling point, lower the heat and simmer for 20 more minutes.

3. Add the pasta and spinach leaves and cook for 20 more minutes, then serve.

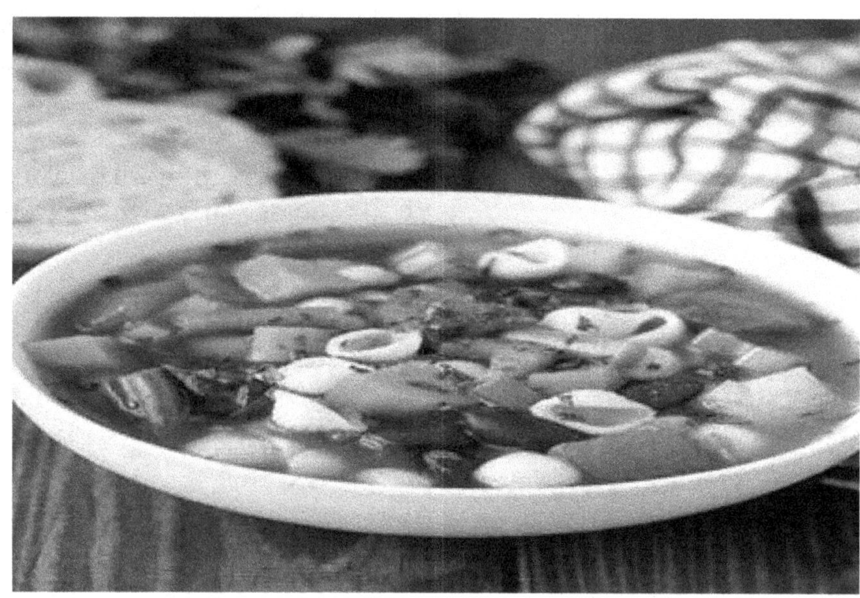

Nutrition

Calories: 262 Fat: 13g Carbs: 16g Protein: 25g

Preparation Time: 15' *Cooking Time: 1 h 20'* *Serves: 8*

136. Olive Garden's Vegetarian Soup

Ingredients

- *3 tablespoons olive oil*
- *1 medium onion, diced*
- *1 small zucchini, chopped*
- *1 (14-ounce) can Italian-style green beans*
- *1 stalk celery, diced*
- *4 teaspoons garlic, minced*
- *1 quart vegetable broth*
- *2 (15-ounce) cans red kidney beans, drained*
- *2 (15-ounce) cans great northern beans, drained*
- *1 (14-ounce) can diced tomatoes with juice*
- *½ cup carrot, shredded*
- *½ cup dry red wine (optional)*
- *½ cup tomato paste*
- *1 teaspoon oregano*
- *1 teaspoon basil*
- *½ teaspoon onion powder*
- *½ teaspoon garlic powder*
- *¼ teaspoon thyme*
- *1 bay leaf*
- *3 cups hot water*
- *4 cups fresh spinach*
- *1½ cups shell pasta*
- *Salt and pepper to taste*

Directions

1. Heat olive oil and sauté onion, celery, zucchini and carrots over medium heat.
2. Stir in garlic, green beans, and tomato paste. Then add broth, red wine, hot water, tomatoes, green beans, oregano, basil, onion powder, garlic powder, thyme, and bay leaf.
3. Bring soup to a boil and cover. Let it simmer for 45 minutes. Remove bay leaf.
4. Mix in spinach and pasta. Cook for 30 minutes. Serve.

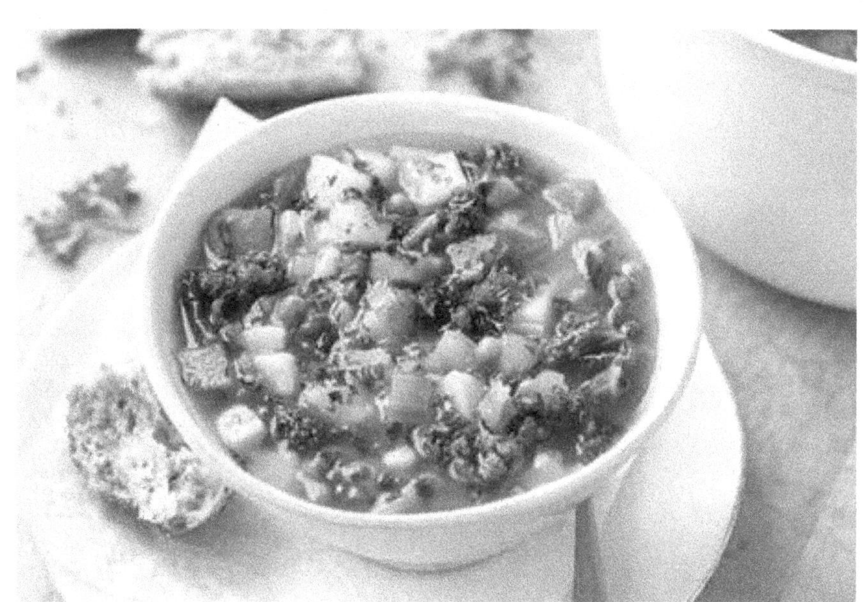

Nutrition

Calories: 199 Fat: 14g Carbs: 20g Protein: 31g

Preparation Time: 20' *Cooking Time: 45'* *Serves: 10*

137. Panera's Squash Soup

Ingredients

- ***2 pounds butternut squash; peeled & cut into 1" cubes***
- ***½ teaspoon cinnamon***
- ***1 cup white onion, chopped***
- ***15 ounces pumpkin***
- ***2 cups vegetable stock***
- ***1 tablespoon honey***
- ***2 teaspoons curry powder or to taste***
- ***1 cup apple juice***
- ***2 tablespoon vegetable oil, divided***
- ***1 tablespoon pumpkin seeds***
- ***½ cup heavy cream***

Directions

1. Preheat your oven to 350°F. Drizzle 1 tablespoon of vegetable oil on top of the butternut squash; stir until coated well.
2. Bake the butternut squash until the squash is fork-tender, for 30 minutes. Do not let the squash brown.
3. Heat 1 tablespoon the vegetable oil over moderate heat in a large stock-pot & sauté the onions for a couple of minutes, until translucent. As you sauté the onions; sprinkle a small amount of salt on top of them. When done; immediately add in the butternut squash, pumpkin, curry powder, vegetable stock, apple juice, cinnamon, & honey. Heat through.
4. Make the soup smooth using an immersion blender. Add cream to the soup; give everything a good stir.
5. Toast the pumpkin seeds over moderate heat in a small skillet. Heat through until fragrant, for a few minutes.
6. Immediately remove from heat. Serve and enjoy.

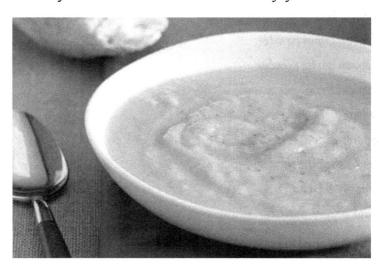

Nutrition

Calories: 110 Fat: 2.5g Carbs: 22g Protein 2g

Preparation Time: 5' *Cooking Time: 4 h 15'* *Serves: 8*

138. Chicken Soup with Egg Noodles

Ingredients

- ***2 boneless, skinless chicken breasts***
- ***1 cup egg noodles***
- ***2 cups water or as required onion, small, diced***
- ***2 cans chicken broth***
- ***1 teaspoon thyme***
- ***2 cups celery, diced***
- ***1 bay leaf***
- ***2 cups carrots, diced***
- ***1 teaspoon minced garlic or garlic salt***
- ***Pepper and salt to taste***

Directions

1. Place the entire ingredients (except the egg noodles) in the bottom of your crock pot; give everything a good stir until evenly combined.
2. Cook for 3 to 4 hours on high-heat or 6 to 8 hours on low-heat.
3. Just 30 minutes before you serve this soup, remove the chicken pieces and shred.
4. Place them to the pot again. Turn on the high of your crock pot & add in the egg noodles; let cook for half an hour.
5. Serve immediately and enjoy.

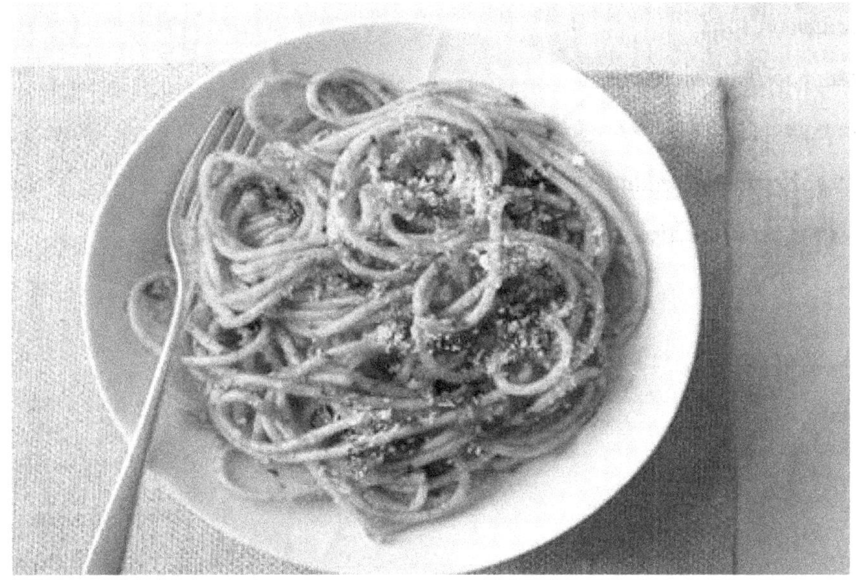

Nutrition

Calories: 124 Fat: 4.7g Carbs: 15g Protein: 23g

Preparation Time: 10' *Cooking Time: 30'* *Serves: 6*

139. Chili's Chicken Enchilada Soup

Ingredients

- *1 tablespoon olive oil*
- *1 onion, chopped*
- *3 cloves garlic, minced*
- *5 cups chicken broth*
- *1 cup masaharina*
- *2 cups water*
- *1 cup enchilada sauce*
- *1 pound Velveeta®, cubed*
- *2 cups shredded chicken*
- *1 teaspoon chili powder*
- *½ teaspoon ground cumin*
- *½ teaspoon salt*
- *½ teaspoon black pepper*
- *½ cup shredded Monterey Jack*
- *½ cup shredded cheddar*
- *Crushed tortilla chips, for topping*

Directions

1. Pour the oil in a pot and then add the onion and cook until it is softened. Add the garlic.
2. Mix the chicken broth and let it boil.
3. In a separate bowl, combine the masaharina with the water and mix until smooth. Whisk the mixture into the broth.
4. Stir in the enchilada sauce and Velveeta. Stir occasionally until the soup thickens and the cheese is melted.
5. Add the chicken, chili powder, cumin, salt, and pepper. Cook to heat through.
6. Serve garnished with a blend of the cheeses and a generous topping of tortilla chips.

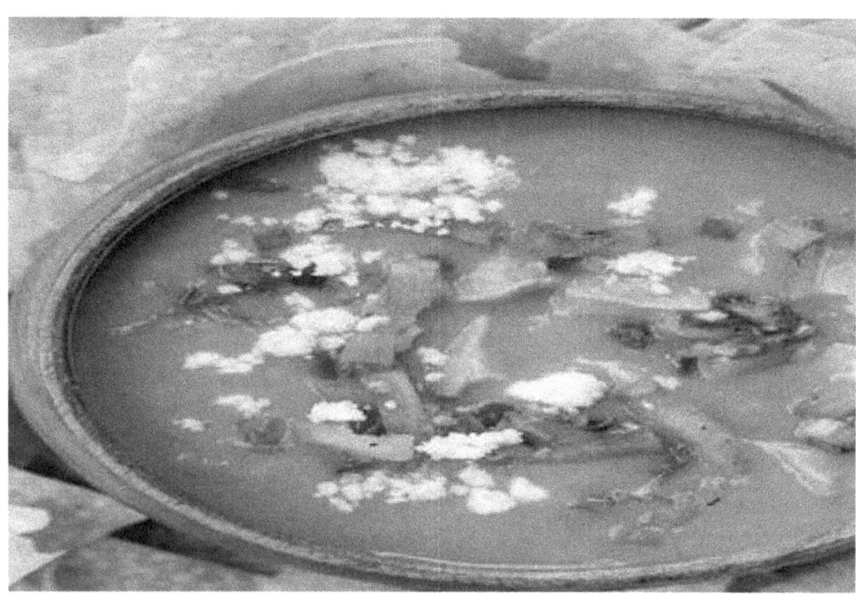

Nutrition

Calories: 410 Carbs: 24g Fat: 26g Protein: 20g

Preparation Time: 10' *Cooking Time: 25'* *Serves: 4*

140. Pappasito's Cantina Tortilla Soup

Ingredients

- *1 large white onion, diced*
- *3 medium carrots, sliced*
- *1 tablespoon jalapeño pepper, minced*
- *1 cup yellow squash, sliced*
- *1 tablespoon salt*
- *1 cup Roma tomatoes, diced*
- *2 quarts chicken broth*
- *1 cup zucchini, sliced*
- *To garnish:*
- *4 cups crispy corn tortilla chips*
- *1 ½ cups shredded Monterey Jack cheese*
- *2 cups corn kernels*

Directions

1. Mix the chicken stock, onion and carrots and let it simmer and cook for 10 minutes.
2. Add the jalapeño, zucchini, squash, and salt. Simmer until all the vegetables are tender.
3. Add the tomatoes and cook to heat through.
4. Serve garnished with tortilla chips, corn and shredded cheese.

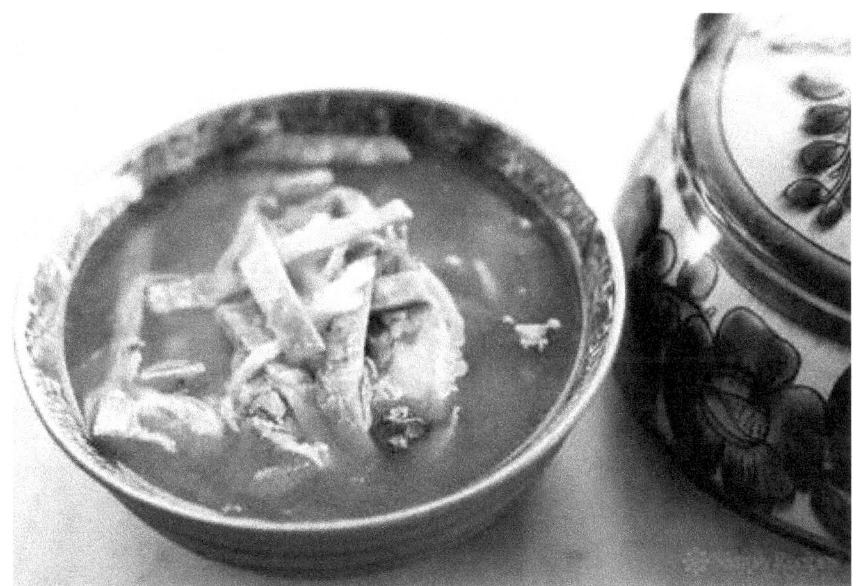

Nutrition

Calories: 300 Carbs: 0g Fat: 10g Protein: 0g

Chapter 10
Snacks and Desserts

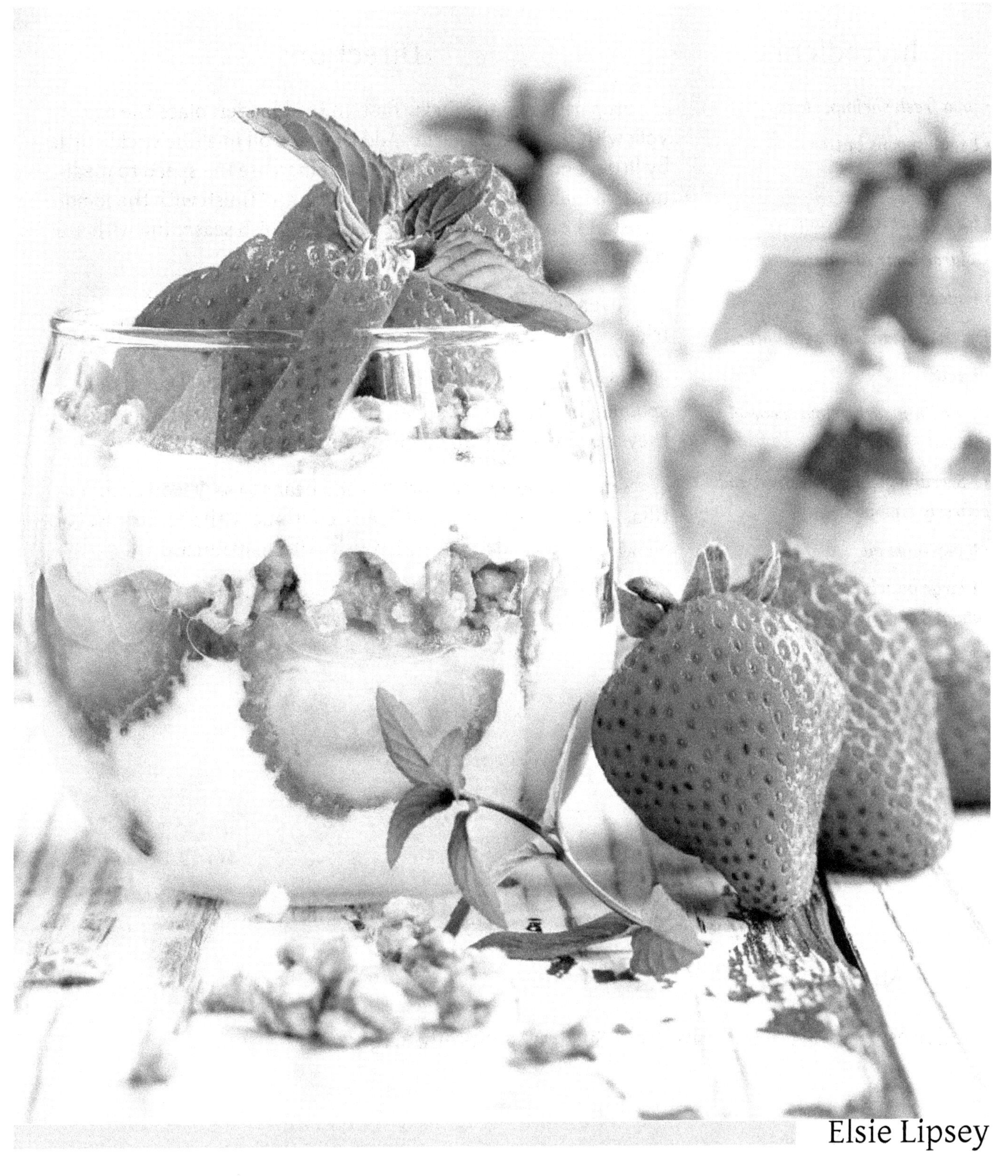

Preparation Time: 10' *Cooking Time: 15'* *Serves: 6*

141. Chili's Spicy Shrimp Tacos

Ingredients

- ***500g fresh shrimp, clean***
- ***1 tablespoons butter***
- ***Sea salt to taste***
- ***1 ½ cups refried beans***
- ***6 large flour tortillas***
- ***1 sliced avocado***

For the coriander mayonnaise:

- ***1 yolk***
- ***1 medium garlic clove, coarsely minced***
- ***1 Serrano pepper, deveined and coarsely chopped***
- ***¾ cup olive oil***
- ***1 large bunch coriander leaves (about 1 ½ cups leaves)***
- ***2 to 3 tablespoons of lemon juice***

Directions

1. Prepare the mayonnaise first. In the blender, place the egg yolk with the minced garlic. Add the olive oil in a fine trickle little by little. Add the serrano pepper and increase the speed to medium. Gradually add the coriander leaves and finish with the lemon juice (add 2 or 3 tablespoon as needed). Finish seasoning with sea salt to taste.

2. Cover with plastic wrap. If prepared in advance, keep in the fridge.

3. Heat a large, low skillet over medium-high heat. Add a tablespoon of butter and sauté half the shrimp with a little salt until they are pink and firm. Remove from heat immediately.

4. Simultaneously heat tortillas and beans to serve: on each tortilla, add two tablespoons of beans, continue with the shrimp, two slices avocado and finish generously with mayonnaise.

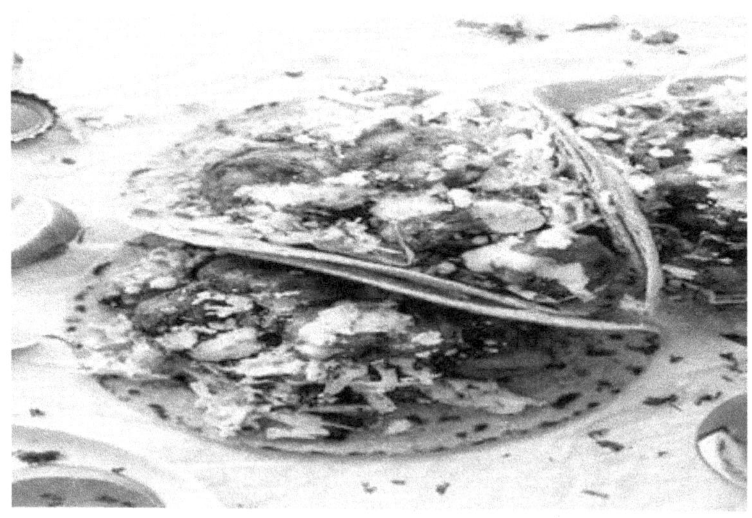

Nutrition

Calories: 242.8 Fat: 6.6g Carbs: 38.4g Sugars: 3g Protein: 8.4g

Preparation Time: 15' *Cooking Time: 40'* *Serves: 4*

142. Mesa Grill's Honey Glazed Salmon

Ingredients

- *4 pieces salmon steaks*
- *3 tablespoons olive oil*
- *5 tablespoon lemon juice*
- *2 tablespoon balsamic vinegar*
- *3 pieces carlic cloves*
- *1 tablespoon ginger root*
- *2 bunch cilantro*
- *4 tablespoon honey*
- *2 tablespoon mustard*

Directions

1. Mix 2 tablespoons of olive oil, lemon juice, balsamic vinegar, chopped garlic, ginger, and cilantro (set aside 3 tablespoons of greens). Marinate the fish in the resulting mixture for 1–2 hours.

2. For the glaze, mix honey, mustard, leftover olive oil, and cilantro. Preheat the oven in grill mode.

3. Cook the fish in the oven for 8-9 minutes, periodically pouring marinade. A few minutes before the end of cooking, grease the fish on both sides with icing. It should turn into a crust, but not burn.

4. On the side, grilled vegetables and a glass of chilled white wine are perfect. Serve and enjoy!

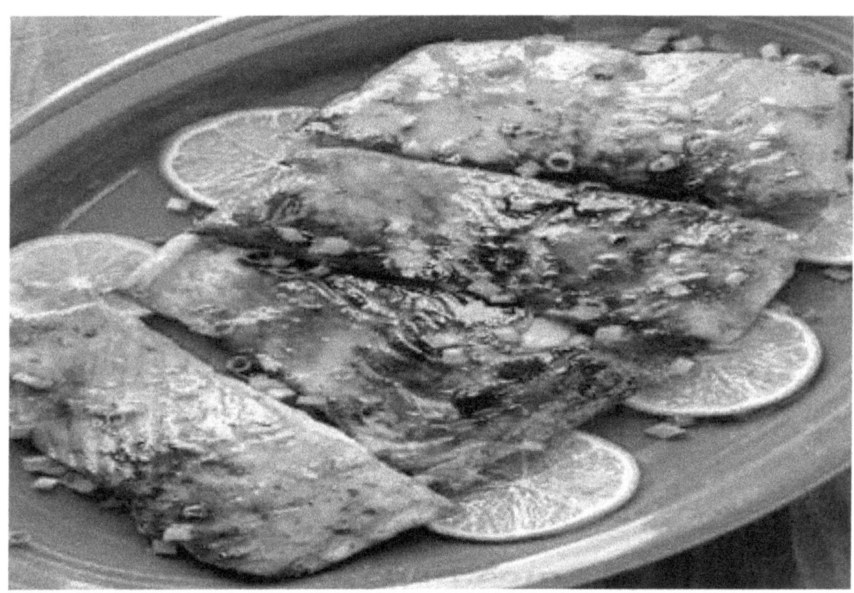

Nutrition

Calories: 150 Fat: 4.2g Carbs: 40g Sugars: 1g Protein: 9g

Preparation Time: 10' *Cooking Time: 20'* *Serves: 5*

143. El Ranchoro's Grande Baja Fish Tacos

Ingredients

- *½ cup (125 ml) mayonnaise*
- *2 c. (30 ml) water*
- *1 Restaurant Baja Fish Soft Taco Set*
- *400g white fish fillets, thawed if frozen (about ¾ to 1 lb.)*
- *Suggested garnishes: finely grated cabbage, fresh coriander, a touch of lemon or lime juice*

Directions

1. Mix the contents of the seasoning bag for Baja sauce (all) with mayonnaise and water until well blended; Reserve.

2. Pour the contents of the fish seasoning packet (from the set) into a shallow dish or bowl. If the fish is dry, wet it lightly with a damp paper towel. Place the fish fillets on the seasoning, then turn them so that they are very lightly coated on both sides.

3. Light the barbecue with gas or charcoal. Before cooking the fish, while the grill is clean, grill the soft flour tortillas (from the set) directly on the grill for 15 to 20 seconds on each side (or until they are lightly browned and toasted); wrap the tortillas in aluminum foil to keep them warm until ready to assemble.

4. Brush the grill with vegetable oil or use a grill basket for the fish (generously coat the basket with cooking spray or brush with oil). Grill the fish over medium-high heat for 3 to 4 minutes on each side (note: thicker fish fillets may require more cooking time). Remove it from the griller and let it sit for 4 to 5 minutes.

5. Divide the fish into 10 portions and divide over the hot and toasted tortillas. Add grated cabbage, Baja sauce, and cilantro and squeeze a little lemon or lime juice over it.

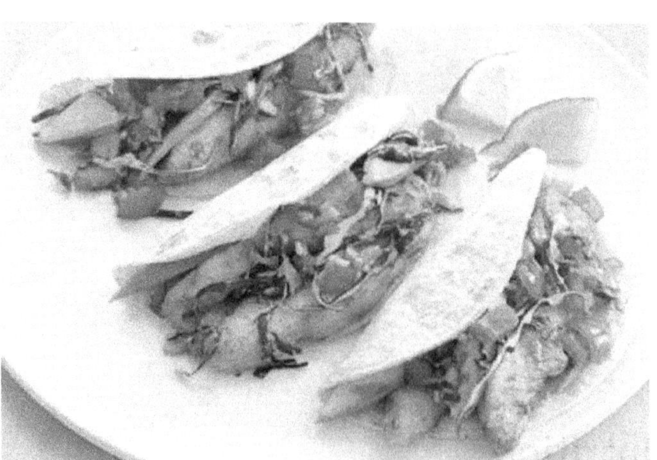

Nutrition

Calories: 100 Fat: 3g Carbs: 21g Sugars: 10g Protein: 5g

Preparation Time: 35' *Cooking Time: 8'* *Serves: 12*

144. Chipotle's Carnitas Tacos

Ingredients

- *½ cup salsa*
- *3 bay leaves*
- *1 tablespoon salt*
- *2 teaspoonful ground cumin*
- *2 teaspoonful dried oregano*
- *2 teaspoonful pepper*
- *1½ teaspoonful garlic powder*
- *4 whole cloves*
- *1¼ cups water*
- *2 medium onions, sliced*
- *1 bone-in pork shoulder roast*
- *24 corn tortillas*
- *Optional toppings: Cheese, sour cream and chopped tomato, celery, and onion*

Directions

1. Mix the first 9 ingredients. Place onions in a 6-qt. Oval toaster. Put roast onions; pour salsa mixture over roast. Cook, covered, on low till pork is tender, 8-10 hours.
2. Remove roast; remove and discard bone. Shred pork with two forks. Serve in tortillas with toppings as desired.
3. Freeze alternative: Freeze chilled pork mix in freezer. To use, partly thaw in fridge overnight. Microwave, covered, on high at a microwave-safe dish until warmed through, stirring occasionally; include broth or water if needed.

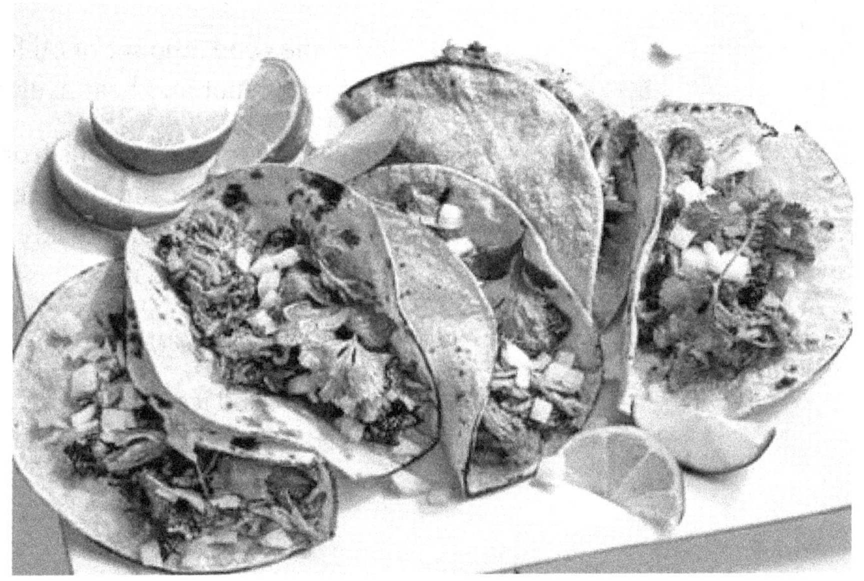

Nutrition

Calories: 178 Total Fat: 15g Carbs: 50g Sugars: 8g Protein: 9g

Preparation Time: 55' *Cooking Time: 5'* *Serves: 1*

145. Chi Chi's Fried Ice Cream

Ingredients

- *Ice cream*
- *2 slices crust less white bread for each scoop of ice cream*
- *1 ½ cups cow's milk*
- *1 and a half cups flour*
- *1 egg*
- *Oil for frying*
- *Chocolate, honey or cream syrup (optional)*

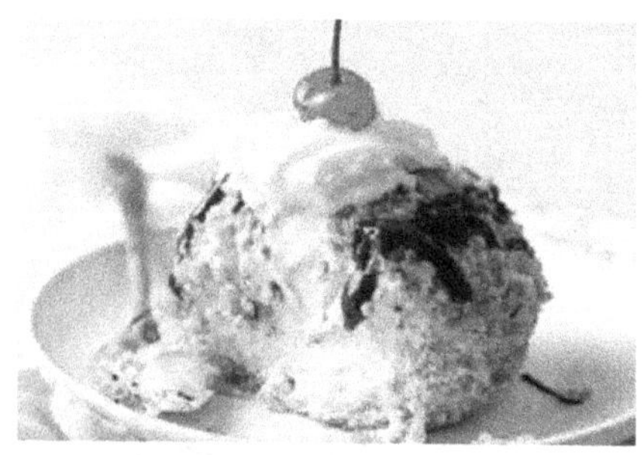

Directions

1. Choose the ice cream flavor that you like the most.

2. Serve half cup the milk of your choice in a container. Then grab a scoop of ice cream and place a slice of bread on top and another on the bottom, like you want to make an ice cream sandwich.

3. Very delicately wrap the ice cream ball in the bread. Then you must seal the union between the two slices bread with a little milk.

4. Once the scoop of ice cream is done, wrap it in aluminum foil and put it in the freezer for 24 hours. You will have to repeat the previous procedure with how many scoops of ice cream you want to fry, the normal thing is to consume one per person.

5. Once the freezing time has passed, you will need to prepare the mixture to coat the fried ice cream. In a bowl, combine the cup sifted flour, the cup milk, and the egg. Whisk until smooth.

6. Add some good amount of oil for frying to a non-stick frying pan or to a high pot and heat over high heat.

7. Remove the ice cream balls from the freezer. Coat in the flour, milk, and egg mixture and fry when the oil is very hot. When it has obtained brown color, quickly remove it from the heat. Then place on an absorbent paper.

8. Repeat the procedure you have done for all the balls.

9. Serve the fried ice cream with a little chocolate syrup, honey, or whipped cream.

Nutrition

Calories: 150 Fat: 20g Carbs: 50g Sugars: 9g Protein: 15g

Preparation Time: 15' *Cooking Time: 30'* *Serves: 8*

146. Frontera Grill's Chocolate Pecan Pie

Ingredients

Pastry:

- ***¾ cup unbleached all-purpose flour***
- ***40g (3 tablespoon) sugar***
- ***1 pinch salt***
- ***75g (1/3 cup) cold unsalted butter, diced***
- ***15ml (1 tablespoon) ice water***
- ***15ml (1 tablespoon) White vinegar***

Garnish:

- ***¼ cup (55g) unsalted butter***
- ***180ml (¾ cup) corn syrup***
- ***¾ cup (160g) lightly packed brown sugar***
- ***170g (6 ounces) dark chocolate, chopped***
- ***4 eggs, beaten***
- ***1 ½ cups (150g) pecans, lightly toasted***

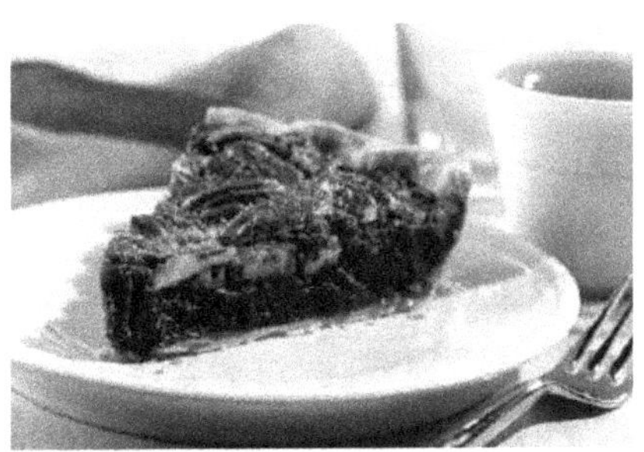

Directions

Pastry:

1. In a blender, mix the flour, sugar, and salt. Add the butter and mix, a few seconds at a time, until the mixture has a grainy texture. Add ice water and vinegar. Mix again, adding a little water if necessary, until the dough begins to form a ball. Remove the dough and form a disc.
2. On a plain surface, roll out the dough and darken a pie plate 23 cm (9-inch) in diameter. Refrigerate 30 minutes.
3. Put the grill in the oven. Preheat the oven to 190° C.

Garnish:

1. Melt the butter. In a saucepan over medium heat,
2. Add the corn syrup and brown sugar. Reheat, then remove from heat. Stir in chocolate and mix until melted. Add the eggs, whisking. Divide the filling into the cold dough. Place the pecans on the garnish.
3. Bake until the filling is firm. Let cool completely on a wire rack.
4. Serve or freeze at this stage.

Nutrition

Calories: 160 Total Fat: 10g Carbs: 50g Sugars: 6g Protein: 12g

Preparation Time: 10' *Cooking Time: 50'* *Serves: 6-8*

147. Z'tejas' Spicy Blackberry Fruit Cobbler

Ingredients

- ***1 ¼ cup divided granulated sugar***
- ***1 cup all-purpose flour***
- ***1 ½ teaspoons of baking powder***
- ***½ teaspoon of salt***
- ***1 cup whole milk***
- ***½ cup unsalted butter, melted***
- ***3 cups fresh blackberries***

Directions

1. Place the oven stand in the middle position and preheat the oven to 350 degrees. Grease a 9-inch round baking dish with a non-stick spray.
2. Combine 1 cup sugar, flour, yeast, and salt. Add milk and mix until smooth.
3. Add melted butter and mix until smooth.
4. Put the dough into a greased baking dish. Lay the berries on top. Sprinkle ¼ cup sugar on top evenly.
5. Bake until the edges are golden and crispy, 50–60 minutes.
6. Serve hot with whipped cream or ice cream, if necessary.

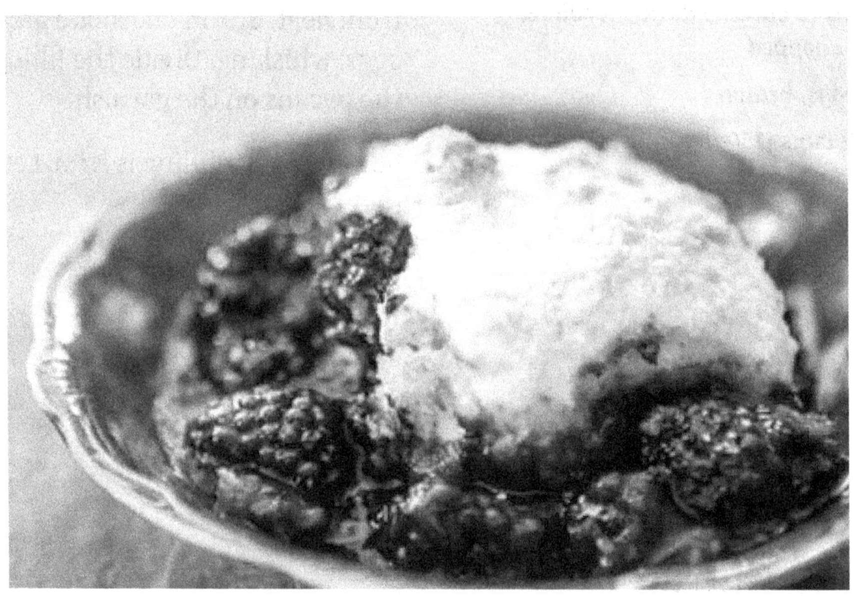

Nutrition

Calories: 140 Fat: 8g Carbs:30 Sugars: 10g Protein: 25g

Preparation Time: 5' *Cooking Time: 0'* *Serves: 5*

148. Abuelo's Sangria Roja

Ingredients

- ***1-liter sangria wine***
- ***¾ cup white Zinfandel***
- ***¼ cup Peach Schnapps***
- ***½ cup Triple Sec***
- ***1 cup Sprite***
- ***1 ½ cups orange soda***
- ***¼ cup brandy***
- ***½ cup raspberry puree***
- ***1-ounce rum***

Directions

1. Combine all ingredients well and serve over fruits of choice: oranges, lemon, lime, peaches, etc.

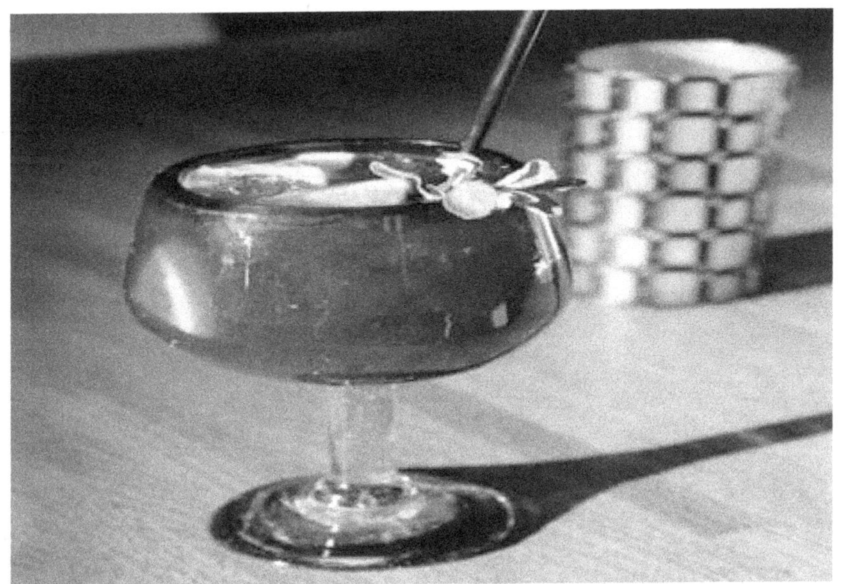

Nutrition

Calories 11 Fat 14g Carbs 78g Sugars 9g Protein 8g

Preparation Time: 15' Cooking Time: 2' Serves: 10 Chilling: 6h

149. Reese's Peanut Butter Cups

Ingredients

- ***Salt, pinch***
- ***1½ cups peanut butter***
- ***1 cup confectioners' sugar***
- ***20 ounces milk chocolate chips***

Directions

1. Take a medium bowl and mix the salt, peanut butter, and sugar until firm.
2. Place the chocolate chips in a microwave-safe bowl and microwave for 2 minutes to melt.
3. Grease the muffin tin with oil spray and spoon some of the melted chocolate into each muffin cup.
4. Take a spoon and draw the chocolate up to the edges of the muffin cups until all sides are coated.
5. Cool in the refrigerator for few hours.
6. Once chocolate is solid, spread about 1 teaspoon of peanut butter onto each cup.
7. Leave space to fill the edges of the cups.
8. Create the final layer by pouring melted chocolate on top of each muffin cup.
9. Let sit at room temperature until cool.
10. Refrigerate for a few hours until firm.
11. Remove the cups and serve.

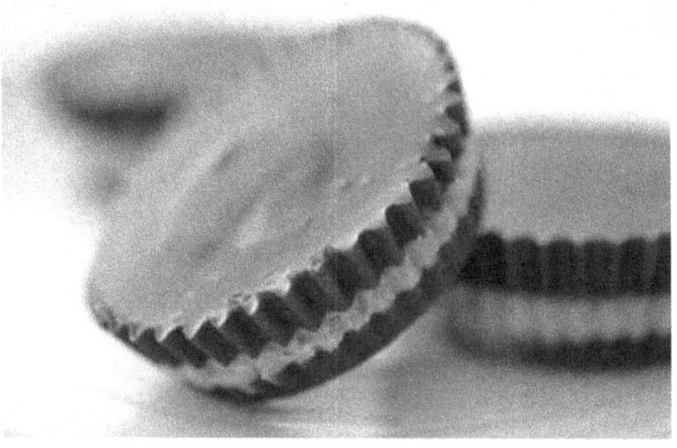

Nutrition

Calories: 455 Total Fat: 21.7g Carbs: 59 g Protein: 9.7g Sodium: 384mg

Preparation Time: 15' Cooking Time: 2' Serves: 6 Chilling: 3h 30'

150. Cadbury's Cream Egg

Ingredients

- ***1/3 cup light corn syrup***
- ***1/3 cup butter***
- ***2 teaspoons vanilla***
- ***1/3 teaspoon salt***
- ***3½ cups white sugar, ground and sifted***
- ***3 drops yellow food coloring***
- ***2 drops red food coloring***
- ***16 ounces chocolate chips, milk***
- ***3 teaspoons vegetable shortening***

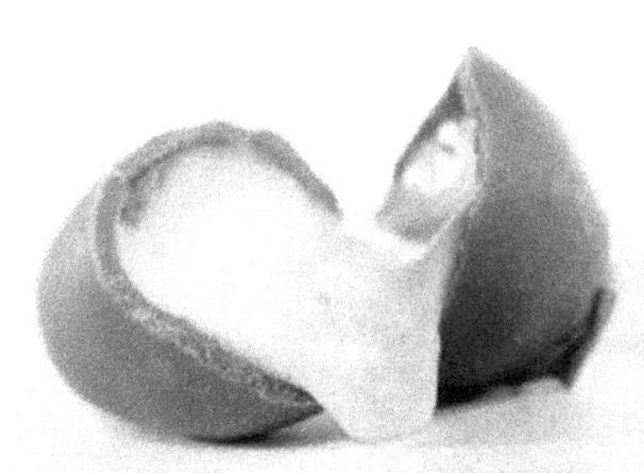

Directions

1. Take a bowl and combine corn syrup, butter, vanilla, salt and powdered sugar.
2. Mix all the ingredients well with a beater.
3. Reserve □ of the mixture in a separate bowl, then add food coloring.
4. Chill both portions in the refrigerator for 2 hours.
5. Form rolls from the orange filling, about ¾-inch in diameter.
6. Wrap the orange rolls with white filling.
7. Repeat until all of the mixture is consumed.
8. Form in the shape of eggs.
9. Let sit in the refrigerator for 1 hour.
10. Melt the chocolate chips in the microwave.
11. Dip each egg roll in the melted chocolate.
12. Cool in the refrigerator for 30 minutes.
13. Once solid, serve and enjoy.

Nutrition

Calories: 104 Total Fat 34.8g Carbs: 174g Protein: 5.9g Sodium: 261mg

Preparation Time: 10' *Cooking Time: 10'* *Serves: 4*

151. Texas Roadhouse's Deep Fried Pickles

Ingredients

- ***Vegetable oil***
- ***¼ cup flour***
- ***1¼ teaspoons Cajun seasoning***
- ***¼ teaspoon oregano***
- ***¼ teaspoon basil***
- ***1/8 teaspoon pepper***
- ***Salt***
- ***2 cups dill pickles***
- ***¼ cup mayonnaise***
- ***1 tablespoon horseradish***
- ***1 tablespoon ketchup***

Directions

1. Preheat oil in a large pot at 375°F.
2. Create the coating by mixing the 1 teaspoon Cajun seasoning, flour, basil, oregano, pepper, and salt.
3. Dip the pickle slices in flour mixture, then carefully lower into hot oil. Work in batches and deep fry for about 2 minutes or until lightly brown.
4. Using a slotted spoon, transfer pickles to a plate lined with paper towels to drain.
5. While pickles drain and cool, add mayonnaise, horseradish, ketchup, and remaining Cajun seasoning in a bowl. Mix well.
6. Serve immediately with dip on the side.

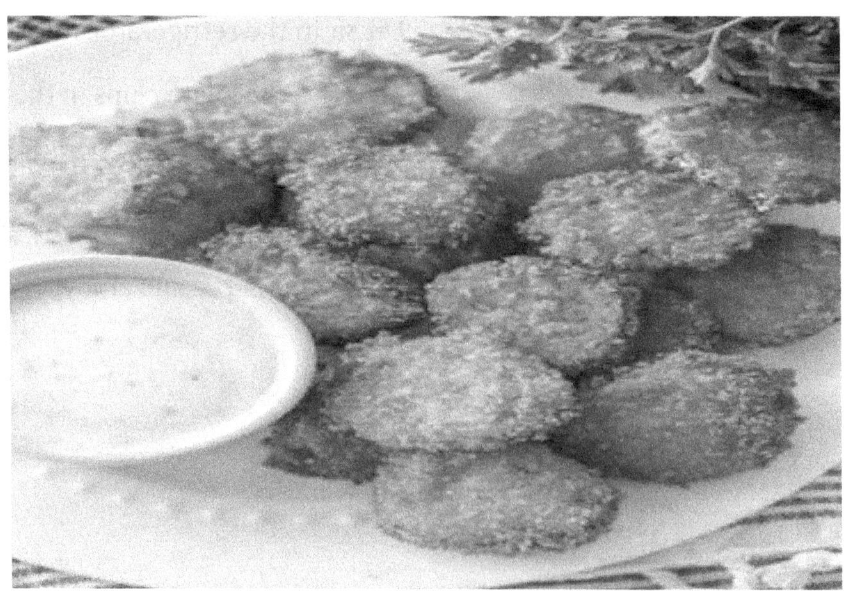

Nutrition

Calories: 296 Total Fat 28g Saturated Fat: 14g Carbs: 12g Sugar: 4g Fibers: 0g Protein: 1g

Preparation Time: 20' *Cooking Time: 30'* *Serves: 8*

152. Starbucks'Cinnamon Rolls

Ingredients

Batter:

- *2 packs dry yeast*
- *Half cup warm water*
- *1/3 cup sugar*
- *½ teaspoon sugar*
- *4-5 cups all-purpose flour,*
- *1 teaspoon salt*
- *1 cup milk, singed and cooled to 110 degrees*
- *1-3 cup vegetable oil*
- *2 eggs,*
- *½ cup butter or margarine, Full*
- *1 cup colored sugar*
- *2 tablespoons cinnamon Icing:*
- *1 cup confectioners' sugar*
- *2-3 tablespoons warm milk*
- *1 teaspoon vanilla*

Directions

1. For the batter, break down yeast in water with ½ teaspoon sugar. Let stand for 5 minutes. In blending bowl, join 3 cups flour, □ cup sugar, and salt. At low speed, progressively beat in milk, oil, eggs, and yeast blend; beat until all-around mixed. Beat in extra flour until batter pulls from sides of the bowl.

2. On a floured surface, massage batter until smooth and versatile, 8-10 minutes. A spot in a lubed bowl, going to oil top. Spread and let ascend in the warm, draft-free territory until multiplied in mass, around 60 minutes.

3. For the filling, beat all fixings together until smooth.

4. Put in a safe spot. Oil 2 (9-inch) round cake skillet. On a daintily floured surface, fold batter into an 18 X 10-inch square shape. Spread with filling. Roll firmly from the long side. Cut into 14 (¼-inch) cuts. Spot 1 move cut side up in the focus of each dish. Orchestrate

5. Spread and let ascend until multiplied in mass, 30 to 40 minutes. Preheat stove to 350ºC. Prepare 25 to 30 minutes, until brilliant earthy colored. Cool in skillet 10 minutes.

6. For the icing, whisk all fixings until smooth.

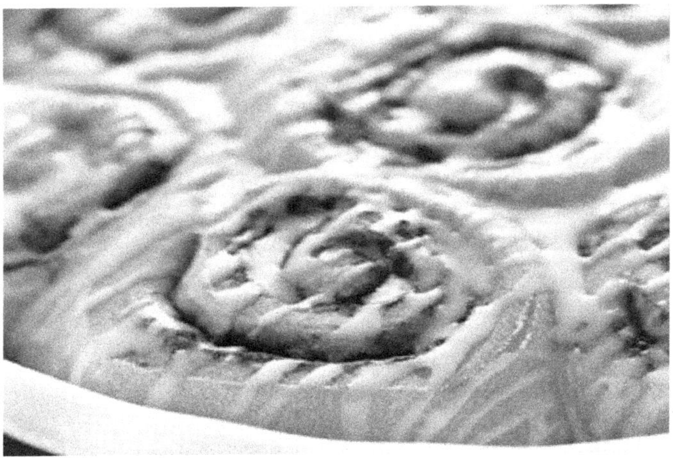

Nutrition

Calories: 160 Fat: 10g Carbs: 50g Sugars: 6g Protein: 12g

Preparation Time: 15' *Cooking Time: 40'* *Serves: 5*

153. York's Peppermint Patties

Ingredients

- ***14 ounces Condensed Milk***
- ***1 tablespoon peppermint extricate green or red food shading, discretionary***
- ***6 cups confectioners' sugar***
- ***1-16 ounces sack semi-sweet chocolate chips***

Directions

1. In a huge blender bowl, consolidate Eagle Brand, concentrate, and food shading whenever wanted. Include 6 cups sugar; beat on low speed until smooth and very much mixed. Turn blend onto a surface sprinkled with confectioners' sugar.
2. Massage gently to frame smooth ball. Shape into 1-inch balls. Spot 2 inches separated on wax paper-lined preparing sheets. Level each ball into a ½ inch patty. Let dry 1 hour or more.
3. Liquefy the chocolate contributes a microwave set on high for 2 minutes. Mix part of the way through the warming time. Dissolve completely, however, don't overheat. Dissolving the chocolate chips should likewise be possible utilizing a double-boiler over low warmth. With a fork, plunges every patty into warm chocolate.

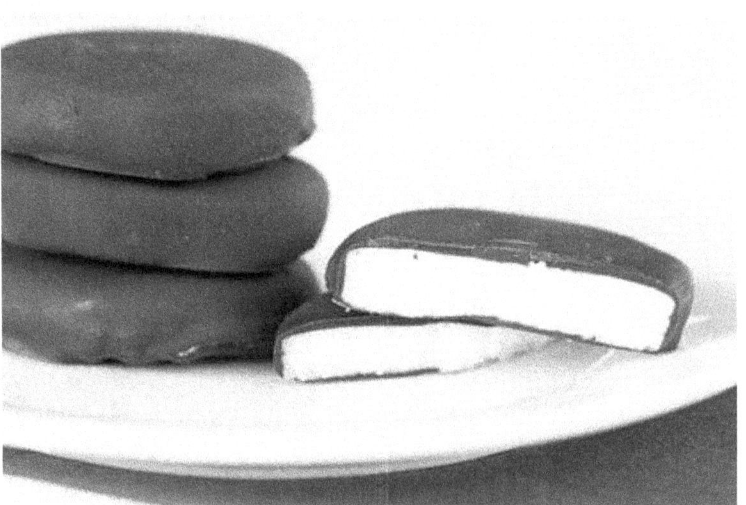

Nutrition

Calories: 140 Fat: 8g Carbs: 30 Sugars: 10g Protein: 25g

Preparation Time: 10' *Cooking Time: 15'* *Serves: 14*

154. Red Lobster's Cheddar Bay Biscuits

Ingredients

- ***1 tablespoon granulated sugar***
- ***2 cups all-purpose flour (2 cups)***
- ***1 teaspoons kosher salt***
- ***1 tablespoon baking powder***
- ***1 tablespoon garlic powder***
- ***8 tablespoon melted unsalted butter, divided***
- ***1 cup whole milk***
- ***8 ounces shredded Mild cheddar cheese***

Directions

1. Heat the oven at 400° Fahrenheit. Cover a baking tray using a sheet of parchment baking paper.
2. Sift the garlic powder, ½ teaspoon of salt, flour, baking powder, and sugar into a hefty-sized mixing container.
3. Melt one stick of butter with the milk and cheddar cheese - don't over mix.
4. Drop 14 biscuits onto the prepared baking sheet. Bake until the biscuits are browned (10–12 min.)
5. Mix the remaining butter, salt, and parsley to brush the tops of the biscuits before serving.

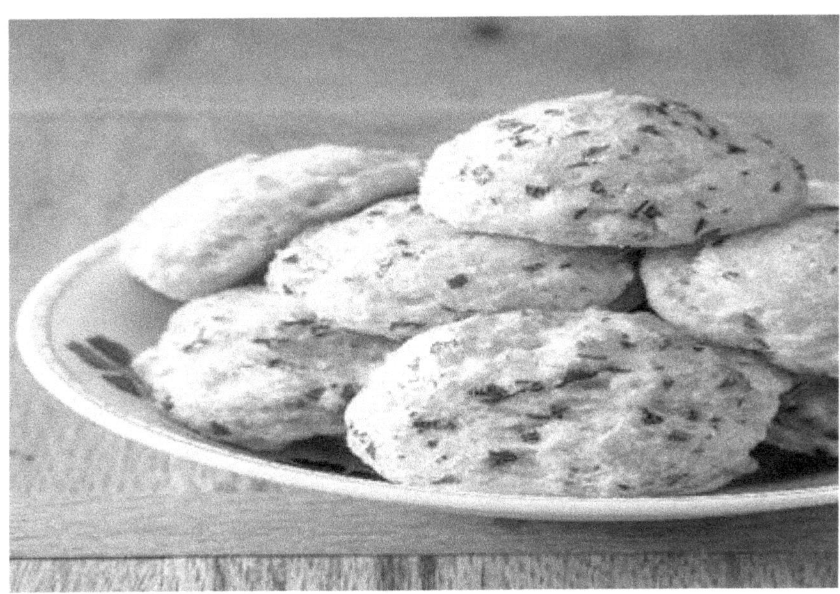

Nutrition

Calories: 140 Fat: 8g Carbs: 30 Sugars: 10g Protein: 25g

Preparation Time: 30' *Cooking Time: 5'* *Serves: 4*

155. Popeye's Pecan Caramel Candies

Ingredients

- ***54 pretzels***
- ***54 rolls of bullets (about 11 ounces)***
- ***54 walnut halves***

Directions

1. Preheat the oven to 250°. Divide the pretzels by 2.5
2. cm and place on a foil-lined baking sheet. Cover each with sweet rolls.
3. Bake for three to four minutes, or until the candle is soft. (The scroll bar still keeps its shape.) Immediately cover with nuts and squeeze out the candy on the crease. Leave until ready.

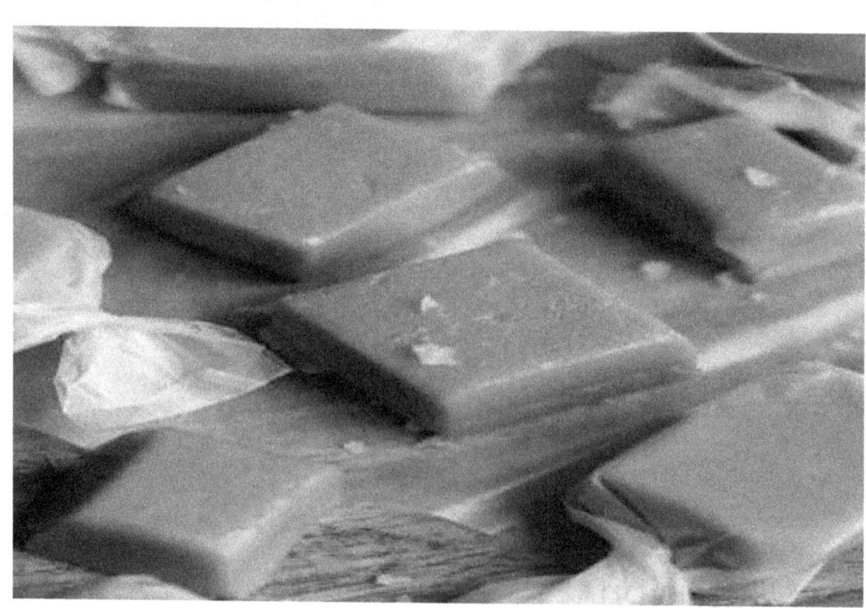

Nutrition

Calories: 150 Fat: 20g Carbs: 50g Sugars: 9g Protein: 15g

Preparation Time: 25' *Cooking Time: 5'* *Serves: 12t*

156. Popeye's Make-ahead Tiamisu

Ingredients

- *½ cup espresso*
- *2 tablespoons coffee liqueur*
- *16 grams of soft cheese, softened*
- *²/³ cup sugar*
- *2 cups sour cream*
- *¼ cup 2% milk*
- *½ teaspoon vanilla extract*
- *2 packs (3 grams each) of gingerbread, sliced into thin slices*
- *1 tablespoon cocoa powder*

Directions

1. Mix coffee and drinks in a small bowl; it was left out.
2. In a large bowl, beat cream cheese and sugar until smooth. Stir the cream, milk and vanilla together until they are combined.
3. Grab a layer of grease on an 11x7 inch piece of finger, in a skottel; brush with half of the coffee mixture. Pour on top half of the cream cheese mixture. Repeat each layer (full board).
4. Cover and refrigerate for 8 hours or overnight.
5. Sprinkle cocoa powder before eating.

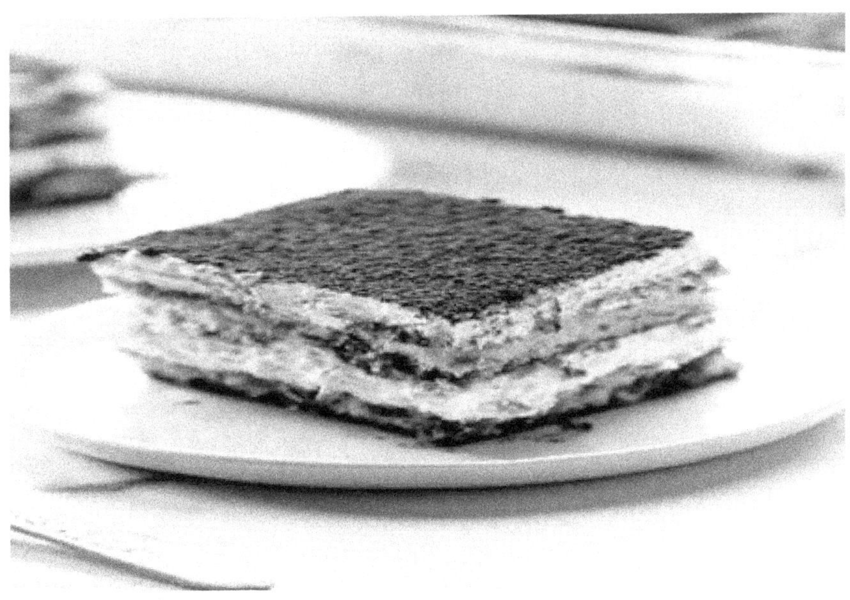

Nutrition

Calories: 160 Fat: 10g Carbs: 50g Sugars: 6g Protein: 12g

Preparation Time: 15’ *Cooking Time: 12’* *Serves: 36*

157. Popeye’s White Chocolate Cereal Bars

Ingredients

- ***4 cups mini jellyfish***
- ***White oven shards (about 1-1/3 cups)***
- ***¼ cup butter***
- ***6 cups crispy rice***

Directions

1. In a large bowl, whisk butter, butter and sugar until fluffy. Add 1 egg at a time, and mix well after each addition. Beat vanilla. Mix flour, baking soda and salt; gradually add to cream mixture and mix well.
2. Stir with the remaining ingredients.
3. Place 3 tablespoons of tablespoons on an unpainted baking sheet. Bake in a 350°C oven until light brown for 10-12 minutes. Refrigerate for 2-3 minutes, then move to a shelf to cool completely.

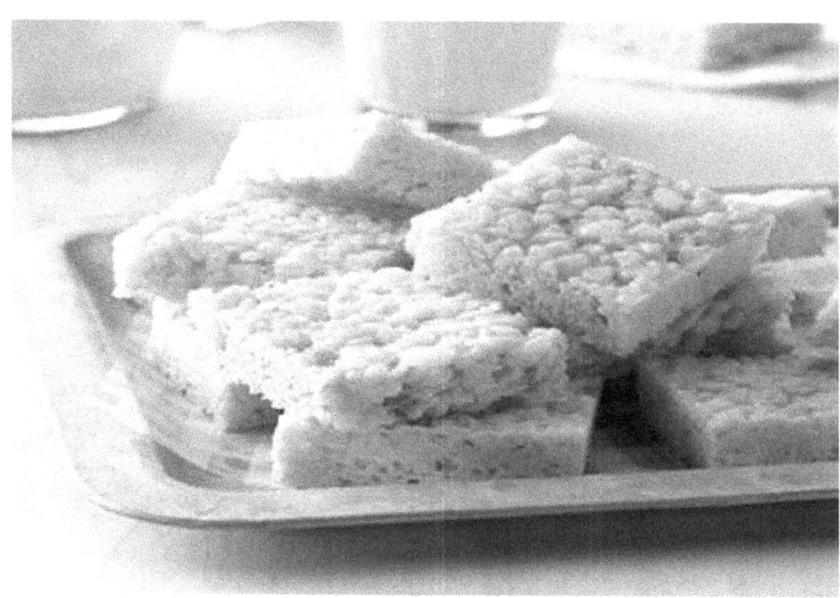

Nutrition

Calories: 140 Fat: 8g Carbs: 30 Sugars: 10g Protein: 25g

Preparation Time: 20' *Cooking Time: 10'* *Serves: 18t*

158. Popeye's Easy Oatmeal Cream Pies

Ingredients

- ***¾ cup butter, softened***
- ***2 large eggs at room temperature***
- ***1 packet of spice cake mix (normal size)***
- ***1 cup fast-cooked oatmeal***
- ***1 can (16 grams) vanilla icing***

Directions

1. Beat butter and eggs together until well mixed. Mix cake and oatmeal mixture. Although the dough is still quite soft, keep it refrigerated and cover for 2 hours or until it is firm enough to roll.
2. Preheat the oven to 350°. Roll half of the dough onto the full surface of the flour to ¼-inch thickness. Cut at 2-½ Flour. Round cookie cutter. Bake for 8 minutes until finished. Remove the shelf from the shelf and allow it to cool completely. Repeat the remaining dough.
3. Sprinkle icing sugar on half of the cookies; add other cookies.
4. Freezing option: freeze the sandwich biscuits installed in the freezing container, and separate the layers with wax paper. Defrost before serving.

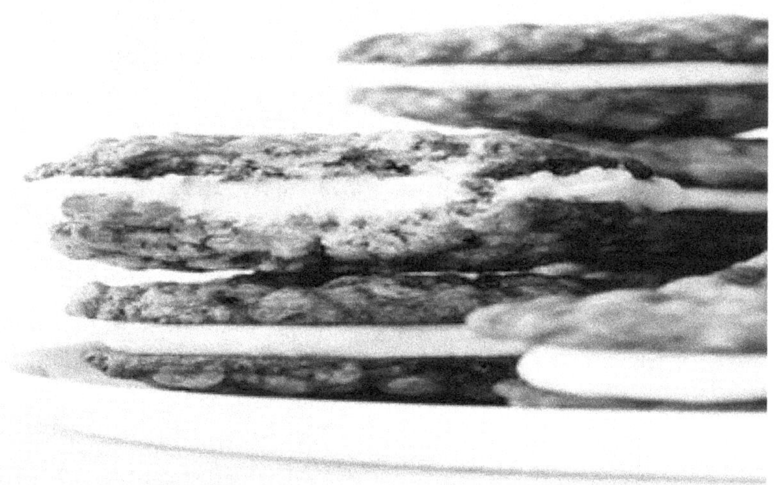

Nutrition

Calories: 178 Fat: 15g Carbs: 50g Sugars: 8g Protein: 9g

Preparation Time: 10' *Cooking Time: 20'* *Serves: 2*

159. Taco Bells's AM Crunchwrap

Ingredients

- ***Flour tortillas (2 large)***
- ***Whisked eggs (3-4) + Milk (1 tablespoon)***
- ***Shredded sharp cheddar cheese (2-4 tablespoon)***
- ***Shredded hash browns (heaping 5 cup)***
- ***Hot sauce - mild - your choice (4 tablespoon)***
- ***Bacon (4 crispy)***
- ***Cooking oil spray***
- ***Taco Bell sauce***

Directions

1. Lightly spritz a skillet using cooking oil spray and warm using the medium temperature setting.
2. Whisk and add the eggs, salt, and pepper into a skillet. Whisk until they are fluffy and set them aside.
3. Warm a skillet and heat the tortillas for about half of a minute. Prepare and close them, placing them in a skillet to cook for about 30 to 40 seconds using the medium temperature setting.
4. Serve with sauce as desired.

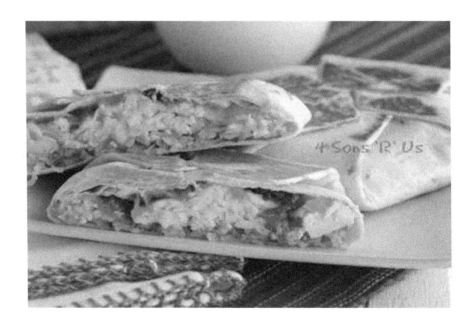

Nutrition

Calories: 255 Carbohydrates: 16g Protein: 15g Fat: 14g Sugars: 2g

Preparation Time: 15' *Cooking Time: 15'* *Serves: 24*

160. Taco Bells's Cinnabon Delights

Ingredients

- ***24 ounces Pillsbury™ refrigerated cinnamon rolls with icing***
- ***2 teaspoons Cinnamon***
- ***¾ cup Granulated sugar***
- ***¼ cup Butter***
- ***¼ cup warmed caramel ice cream topping***
- ***¼ cup Betty Crocker™ Rich & Creamy white frosting***

Directions

1. Heat the oven at 350° Fahrenheit. Prepare a baking tray using a layer of parchment baking paper. Open the rolls and slice each one into three pieces. Roll each one into a ball.
2. Melt the butter in the microwave. Whisk the sugar and cinnamon in another bowl.
3. Roll the dough balls through the butter, then the cinnamon and sugar. Arrange them on the baking tin. Bake them until nicely browned (10min.) and cool for another ten minutes.
4. Warm the frosting for about ten seconds in the microwave to soften it slightly for piping. Scoop the filling into the piping bag.
5. Squirt in the frosting into the ball until it puffs. Garnish them using the sauce and serve.

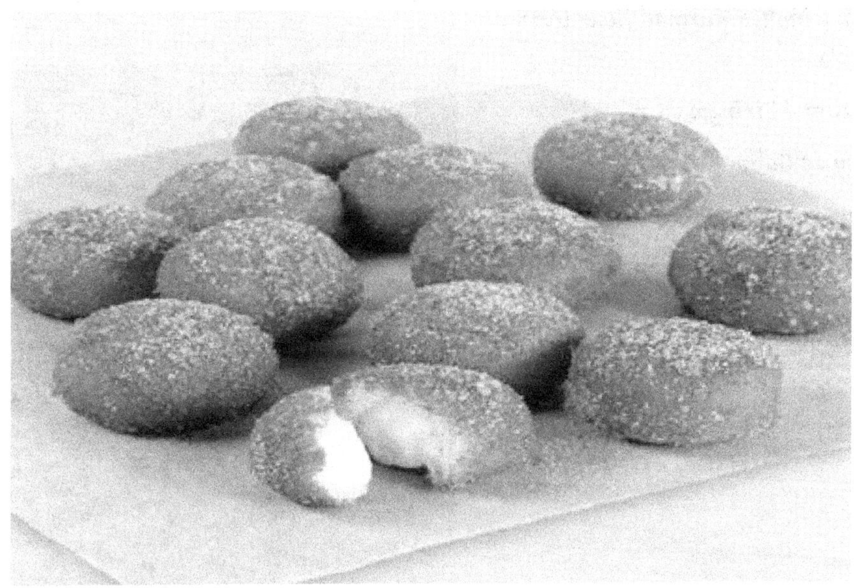

Nutrition

Calories: 62.1 Protein: 0.1 grams Fat Content: 2.3 grams Carbohydrates: 10.7 grams Sugars: 7.8 grams

Preparation Time: 10' *Cooking Time: 15'* *Serves: 8*

161. Taco Bells's Dressed Egg Taco

Ingredients

- *1/3 cup black beans*
- *1/3 cup Pico de Gallo*
- *1/3 cup cubed avocado*
- *1 tablespoon Lime juice*
- *1 cup frozen, thawed potatoes*
- *½ lb. bulk pork sausage*
- *6 large eggs*
- *2 tablespoon milk*
- *½ cup Monterey Jack shredded cheese*
- *8 @ 6 inches warmed flour tortillas*
- *Optional Fixings:*
- *Pico de Gallo*
- *Sour cream*
- *Freshly chopped cilantro*

Directions

1. Rinse and drain the beans.
2. Gently mix the avocado, beans, pico de gallo, and lime juice.
3. Cook the potatoes and crumbled sausage using the medium temperature setting until the sausage is no longer pink (6-8 min.)
4. Whisk the eggs and milk. Pour them into the skillet, stirring over medium heat until the eggs are thickened, and no liquid egg remains.
5. Stir in the cheese.
6. Put a spoonful of the egg mixture into each of the tortillas, and top with the bean mixture. Garnish them to your liking.

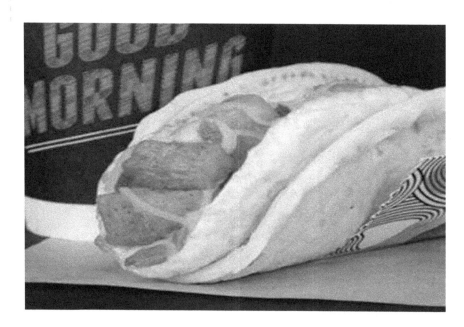

Nutrition

Calories: 291 Protein: 13g Fat: 16g Carbohydrates: 22g Sugars: 1g

Preparation Time: 10' *Cooking Time: 20'* *Serves: 12*

162. Taco Bells's Delicious Tacos

Ingredients

- *1 ½ tablespoon golden MasaHarina corn flour, ex. Bob's Red Mill*
- *1.33 lb. ground chuck*
- *4-5 teaspoons chili powder*
- *¼ teaspoons sugar*
- *¼ teaspoons ground cumin*
- *1 teaspoons dried minced onion*
- *5 teaspoons spices*
- *Onion powder*
- *Seasoning salt*
- *Garlic powder*
- *Paprika*
- *Garlic salt*
- *Beef bouillon powder*
- *To Serve:*
- *12 taco shells*
- *Shredded Iceberg lettuce*
- *2 Diced Roma tomatoes*
- *1 cup shredded cheddar cheese*
- *Optional: Sour cream*

Directions

1. Combine all of the 'beef filling' fixings except for the meat. Combine the spice mix - blending thoroughly.
2. Cook the beef until browned. Transfer it from the burner and dump the meat into a strainer to rinse with hot water.
3. Toss the beef into the pan and stir in the spice mix with water (75–1 cup). Simmer using the med-low temperature setting to cook away most of the liquids (20 min.)
4. Prepare the tacos. Pop the shells into a 350° Fahrenheit oven for 7–10 minutes.
5. Assemble them with the meat, lettuce, tomatoes, sour cream, and cheese to your liking.
6. Serve them promptly.

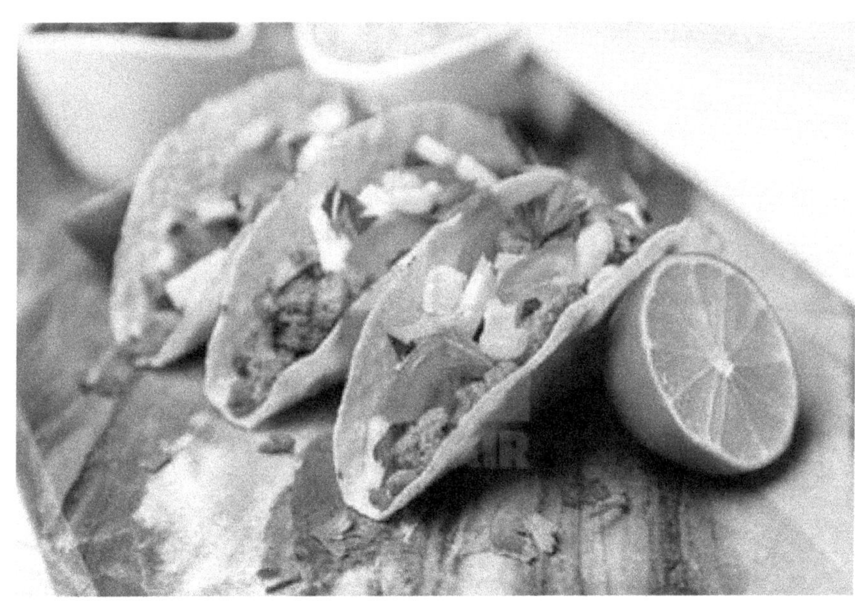

Nutrition

Calories: 236 Protein: 12g Fat: 15g Carbohydrates: 10g Sugars: 1g

Preparation Time: 15' *Cooking Time: 20'* *Serves: 6*

163. Taco Bells's Chalupa Supreme

Ingredients

- *6 inches Corn tortillas*
- *2 teaspoons olive oil*
- *1/3 cup Shredded part-skim mozzarella cheese*
- *2 cups Cooked chicken breast*
- *Diced tomatoes with green chiles*
- *1 teaspoons ground cumin*
- *1 teaspoons garlic powder*
- *¼ teaspoons black pepper and salt*
- *1 teaspoons Onion powder*
- *½ cup finely shredded cabbage*

Directions

1. Warm the oven in advance at 350°F. Arrange the tortillas on an ungreased baking sheet. Brush them using a bit of oil and a sprinkle of cheese.

2. Chop and toss the chicken, tomatoes, and seasonings in a large skillet. Simmer and stir using the medium temperature setting (6–8 min.) or until most of the liquid is evaporated.

3. Spoon the delicious mixture over the tortillas.

4. Bake it for 15–18 minutes until the tortillas are crisp and cheese is melted. Garnish with the cabbage.

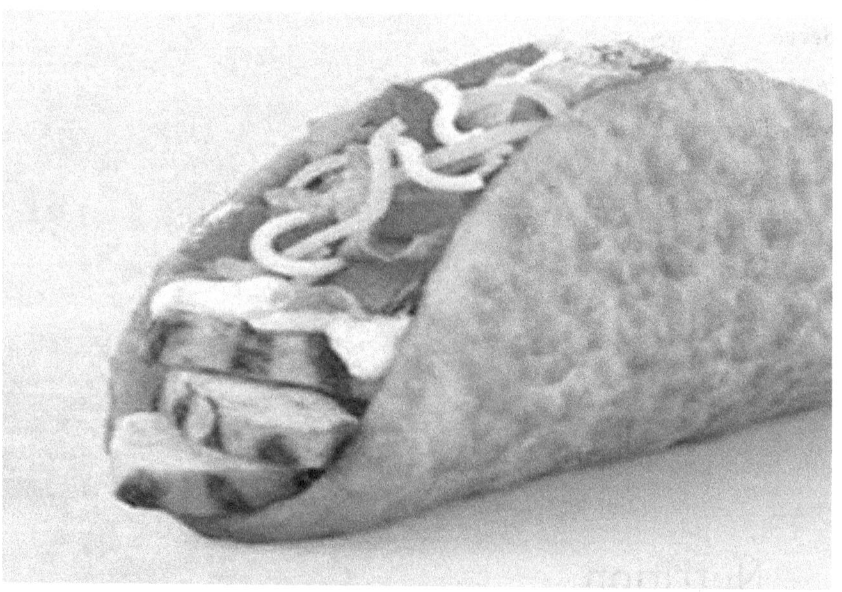

Nutrition

Calories: 206 Carbohydrates: 17g Protein: 19g Fat: 6g Sugars: 3g

Preparation Time: 10’ *Cooking Time: 20’* *Serves: 6*

164. Taco Bells’s Grilled Steak Soft Tacos

Ingredients

- ***The Salsa:***
- ***2 large tomatoes***
- ***½ cup red onion***
- ***¼ cup lime juice***
- ***1 Jalapeno pepper***
- ***3 tablespoon fresh cilantro***
- ***1/3 teaspoons salt, divided***
- ***2 teaspoons ground cumin, divided***
- ***1.5 lb. beef flank steak***
- ***1 tablespoon canola oil***
- ***6 @ 8 inches whole wheat tortillas***
- ***1 onion***
- ***Optional: lime wedges & sliced avocado***

Directions

1. Deseed and chop the tomatoes and jalapeno. Dice the onion and cilantro.
2. Combine the first five fixings (before the line). Stir in one teaspoon cumin and ¼ teaspoon salt. Set it to the side for now.
3. Sprinkle the steak using the rest of the salt and cumin.
4. Grill using the medium temperature setting (with a lid on) until the meat is as you like it (med-rare, on an instant-read thermometer, is about 135°F), or 6–8 minutes. Let the cooked meat stand for 5 minutes before slicing.
5. Warm the oil in a skillet using the med-high temperature setting and sauté them until the onion is crisp-tender.
6. Slice steak thinly across the grain and serve on tortillas with onion and salsa.
7. If desired, serve with avocado and lime wedges.

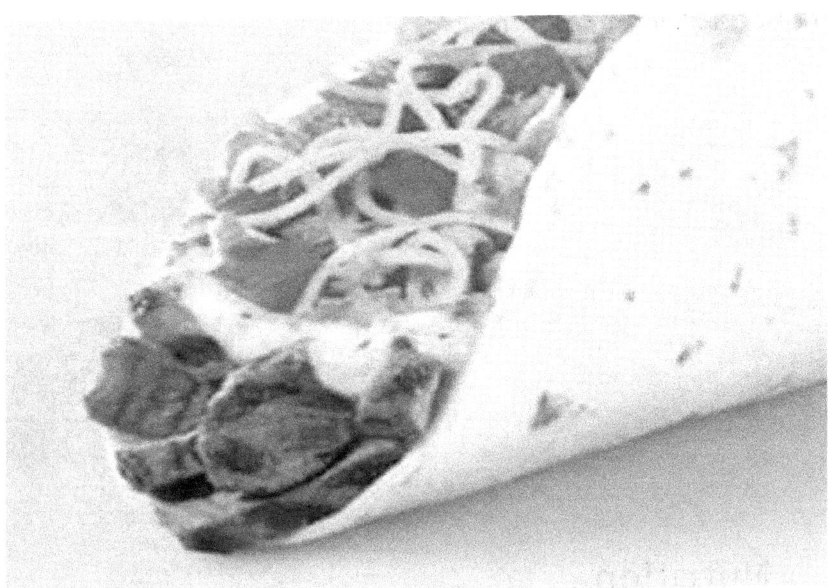

Nutrition

Calories: 329 Protein: 27g Fat: 12g Carbohydrates: 29g Sugars: 3g

Preparation Time: 10' *Cooking Time: 15'* *Serves: 6*

165. Taco Bells's XXL Grilled Stuffed Burrito

Ingredients

- ***1/3 cup black beans***
- ***ounces whole grain rice medley, ex. Santa Fe ready-to-serve***
- ***½ lb. lean ground beef***
- ***1/3 cup frozen corn***
- ***12 ounces salsa of choice***
- ***4 ounces velvetta thinly sliced processed cheese***
- ***6 @ 10-inch flour tortillas***

Optional Toppings:

- ***Torn lettuce leaves***
- ***Sour cream***
- ***Shredded Mexican cheese blend***
- ***Chopped sweet red pepper & onions***
- ***Also Needed: 4-qt. microwave-safe dish***

Directions

1. Measure and add the beans into a colander. Thoroughly rinse and drain them.
2. Warm the rice and crumble beef into the baking dish. Thaw and add in the corn and beans.
3. Microwave, covered, using the high-temperature setting until the beef is no longer pink (4-5 min.) and drain.
4. Stir in salsa and cheese and microwave until the cheese is melted (2-3 min.). Fold in rice.
5. Spoon ¾ cup the beef mixture into the center of each tortilla. Add additional ingredients as desired.
6. Fold the bottom and sides of the tortilla over filling and roll it up. Enjoy them at dinner or anytime!

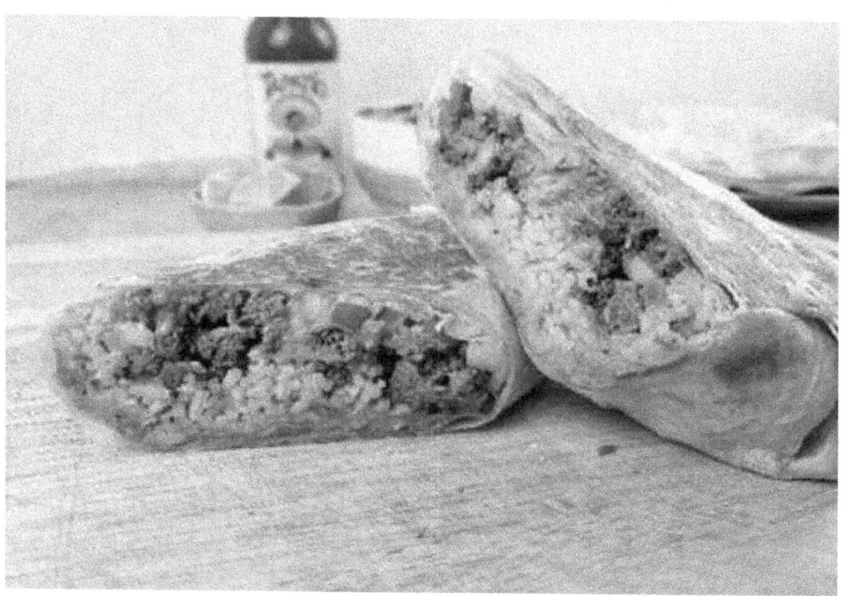

Nutrition

Calories: 452 Protein: 21g Fat: 13g Carbohydrates: 56g Sugars: 4g

Preparation Time: 5' *Cooking Time: 15'* *Serves: 6*

166. Taco Bells's Taco Bell Crispitos

Ingredients

- ***1/8 cup Cinnamon***
- ***½ cup Sugar***
- ***10 Tortillas***
- ***Vegetable oil***

Directions

1. Combine the sugar and cinnamon.
2. Warm a skillet/dutch oven (medium-high/approx. 350° Fahrenheit). Don't let it get "smoking" hot.
3. Use a sharp knife to quarter the tortillas. Deep-fry them two to four at a time for about half a minute per side. Place them onto a paper-lined wire rack to cool.
4. While they are draining, sprinkle them using the sugar-cinnamon mixture and serve.

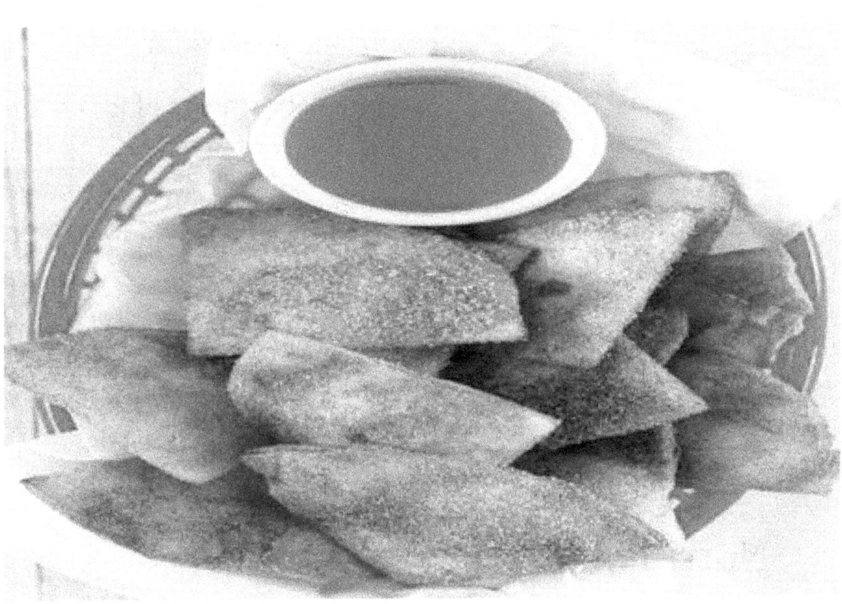

Nutrition

Calories: 443 Protein: 8g Fat: 15g Carbohydrates: 67g Sugars: 21g

Preparation Time: 10' *Cooking Time: 10'* *Serves: 2*

167. Applebee's Apple Chimi's Cheesecake

Ingredients

- *2 (9-inch) flour tortillas*
- *¼ cup granulated sugar*
- *½ teaspoon cinnamon*
- *3 ounces cream cheese, softened*
- *½ teaspoon vanilla extract*
- *1/3 cup apple, peeled and finely chopped*
- *Oil for frying*
- *Vanilla ice cream (optional)*
- *Caramel topping (optional)*

Directions

1. Make sure your tortillas and cream cheese are at room temperature; this will make them both easier to work with.
2. In a small bowl, combine the sugar and cinnamon.
3. Combine the cream cheese and vanilla until smooth. Fold in the apple.
4. Divide the apple and cheese mixture in two and place half in the center of each tortilla.
5. Fold the tortilla top to the middle, then the bottom to the middle, and then roll it up from the sides.
6. Put oil in a skillet in medium heat.
7. Place the filled tortillas into the skillet and fry on each side until they are golden brown. Transfer them to a paper towel lined plate to drain any excess oil, then immediately coat them with the cinnamon and sugar.
8. Serve with a scoop of ice cream.

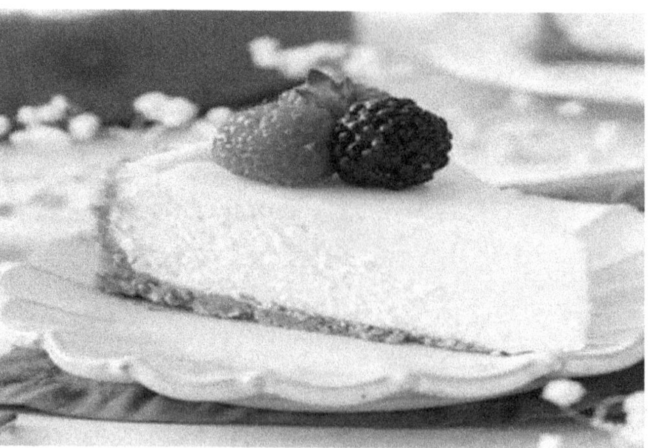

Nutrition

Calories: 267 Fat: 5g Carbs: 15g Protein: 18g Sodium: 276mg

Preparation Time: 1 h *Cooking Time: 30'* *Serves: 8*

168. Applebee's Triple Chocolate Meltdown

Ingredients

- ***2 cups heavy cream, divided***
- ***1 cup white chocolate chips***
- ***1 cup semi-sweet chocolate chips***
- ***1-pound bittersweet chocolate, chopped***
- ***½ cup butter, softened***
- ***6 eggs***
- ***1 ½ cups sugar***
- ***1 ½ cups all-purpose flour***
- ***Ice cream, for serving***

Directions

1. Preheat the oven to 400°F.
2. Prepare 8 ramekins by first coating the inside with butter then sprinkling them with flour so the bottom and sides are covered. Place them on a baking tray.
3. In a saucepan, bring 1 cup heavy cream to a simmer. Remove it from the heat and add the white chocolate chips, stirring until the chocolate is melted and the mixture is smooth. Let it to cool for about a half an hour, stirring occasionally.
4. Repeat with the other cup cream and the semi-sweet chocolate chips.
5. In a double boiler, combine the bittersweet chocolate with the softened butter and stir until the chocolate is melts and becomes smooth and remove the bowl from the heat and allow it to cool for about 10 minutes
6. In a bowl, beat the eggs and the sugar together for about 2 minutes, or until the mixture is foamy. Fold in the bittersweet chocolate mixture.
7. Beat in flour half a cup at a time in the blender, being careful not to overmix the batter.
8. Pour the batter evenly and place the baking tray in oven. Bake for about 18 minutes.
9. When done, the cakes should have a slight crust but still be soft in the middle. Remove them from oven when they have reached this look. If you cook them too long you won't get the lava cake effect.
10. Let the ramekins sit on the tray for 2–3 minutes and then invert them onto serving plates.
11. Drizzle some of both the semi-sweet and white chocolate sauces over the top and serve with a scoop of ice cream.

Nutrition

Calories: 421 Fat: 13g Carbs: 22g Protein: 24.0g Sodium: 311mg

Preparation Time: 1 h *Cooking Time: 0’* *Serves: 8t*

169. Applebee’s Chocolate Mousse Dessert Shooter

Ingredients

- ***2 tablespoons butter***
- ***6 ounces’ semi-sweet chocolate chips (1 cup), divided***
- ***2 eggs***
- ***1 teaspoon vanilla***
- ***8 oreo cookies***
- ***½ cup prepared fudge sauce***
- ***2 tablespoons sugar***
- ***½ cup heavy cream***
- ***Canned whipped cream***

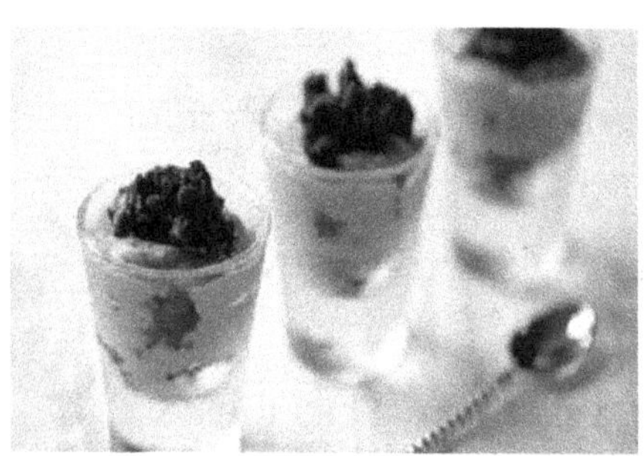

Directions

1. Melt the butter and all but 1 tablespoon of the chocolate chips in a double boiler.
2. When they are melted, stir in the vanilla and remove from the heat.
3. Whisk in the egg yolks.
4. Beat the egg whites and pour them into the chocolate mixture.
5. Beat the sugar and heavy cream in a separate bowl until it forms stiff peaks or is the consistency that you desire. Fold this into the chocolate mixture.
6. Crush the remaining chocolate chips into small pieces and stir them into the chocolate.
7. Crush the oreos. (You can either scrape out the cream from the cookies or just crush the entire cookie.)
8. Put some of the cookie crumbs into the bottom of your cup and pat them down. Layer the chocolate mixture on top. Finish with whipped cream and either more chocolate chips or oreo mixture.
9. Store in the refrigerator until ready to serve.

Nutrition

Calories: 389 Fat: 11.6g Carbs: 25. 2g Protein: 39.0g Sodium: 222mg

Preparation Time: 15' *Cooking Time: 25'* *Serves: 4-6*

170. Applebee's Cinnamon Apple Turnover

Ingredients

- ***1 large Granny Smith apple***
- ***½ teaspoon cornstarch***
- ***¼ teaspoon cinnamon***
- ***Dash ground nutmeg***
- ***¼ cup brown sugar***
- ***¼ cup applesauce***
- ***¼ teaspoon vanilla extract***
- ***1 tablespoon butter, melted***
- ***1 sheet puff pastry, thawed***
- ***Whipped cream***

Directions

1. Preheat the oven to 400°F.

2. Spray the baking sheet with some non-stick cooking spray or using a bit of oil on a paper towel.

3. In a mixing bowl, mix together the apples, cornstarch, cinnamon, nutmeg, and brown sugar. Stir to make sure the apples are well covered with the spices. Then stir in the applesauce and the vanilla.

4. Cur the pastries into squares. You should be able to make 4 or 6 depending on how big you want your turnovers to be and how big your pastry is.

5. Place some of the apple mixture in the center of each square and fold the corners of the pastry up to make a pocket. Pinch the edges together to seal. Then brush a bit of the melted butter over the top to give the turnovers that nice brown color.

6. Put pastry onto the prepared baking pan and transfer to the preheated oven. Bake 20–25 minutes, or until they become a golden brown in color.

7. Serve with whipped cream on top or vanilla ice cream.

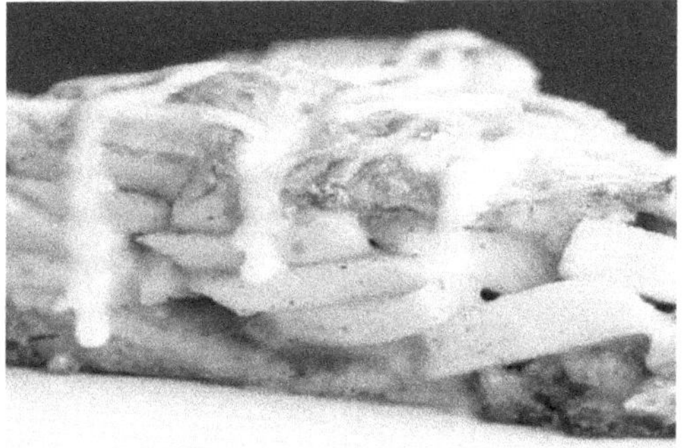

Nutrition

Calories: 235 Fat: 15.8g Carbs: 20. 5g Protein: 26g Sodium: 109mg

Preparation Time: 10' *Cooking Time: 45'* *Serves: 8*

171. Applebee's Cherry Chocolate Cobbler

Ingredients

- ***1½ cups all-purpose flour***
- ***½ cup sugar***
- ***2 teaspoons baking powder***
- ***½ teaspoon salt***
- ***¼ cup butter***
- ***6 ounces' semisweet chocolate morsels***
- ***¼ cup milk***
- ***1 egg, beaten***
- ***21 ounces' cherry pie filling***
- ***½ cup finely chopped nuts***

Directions

1. Preheat the oven to 350°F.
2. Mix and combine the flour, sugar, baking powder, salt and butter in a large mixing bowl. Cut the mixture until there are lumps the size of small peas.
3. Melt the chocolate morsels. Let cool for approximately 5 minutes, then add the milk and egg and mix well. Beat into the flour mixture, mixing completely.
4. Spread the pie filling in a 2-quart casserole dish. Randomly drop the chocolate batter over the filling, then sprinkle with nuts.
5. Bake for 40–45 minutes.
6. Serve with vanilla ice cream if desired.

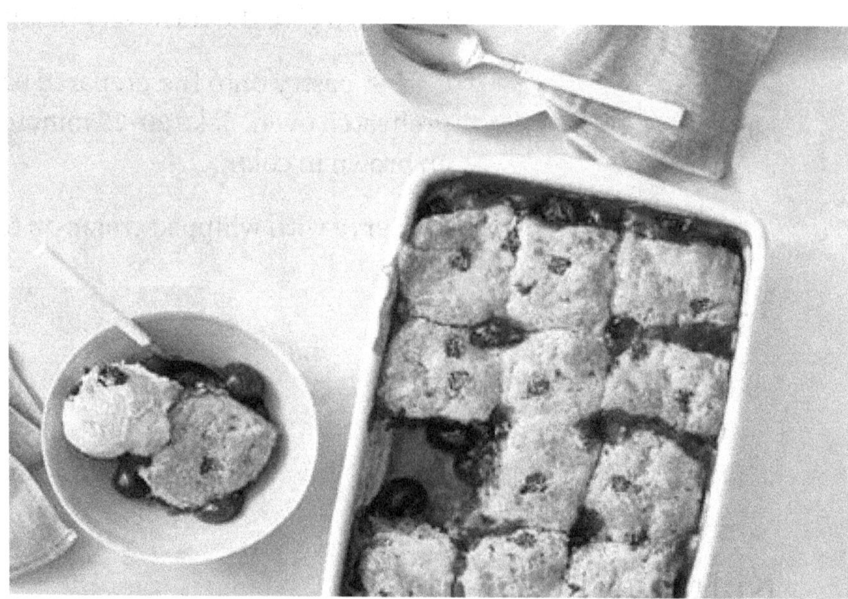

Nutrition

Calories: 502 Fat: 1.8g Carbs: 10. 2g Protein: 19.0g Sodium: 265mg

Preparation Time: 10' *Cooking Time: 50'* *Serves: 8*

172. Applebee's Chocolate Pecan Pie

Ingredients

- ***3 eggs***
- ***½ cup sugar***
- ***1 cup corn syrup***
- ***½ teaspoon salt***
- ***1 teaspoon vanilla extract***
- ***¼ cup melted butter***
- ***1 cup pecans***
- ***3 tablespoons semisweet chocolate chips***
- ***1 unbaked pie shell***

Directions

1. Preheat the oven to 350°F.
2. Beat the eggs and mix the sugar in a mixing bowl, then add the corn syrup, salt, vanilla and butter.
3. Put the chocolate chips and pecans inside the pie shell and pour the egg mixture over the top.
4. Bake for 50–60 minutes or until set.
5. Serve with vanilla ice cream.

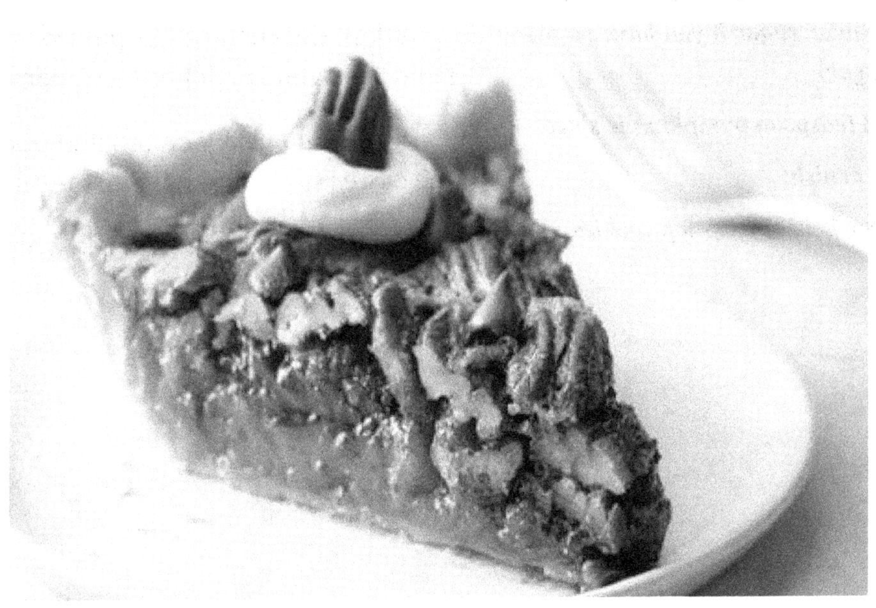

Nutrition

Calories: 483 Fat: 13.8g Carbs: 22. 2g Protein: 29.7g Sodium: 154mg

Preparation Time: 30' *Cooking Time: 35'* *Serves: 8*

173. Applebee's Pumpkin Custard with Gingersnaps

Ingredients

- ***Custard***
- ***8 egg yolks***
- ***1¾ cups (1 15-ounce can) pure pumpkin puree***
- ***1¾ cups heavy whipping cream***
- ***½ cup sugar***
- ***1½ teaspoons pumpkin pie spice***
- ***1 teaspoon vanilla***

Topping:

- ***1 cup crushed gingersnap cookies***
- ***1 tablespoon melted butter***

Whipped Cream:

- ***1 cup heavy whipping cream***
- ***1 tablespoon superfine sugar (or regular sugar if you have no caster sugar)***
- ***½ teaspoon pumpkin pie spice***
- ***Garnish:***
- ***8 whole gingersnap cookies***

Directions

1. Preheat the oven to 350°F.
2. Separate the yolks from 8 eggs and whisk them together in a large mixing bowl until they are well blended and creamy.
3. Add the pumpkin, sugar, vanilla, heavy cream and pumpkin pie spice and whisk to combine.
4. Cook the custard mixture, stirring until it has thickened enough that it coats a spoon.
5. Put some of the mixture into custard cups or an 8×8-inch baking pan and bake for about 20 minutes if using individual cups or 30–35 minutes for the baking pan, until it is set, and a knife inserted comes out clean.
6. While the custard is baking, make the topping by combining the crushed gingersnaps and melted butter. Sprinkle the gingersnap mixture over the top.
7. When the custard has passed the clean knife test, remove from the oven and let cool to room temperature.
8. Whisk the heavy cream and pumpkin pie spice together with the caster sugar and beat just until it thickens.
9. Serve the custard with the whipped cream and garnish each serving with a gingersnap.

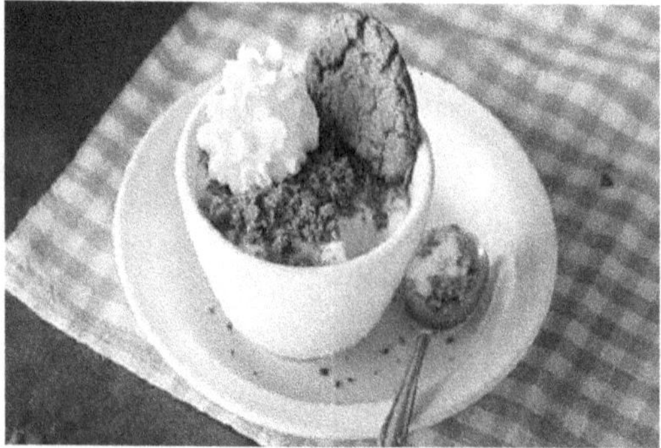

Nutrition

Calories: 243 Fat: 6.8g Carbs: 13. 2g Protein: 17.0g Sodium: 313mg

Preparation Time: 60-90' *Cooking Time: 0'* *Serves: 4*

174. Applebee's Layered Berry Dish

Ingredients

- ***500g mixed berries (e.g. strawberries, raspberries, blueberries, currants; fresh or frozen)***
- ***100g sugar***
- ***3 tablespoon freshly squeezed lemon juice***
- ***3 teaspoonful vegetable binder (e.g. locust bean gum, approx. 10 g)***
- ***8-10 mint leaves***
- ***500g Cream curd***
- ***Grated zest of 1 organic lemon***
- ***2 packets vanilla sugar***
- ***200 g cream***
- ***100 g Cantuccini (Italian almond biscuits)***

Directions

1. Carefully wash and select the berries, clean the strawberries and quarter them. Let the frozen berries thaw. Puree half of the berries with 75 g sugar and lemon juice.

2. Stir in the binding agent with the whisk and continue stirring for 1 min. Rub the mint leaves, cut them into fine strips and set aside 2 tablespoon Place the rest with the remaining berries under the puree.

3. Mix the curd with the lemon zest, vanilla sugar and other sugar. Whip the cream continuously until it turns stiff and fold in.

4. Roughly crush the cantuccini in a freezer bag with a rolling pin. Alternate the curd cream, cookies and berries in 4-6 glasses. Finish with curd and sprinkle with the other berries. Chill the cream for 1 hour.

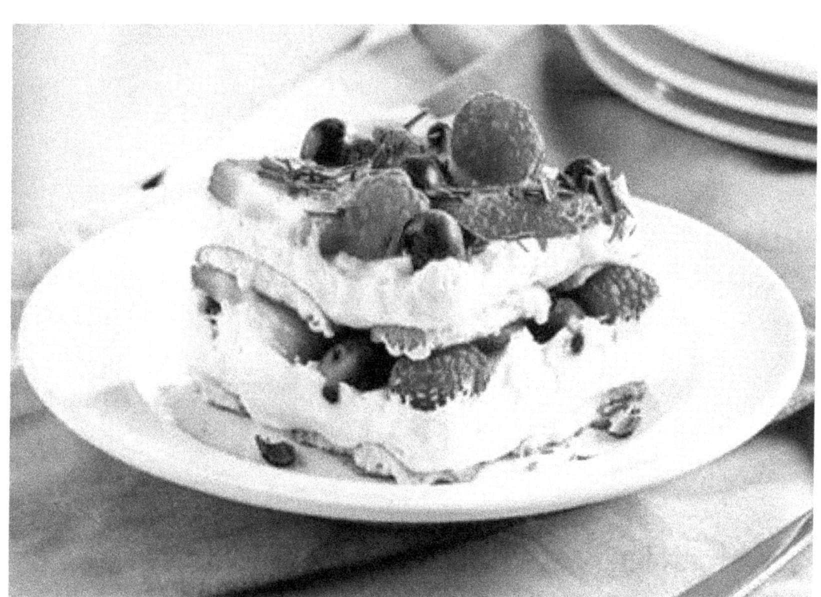

Nutrition

Calories: 178 Fat: 15g Carbs: 50g Sugars: 8g Protein: 9g

Preparation Time: 60-90' *Cooking Time: 0'* *Serves: 4*

175. Magnolia Bakery's Banana Trifle in the Glass

Ingredients

- ***1 small ripe banana***
- ***3 tablespoons Limoncello (lemon liqueur)***
- ***50g low-fat quark***
- ***1 tablespoon Crème fraiche Cheese***
- ***1 teaspoon sugar***
- ***50g chocolate biscuits (finished product)***
- ***1 tablespoon dried banana chips (optionally ¼ teaspoonful unsweetened cocoa powder)***

Directions

1. Peel the banana, cut into slices and drizzles with 1 tablespoon limoncello.
2. Mix the curd with the crème fraîche and the sugar.
3. Crumble half of the chocolate biscuits into a glass of 0.3 l and drizzle with 1 tablespoon limoncello.
4. Put half of the banana slices and the quark cream on each. Crumble the remaining biscuits on top and drizzle with the remaining limoncello. Layer the remaining banana slices and cream. Cover and chill for 1 hour.
5. To serve, either crumbles the banana chips over the dessert (the rest tastes like a sweet snack or in breakfast cereal) or dust the cocoa powder through a small sieve.

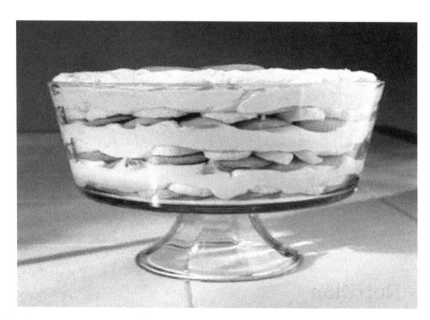

Nutrition

Calories: 100 Fat: 3g Carbs: 21g Sugars: 10g Protein: 5g

Preparation Time: 30' *Cooking Time: 0'* *Serves: 4*

176. Magnolia Bakery's Banana Layer Cream in a Glass

Ingredients

- ***1 ripe banana***
- ***2 tablespoon Lemon juice***
- ***100g cream***
- ***1 teaspoon vanilla sugar***
- ***100g chocolate biscuits (finished product)***
- ***8 tablespoon Marsala (Italian dessert wine; or pineapple juice)***
- ***4 teaspoonful chocolate chips***

Directions

1. Crush the banana finely with a fork, mix immediately with lemon juice. Continuously whip the cream together with vanilla sugar until stiff and pull it into the sauce.
2. Pick up half of the biscuits, place in two glasses and drizzle with 2 tablespoons of Marsala. Add a quarter of the banana cream and sprinkle 1 teaspoonful of chocolate shavings on top.
3. Crumble the remaining biscuits on top, soak with Marsala and spread the rest of the cream on top. Sprinkle with the remaining chocolate chips and chill until ready to serve.

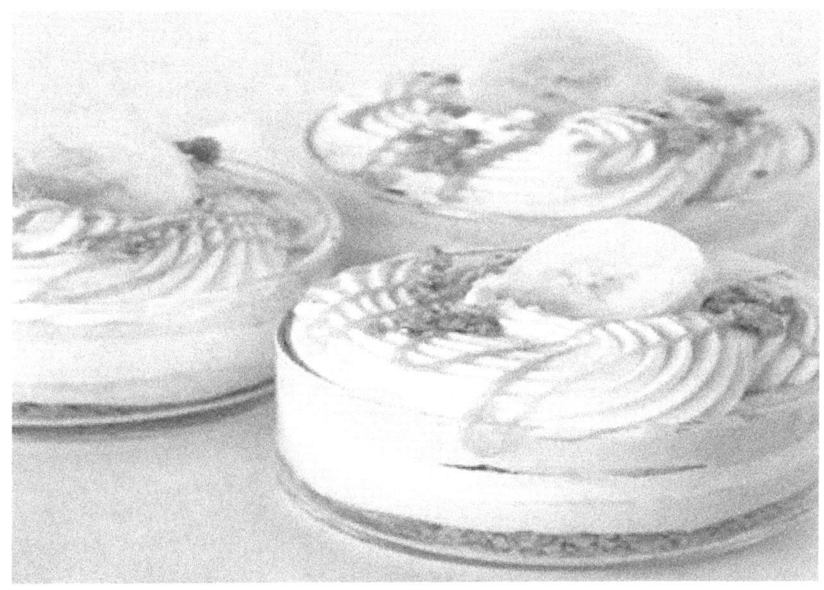

Nutrition

Calories: 150 Fat: 4.2g Carbs: 40g Sugars: 1g Protein: 9g

Preparation Time: 40' *Cooking Time: 0'* *Serves: 4*

177. Amy's Bread's Yogurt Mousse with Poppy Seeds

Ingredients

- ***1 Vanilla bean***
- ***2 tablespoon Poppy seeds***
- ***2 tablespoon sugar***
- ***100g cream***
- ***400g Plain yogurt (3.5% fat)***
- ***250g Seasonal fruits (e.g. strawberries, currants, peaches)***
- ***1 Stalks of lemon balm***
- ***Kitchen strainer plus collecting bowl***
- ***Kitchen towel made of fabric***

Directions

1. Cut the vanilla pod lengthways the evening before and scrape out the pulp. Finely grind the vanilla pulp with poppy seeds and sugar in a blitz chopper. Whip the cream until creamy (not stiff).

2. Mix the yoghurt with the poppy seed mixture and fold in the creamy cream. Line the sieve with the kitchen towel, pour in the yoghurt-cream mixture and cover with the corners of the kitchen towel. Hang the strainer in a bowl and place in the fridge overnight so that the whey can drain off and an airy cream is created.

3. To serve, wash the fruits, peel if necessary, cut them into bite-size pieces and spread them on two plates. Form the yoghurt mousse with two tablespoons and arrange on the fruit. Pluck Melissa leaves, rub and garnish the mousse with them.

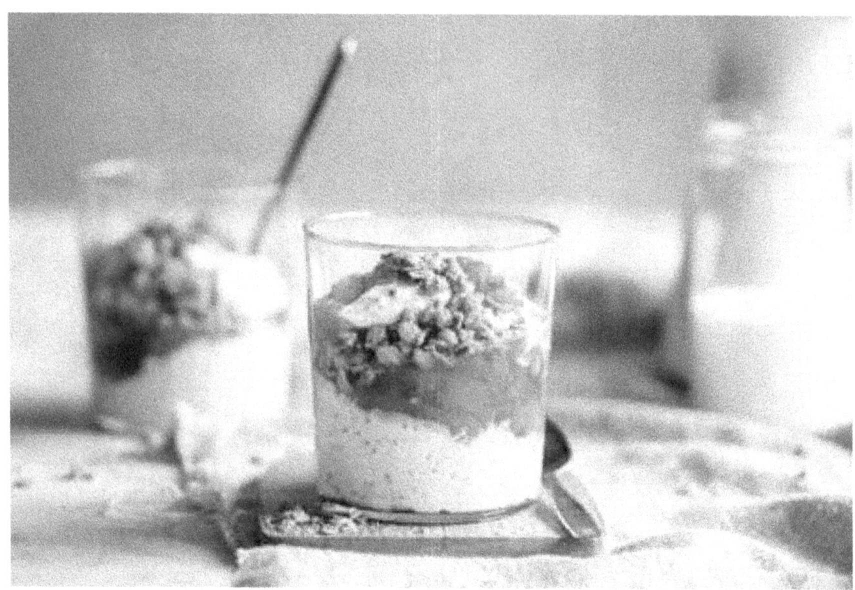

Nutrition

Calories: 242.8 Fat: 6.6g Carbs: 38.4g Sugars: 3g Protein: 8.4g

Preparation Time: 60' *Cooking Time: 90'* *Serves: 0-4*

178. Cheesecake Factory's Frozen Yogurt with Raspberry Puree

Ingredients

- ***600g Plain yogurt (3.5% fat)***
- ***¼ teaspoonful ground vanilla***
- ***30g powdered sugar***
- ***1 organic lime***
- ***2nd Protein (size M)***
- ***Salt***
- ***1 small bunch of lemon balm***
- ***300g Raspberries***
- ***2-3 tablespoon apple syrup***

Directions

1. Place the yoghurt in a strainer covered with gauze and let it drain in the refrigerator for 4–6 hours. This gives about 300 g of yoghurt mass, with a consistency similar to cream cheese.

2. Mix the yoghurt mixture with ground vanilla and powdered sugar. Wash the lime hot and dry. Rub the bowl finely and mix in. Mix the egg whites and add a pinch of salt to a firm snow and fold into the mixture.

3. Put the mixture into a metal bowl and cover with cling film and place in the freezer. Stir every 30 minutes so that no larger crystals form. After about 3 hours you have a creamy mass of ice cream.

4. For the raspberry puree, rinse the lemon balm and pat it dry, put a few leaves aside, finely chop the rest. Read the raspberries, wash and puree with the blender. Swipe through a sieve and mix with apple juice and chopped lemon balm.

5. Spread the raspberry puree on plates and garnish with the lemon balm leaves. Cut the frozen yoghurt with a spoon and arrange on the raspberry puree.

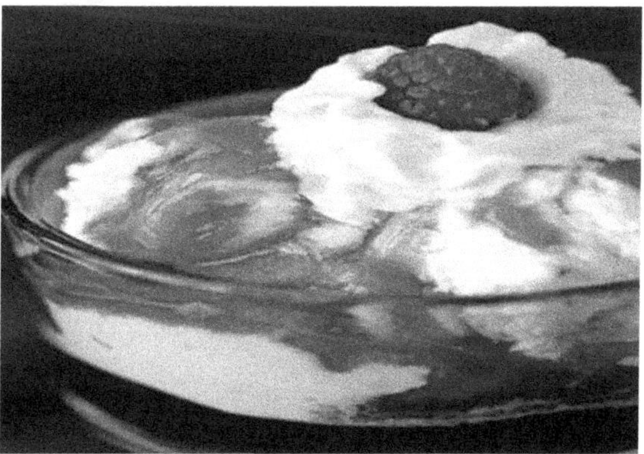

Nutrition

Calories: 147 Fat: 17g Carbs: 87g Sugars: 15g Protein: 14g

Preparation Time: 30' *Cooking Time: 0'* *Serves: 1*

179. Amy's Bread's Greek Yogurt with Honey and Pistachios

Ingredients

- ***150g Greek yogurt (10% fat, alternatively cream yogurt)***
- ***2 tablespoon liquid orange honey (alternatively other honey)***
- ***1 tablespoon unsalted pistachio nuts***
- ***Some seasonal fruit (e.g. 1 small blue fig, 2 strawberries or a few tangerines)***

Directions

1. Whisk the yogurt and 1 tablespoon of honey with a whisk until creamy and pour into a small bowl.
2. Roughly chop the pistachio nuts. Drizzle the remaining honey onto the yoghurt. Sprinkle pistachios over it.
3. Garnish with a quartered fig, halved strawberries or the tangerine wedges.

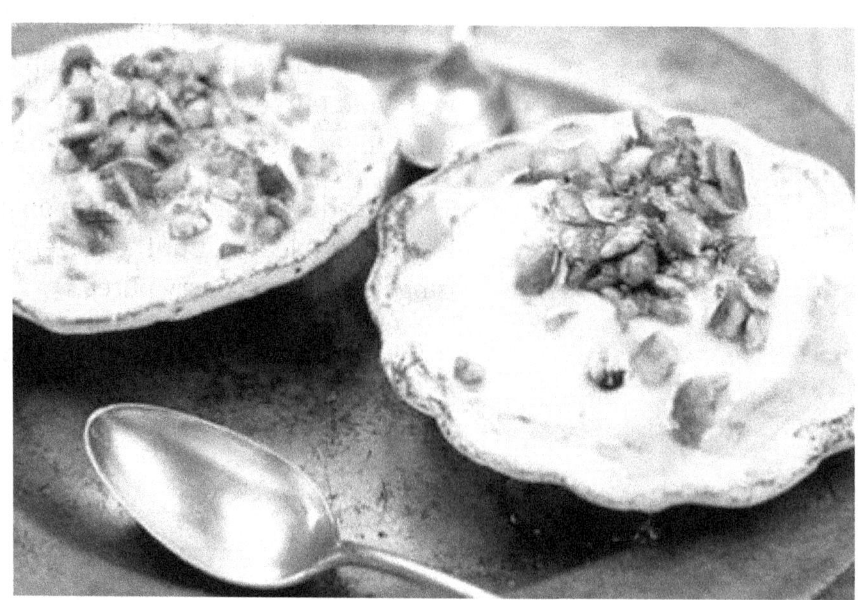

Nutrition

Calories: 184 Fat: 4g Carbs: 57g Sugars: 9g Protein: 12g

Preparation Time: 30' *Cooking Time: 60'* *Serves: 5-4*

180. Denmark's Classic Red Groats

Ingredients

- ***600g mixed berries and red fruits (e.g. sour cherries, strawberries, raspberries, currants)***
- ***½ Vanilla bean***
- ***½ Cherry or black currant juice***
- ***3 tablespoon food starch***
- ***1–2 tablespoon Cassis liqueur (black currant liqueur, as desired) approx.***
- ***3–4 tablespoon sugar***

Directions

1. Wash the fruits, clean them and let them drain on a kitchen towel. Stone the cherries, halve or quarter large strawberries, pluck currants from the panicles. Cut the vanilla pods into half lengthways and scrape out the pulp. Boil the marrow and pod with the fruit juice in a saucepan.

2. Mix the starch with 3–4 tablespoons of water and pour into the boiling fruit juice while stirring. Cook it for 2–3 minutes until the starch binds.

3. Add the prepared fruits and the liqueur as desired. Let the fruits heat up briefly in the brew, boil for a maximum of 1–2 minutes—they should neither become mushy nor crumble.

4. Remove from the heat and sweeten with more or less sugar, depending on your taste. Let the groats cool. Remove the vanilla pod before serving and serve the groats with only lightly whipped cream or the vanilla sauce.

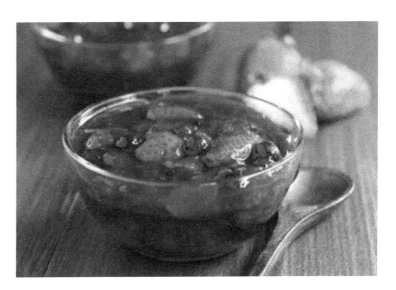

Nutrition

Calories: 119 Fat: 20g Carbs: 76g Sugars: 12g Protein: 10g

Preparation Time: 90' *Cooking Time: 0'* *Serves: 4*

181. Italian's Panna Cotta with Raspberry Sauce

Ingredients

- *2nd Vanilla pods*
- *400ml milk*
- *600g cream*
- *50g sugar*
- *7 sheets white gelatin*
- *500g fresh raspberries (alternatively thawed frozen raspberries)*
- *150g powdered sugar*
- *200g yogurt*
- *6 Small portions or small cups (approx. 180ml content)*

Directions

1. Slice the vanilla pods lengthways, scrape out the pulp. Boil milk, cream, sugar and vanilla pulp briefly in a saucepan, then let simmer over low heat for about 20 minutes.

2. Let the gelatin be soaked in cold water for about 5 minutes, then squeeze it out and dissolve in the hot cream milk (caution: do not let it boil!) While stirring. Fill the cream milk into small portions or small cups. Cover and refrigerate in the refrigerator for approx. 6 hours until the mixture has set.

3. Wash the raspberries, set aside about 3 berries per serving for garnish. Puree the remaining berries with powdered sugar and yoghurt. Pour the panna cotta onto a plate (this works best if you briefly dip the molds in hot water to the edge) and pour the sauce over them. Garnish with raspberries.

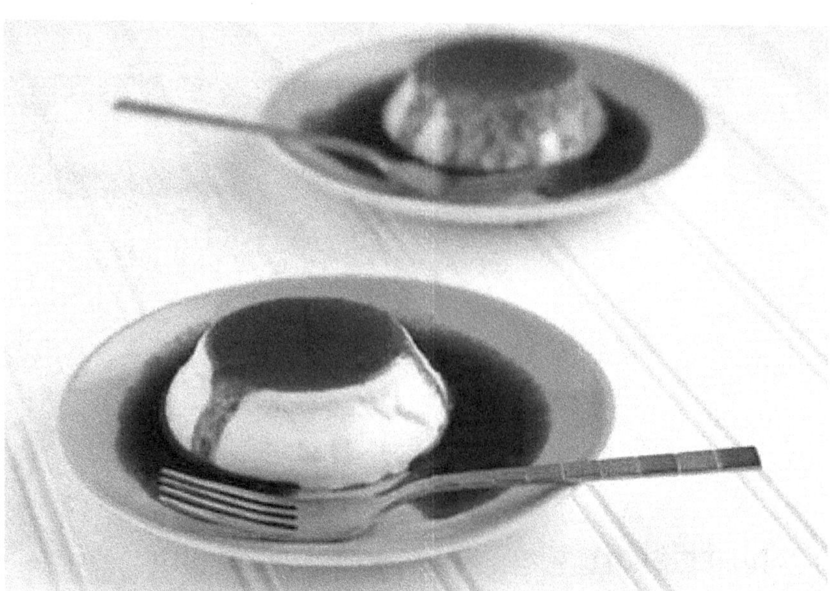

Nutrition

Calories: 178 Fat: 24g Carbs: 123g Sugars: 15g Protein 27g

Chapter 11
Special Drinks

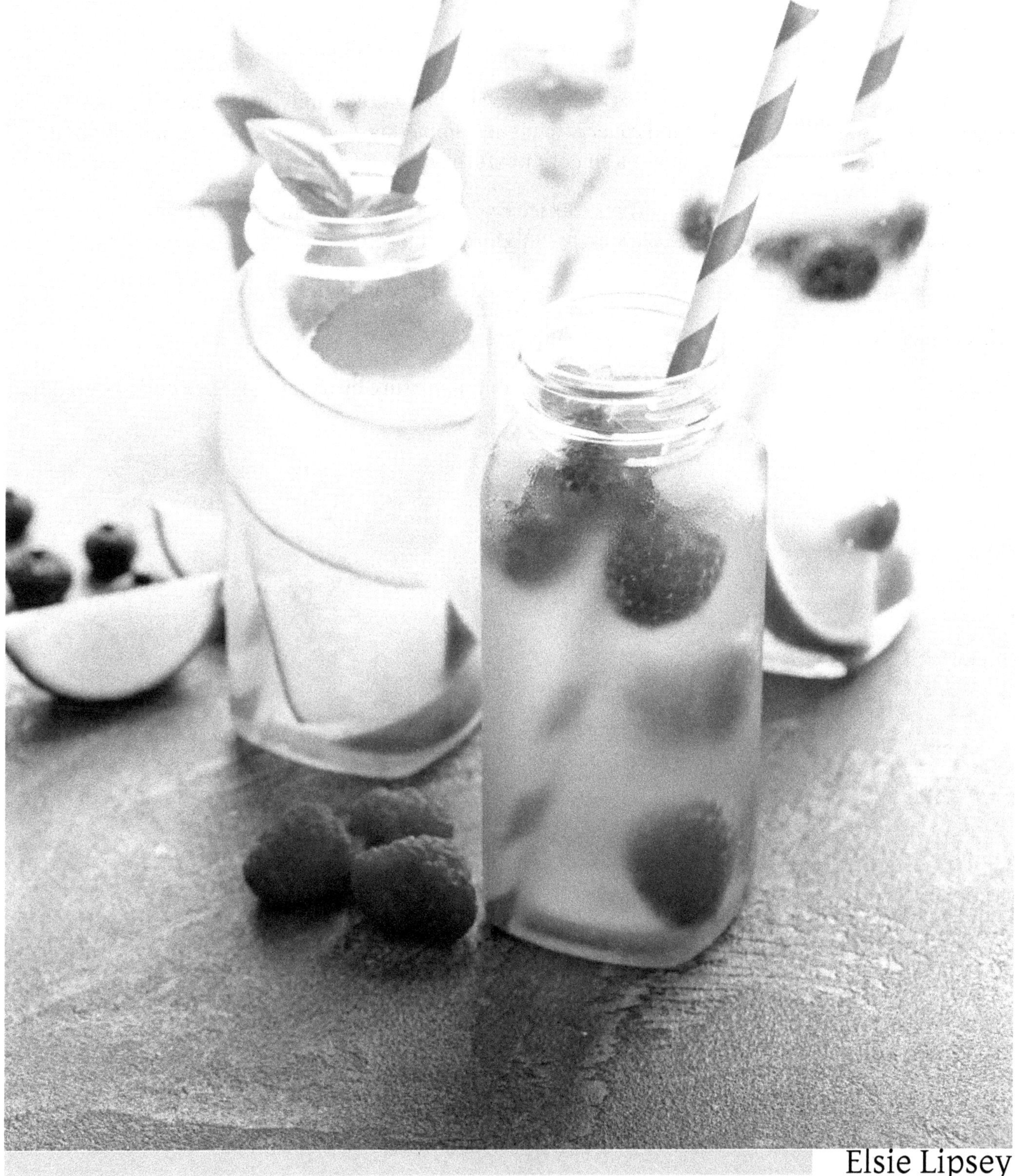

Preparation Time: 10' *Cooking Time: 0'* *Serves: 3*

182. Starbucks' Hazelnut Frappuccino

Ingredients

- *½ cup nutella*
- *2 cups vanilla ice cream*
- *1 cup whole milk*
- *6 ice cubes*
- *4 teaspoonfuls espresso powder (instant)*

For optional:

- *Chocolate curls*

Directions

1. Use a blender for mixing nutella, milk, and espresso powder and cover it to blend completely. Combine ice cubes and blend to make a smooth mixture.
2. Then, mix ice cream and blend the mixture by covering it. Make sure the mixture is smooth.
3. Pour the prepared mixture into glasses.
4. Serve immediately to enjoy it.
5. You can garnish the mixture by using chocolate curls as per your choice.

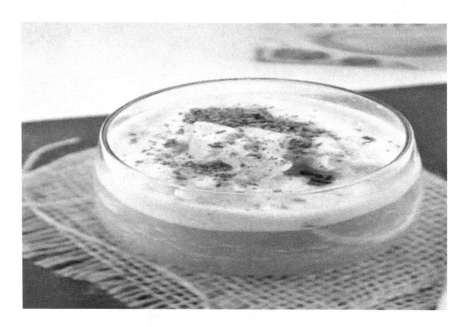

Nutrition

Calories: 474 Protein: 9g Fat: 27g Carbs: 55g Fiber: 2g

Preparation Time: 10' *Cooking Time: 0'* *Serves: 6*

183. Olive Garden's Green Apple Moscato Sangria

Ingredients

- ***8 cups ice***
- ***750ml moscato***

½ a cup each of:

- ***Orange slices***
- ***Strawberries***
- ***Green apple slices***

6 ounces each of:

- ***Apple puree***
- ***Pineapple juice***

Directions

1. Make a mixture of pineapple juice, apple puree, and chilled moscato in a large-sized pitcher.
2. Stir the mixture well.
3. Take several ice cubes in a glass and pour the iced beverage in the glass before serving it.
4. Serve and enjoy it.
5. If you want to have a fun drink at a festive occasion and yet don't want it to contain too much alcohol, then sangria is the drink for you.
6. Add some slices fruits such as blueberries, orange, strawberries, and so on.

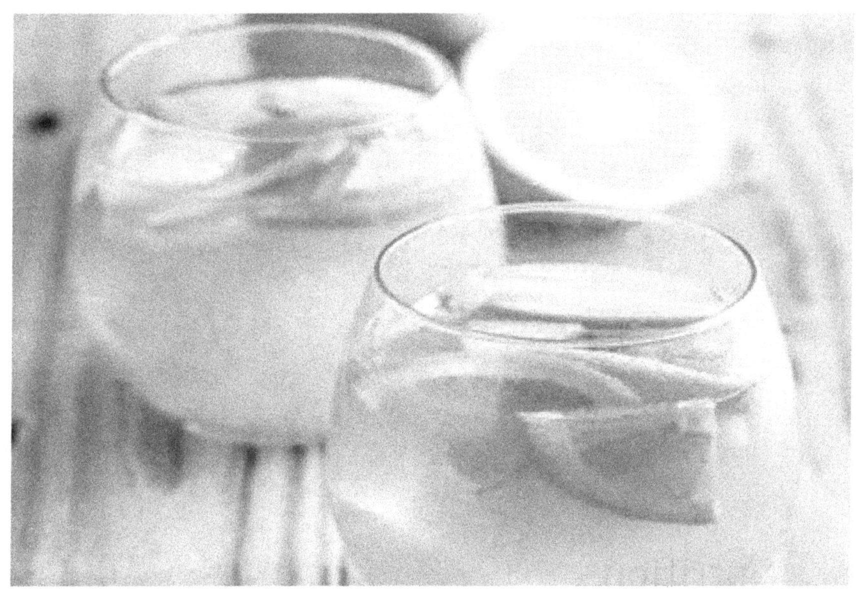

Nutrition

Calories: 210 Protein: 0g Fat: 0g Carbs: 35g Fiber: 0g

Preparation Time: 5' *Cooking Time: 0'* *Serves: 1*

184. Dunkin' Donuts Salted Caramel Hot Chocolate

Ingredients

- ***2–3 teaspoonfuls cocoa powder (unsweetened)***
- ***1 cup whole milk***
- ***1 tablespoon caramel syrup (without sugar)***
- ***2 tablespoons granulated sugar***
- ***½ tablespoon vanilla extract***
- ***Whipped cream***

For Toppings:

- ***½ tablespoon sea salt***

Directions

1. Use a large-sized mug for mixing sea salt, sugar, and cocoa.
2. Maintain a high heat setting in the microwave to heat the milk.
3. Remove the hot milk from microwave and mix vanilla extract in it.
4. Mix the cocoa mixture with the mixture of milk. Stir it to get a smooth mixture.
5. Use whipped cream for toppings and also use caramel syrup for drizzling on the top.
6. Sprinkle a pinch of sea salt as per your choice.
7. Serve the hot beverage and enjoy it.

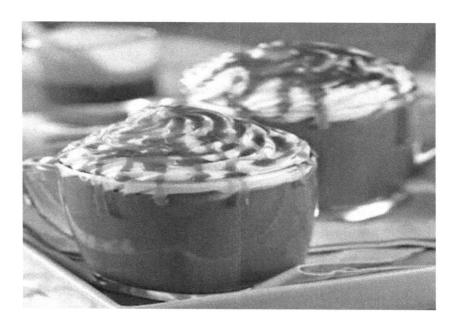

Nutrition

Calories: 360 Protein: 13g Fat: 9g Carbs: 66g Fiber: 2g

Preparation Time: 10' *Cooking Time: 10'* *Serves: 1*

185. Starbucks' Caramel Apple Spice

Ingredients

- ***64 ounces of apple juice (100% pure)***
- ***2 tablespoons flour***
- ***½ each of:***
- ***White sugar***
- ***Brown sugar (packed)***
- ***5 tablespoons powdered sugar***

1 cup each of:

- ***Whipped cream (heavy)***
- ***Water***

½ teaspoons each of:

- ***Vanilla extract***
- ***Cinnamon***
- ***A couple of dashes cinnamon***

For toppings:

- ***Caramel***

Directions

1. Set the oven at medium-low heat and steam the apple juice in a large-sized pot. Be careful to avoid boiling.
2. Take a small-sized pot to mix flour, sugar, and cinnamon in it.
3. Stir the mixture after adding water.
4. Set the oven at the medium-low flame and boil the mixture for two minutes.
5. Heat lightly to make the syrup achieve an appropriate thickness.
6. Remove the mixture from the oven and leave it to cool down. It will increase the consistency of the mixture. Mix the vanilla extract in the mixture.
7. Use cinnamon dolce syrup for pouring over the steamed apple juice. Otherwise, you can keep the syrup in the dispenser to mix individually in the glasses.
8. Apply homemade whipped cream as toppings and drizzle the mixture with caramel toppings.
9. You can fold in a few cinnamon dashes and vanilla as per your preference.
10. Serve it immediately and enjoy it.

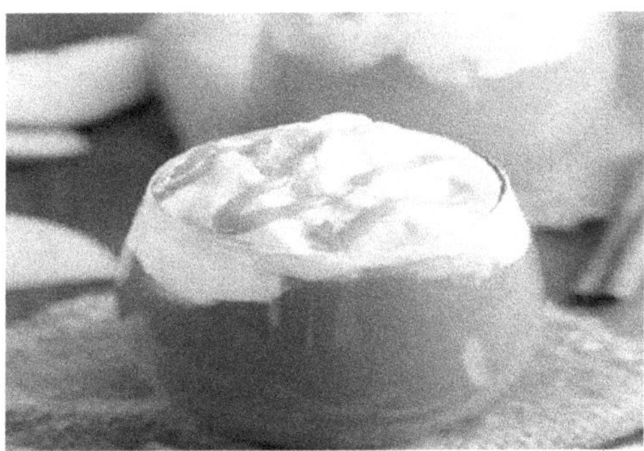

Nutrition

Calories: 210 Protein: 0g Fat: 6g Carbs: 40g Fiber: 0g

Preparation Time: 30' *Cooking Time: 0'* *Serves: 2*

186. Starbucks' Pink Drink

Ingredients

- ***1-2 cups coconut milk (Unsweetened)***
- ***1 cup hot boiling water***
- ***Strawberries (fresh and sliced)***
- ***½ cup grape juice (white)***
- ***4 packs of acai berry tea***
- ***Optional:***
- ***Agave nectar***

Directions

1. Use two cups measuring glass for placing acai berry teas after unwrapping them. Mix hot water in it and leave it to cool down it. Toss the tea packets after squeezing them.
2. Combine grape juice in the prepared tea within the measuring cup.
3. Use ice and one cup tea mixture for filling a cup.
4. Also, use coconut milk as per your choice for the toppings of the drink.
5. You can use slices strawberries and any type of sweetener as per your choice.
6. Serve and enjoy!

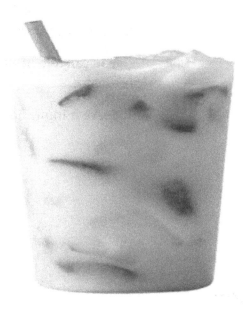

Nutrition

Calories: 124 Protein: 2g Fat: 5g Carbs: 21g Fiber: 2g

Preparation Time: 7' *Cooking Time: 0'* *Serves: 6*

187. Olive Garden's Watermelon Moscato Sangria

Ingredients

- ***4 cups Ice***
- ***750ml. Moscato***
- ***1 orange (sliced)***
- ***6 ounces each of:***
- ***Watermelon syrup***
- ***Ginger ale***
- ***¾ cup strawberries (sliced)***

Directions

1. Wash the fruits and make small-sized slices by cutting them.
2. Use a large-sized pitcher for pouring the moscato.
3. Mix watermelon syrup and ginger ale in the pitcher and stir them for mixing completely.
4. Stir the mixture slowly within the pitcher after the mixing ice.
5. Then, combine sliced strawberries and oranges in the mixture.
6. As per your choice, serve the drink with sliced watermelon.

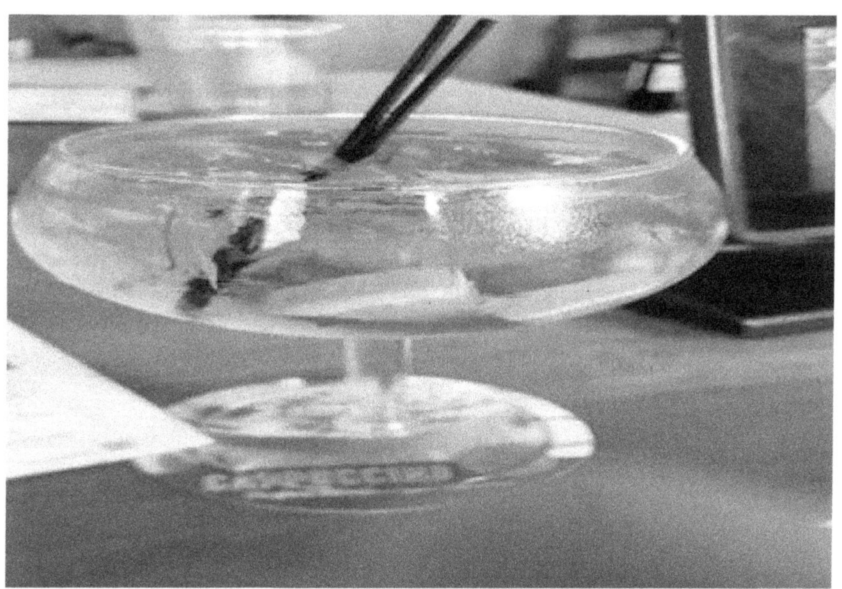

Nutrition

Calories: 204 Protein: 0g Fat: 0g Carbs: 33g Fiber: 0g

Preparation Time: 5' *Cooking Time: 0'* *Serves: 2*

188. Smoothie King's Caribbean Way

Ingredients

- ***1 cup papaya nectar***
- ***1 banana (average)***
- ***1 ½ cups ice***
- ***2 cups strawberries (fresh)***
- ***¼ cup turbinado sugar***

Directions

1. Use a blender for mixing papaya nectar, banana, strawberries, and sugar and make a puree after covering it.
2. Make a smooth mixture by adding ice to the prepared puree.
3. Enjoy it after serving.

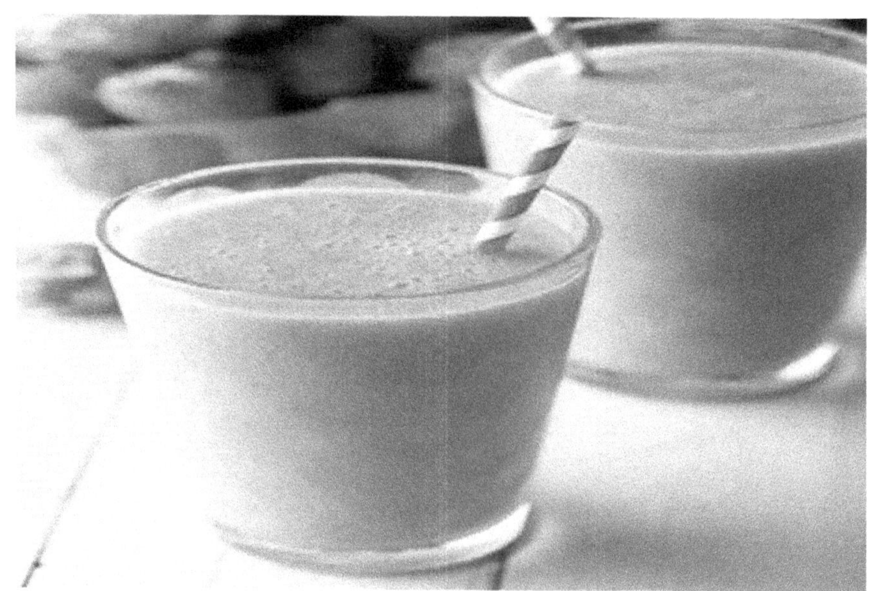

Nutrition

Calories: 261 Protein: 2g Fat: 1g Carbs: 65g Fiber: 5g

Preparation Time: 10 *Cooking Time: 0'* *Serves: 2*

189. Panera's Mango Smoothie

Ingredients

- ***½ banana (medium ripe))***
- ***1 tablespoon honey***
- ***½ cup each of:***
- ***Pineapple juice (unsweetened)***
- ***Plain yogurt (reduced fat)***
- ***2 cups frozen mango (chopped after peeling)***

Directions

1. Mix all the ingredients using a blender and make a smooth mixture.
2. Serve it immediately after pouring the smoothie in chilled glasses.

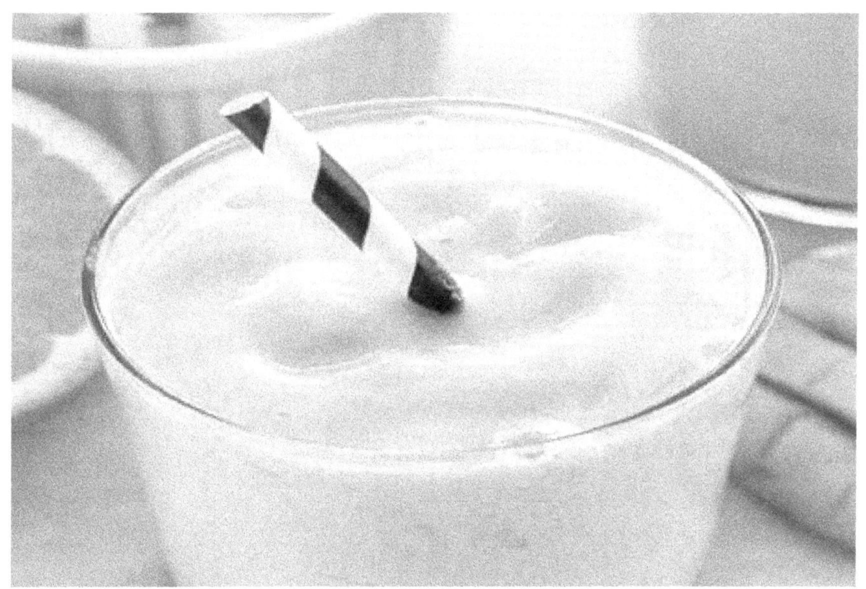

Nutrition

Calories: 237 Protein: 5g Fat: 2g Carbs: 56g Fiber: 4g

Preparation Time: 5' *Cooking Time: 0'* *Serves: 2*

190. Sonic Drive-in's Strawberry Shake

Ingredients

- ***1 ½ ice cream (vanilla)***
- ***1 tablespoon strawberry preserves***
- ***1/3 cup 2% milk***
- ***½ of frozen strawberries (unsweetened)***

Directions

1. Take all the ingredients in a blender and make a smooth mixture.
2. Serve it to enjoy immediately by pouring them in chilled glasses.

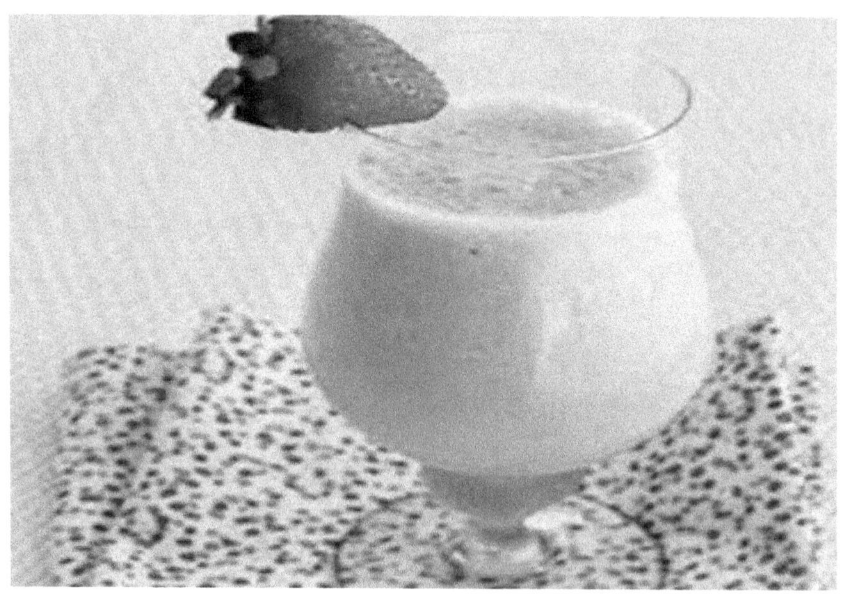

Nutrition

Calories: 257 Protein: 5g Fat: 12g Carbs: 35g Fiber: 1g

Preparation Time: 7' *Cooking Time: 0'* *Serves: 2*

191. Red Robin's Screaming Red Zombie

Ingredients

- *3 ounces orange juice*
- *4 ounces lemon juice*
- *½ ounces each of:*
- *Bacardi Select Ram*
- *Myer's Dark Rum*
- *Grenadine*
- *1 tablespoon sugar*
- *1 ounce of light rum*

Directions

1. Use a bowl to make a mixture of lemon juice and sugar.
2. Then, mix one ounce of rum and orange juice with mixture lemon juice. Stir the mixture to blend completely.
3. Fill the ice into the half part of the cup measuring 16 ounces.
4. Pour the mixture over the ice containing cup.
5. Use a spoon to float to mix all the three ingredients required in half-ounces each.
6. Enjoy the drink immediately after serving it.

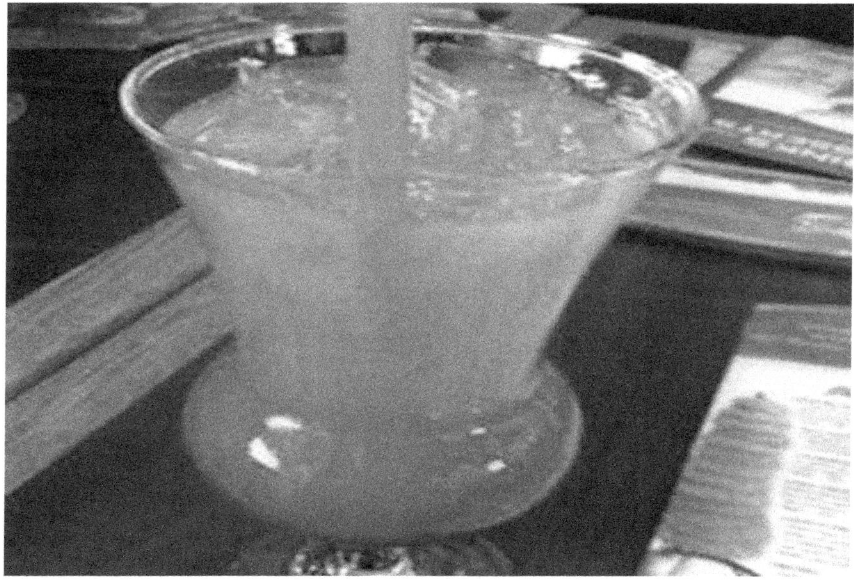

Nutrition

Calories: 278 Protein: 1g Fat: 0g Carbs: 38g Fiber: 0g

Preparation Time: 5' *Cooking Time: 0'* *Serves: 1*

192. Burger King's Lucky Charm Milkshake

Ingredients

- ***1 tablespoon marshmallow cream***
- ***2 cups vanilla ice cream***
- ***¼ cup Lucky Charm Cereal***
- ***½ cup milk***
- ***Optional:***
- ***2 tablespoons whipped cream***

Directions

1. Use a blender to blend milk, vanilla ice cream, and marshmallows cream. Do the blending process for one minute.
2. Then, mix the cereal after tossing them.
3. You can use whipped cream as per your choice on the top of the mixture.
4. Moreover, you can use marshmallows as the topping of the mixture.
5. Serve it and enjoy.

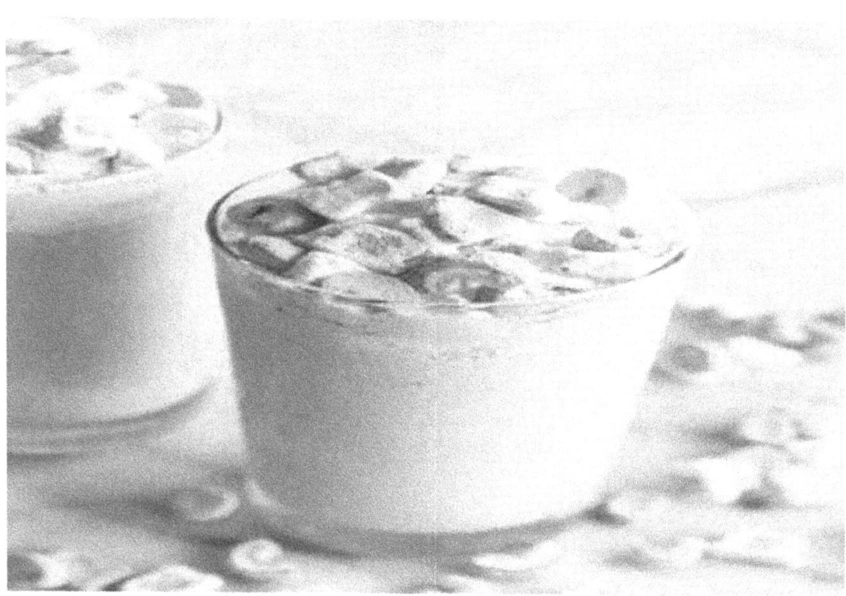

Nutrition

Calories: 696 Protein: 14g Fat: 21g Carbs: 81g Fiber: 2g

Preparation Time: 5' *Cooking Time: 0'* *Serves: 1*

193. The Cheesecake Factory's Piña Colada

Ingredients

½ cup each of:

- ***Pineapple (crushed and canned)***
- ***Vanilla ice cream***
- ***Ground cinnamon***
- ***¼ cup rum (coconut-flavored)***
- ***Maraschino cherry and pineapple wedges***

Directions

1. Take a blender and place pineapple, ice cream, and rum in it. Cover it and blend for 30 seconds to mix them completely.
2. Use chilled glasses and pour the smooth mixture in them.
3. Use cinnamon for sprinkling in it and use pineapple or a cherry for garnishing the smooth mixture.
4. Enjoy the delicious piña colada after serving it immediately.

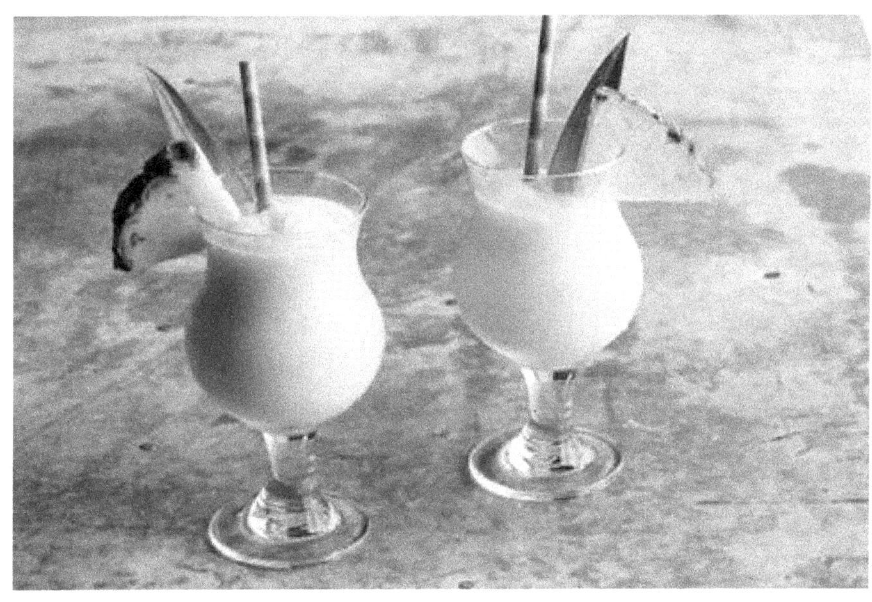

Nutrition

Calories: 360 Protein: 3g Fat: 7g Carbs: 41g Fiber: 1g

Preparation Time: 10' *Cooking Time: 0'* *Serves: 1*

194. Starbucks' Peppermint Mocha

Ingredients

- ***8 packets cocoa mix (instant hot)***
- ***¼ peppermint schnapps liqueur***
- ***4 cups 2% milk***
- ***1 ½ cups brewed espresso***
- ***Optional: Whipped cream***

Directions

1. Take a large-sized saucepan and heat milk in it after setting it on the oven at medium flame. Bubbles will produce around the pan and mix cocoa in the mixture. Whisk the mixture to blend properly.
2. Heat the mixture after adding espresso.
3. Stir the liqueur after removing it from the oven.
4. You can enjoy it with whipped cream as per your choice.
5. You can use the extract of peppermint with an extra three-quarter cup an extra brewed espresso instead of peppermint schnapps liqueur. Moreover, you can use dark roast coffee (double strength) instead of brewed espresso.

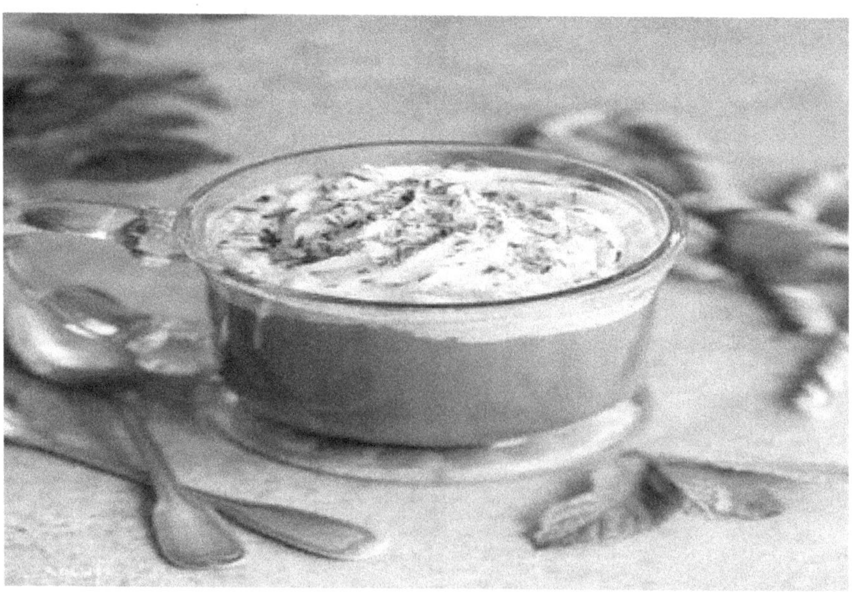

Nutrition

Calories: 197 Protein: 5g Fat: 6g Carbs: 22g Fiber: 1g

Preparation Time: 2h 25' *Cooking Time: 0'* *Serves: 2*

195. Red Lobster's Sparkling Fruit for Brunch

Ingredients

- ***2 servings fresh fruit of choice***
- ***½ cup Sugar***
- ***1 cup white wine/champagne***
- ***½ teaspoons freshly chopped mint***

Directions

1. Choose from melon balls, strawberries (hulled & sliced length-wise, pears, peaches, pears, or nectarines (seeded, peeled, and quartered). Combine the fruit gently in a container with the sugar.

2. Mix and pour the chosen beverage to almost cover the fruit.

3. Let it chill for 1–2 hours in the fridge.

4. Enjoy in a chilled champagne glass with a friend on a lazy day! It's worth the wait!

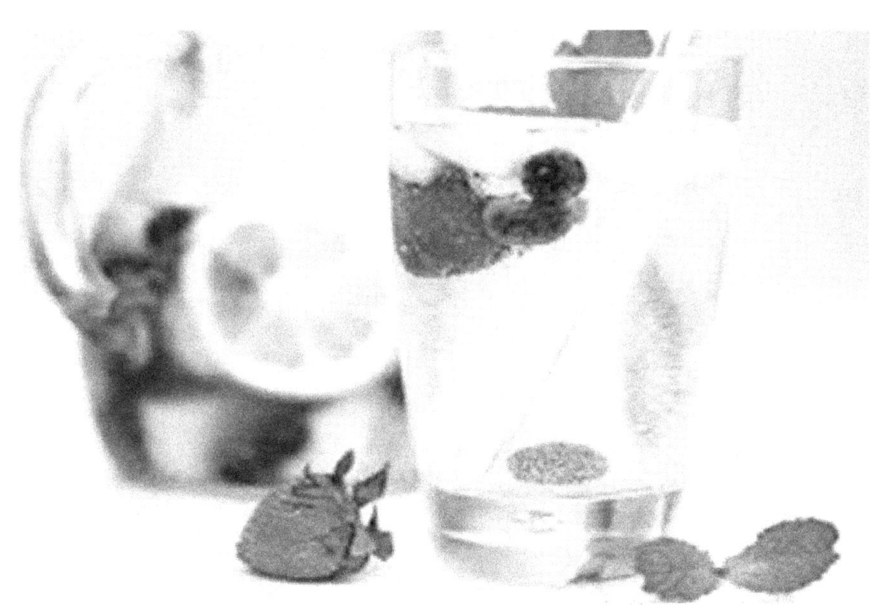

Nutrition

Calories: 80 Fat: 4g Carbs: 20g Sugars: 2g Protein: 15g

Preparation Time: 10' *Cooking Time: 10'* *Serves: 8*

196. Starbucks' Mocha Frappuccino

Ingredients

- *¾ cup chocolate syrup*
- *4 cups milk*
- *¾ cup sugar*
- *3 cups espresso coffee*
- *For Topping:*
- *Chocolate syrup*
- *Whipped cream*

Directions

1. Prepare the coffee as per the directions provided by the manufacturer.
2. Mix hot coffee & sugar in a mixer until the sugar is completely dissolved, for a minute or two, on high settings.
3. Add chocolate syrup & milk; continue to mix for a minute more.
4. For easy storage, pour the mixture into a sealable container. Put inside the refrigerator until ready to use.
5. Now, combine mix & ice (in equal proportion) in a blender & blend until smooth, on high settings & prepare the drink.
6. Pour the drink into separate glasses & top each glass first with the whipped cream & then drizzle chocolate syrup on the top.
7. Serve & enjoy!

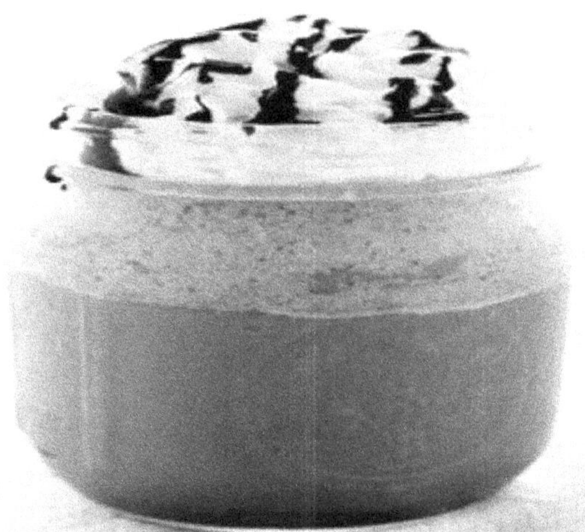

Nutrition

Calories: 197 Protein: 4.54 g Fat: 4.47g Carbohydrates: 35g

Preparation Time: 15' *Cooking Time: 5'* *Serves: 1*

197. Starbucks' Frozen Caramel Macchiato

Ingredients

- ***4 tablespoons whipped topping***
- ***1 cup whole milk, ice cold***
- ***2 fluid ounces original Starbucks whole bean espresso coffee or brewed Starbucks espresso***
- ***2-3 tablespoons buttery rich caramel syrup, thick***
- ***2 tablespoons vanilla syrup***
- ***8 ice cubes***
- ***2 tablespoons half & half***

Directions

1. First brew the Starbucks espresso shot. Then, fill a large glass with ice; leaving approximately 2 inches from the top; add in the whole milk and then pour 2 tablespoons of heavy cream or half & half. After that, add vanilla syrup & brewed Starbucks whole bean espresso on top of the milk.

2. Drizzle the indoor of your glass with thick caramel syrup & top with whipped cream; lastly drizzle a small amount of caramel syrup more over the top.

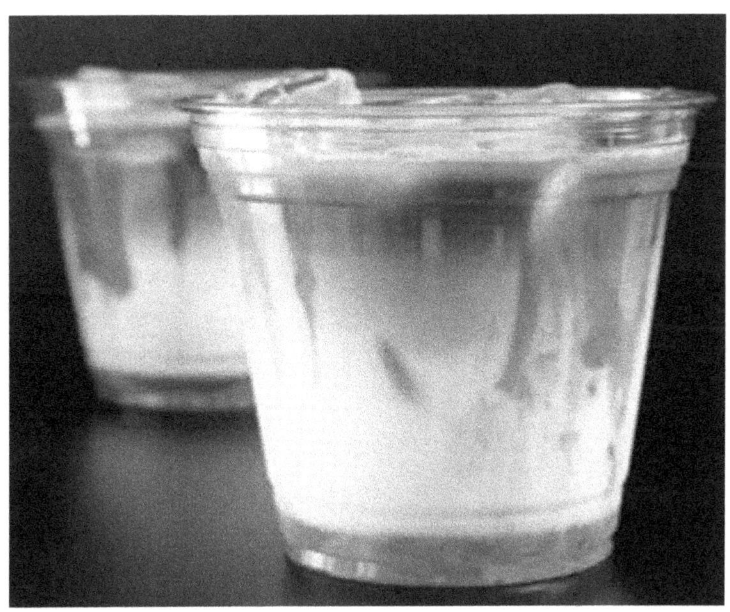

Nutrition

Calories: 365 Protein: 12.58g Fat: 12.58g Carbs: 48.4g

Preparation Time: 6' *Cooking Time: 0'* *Serves: 1*

198. Taco Bells's TB Baja Blast Freeze

Ingredients

- ***8 ounces Mountain Dew***
- ***3 ounces Powerade Berry Blast***
- ***Ice***

Directions

1. Toss each of the fixings into a blender.
2. Pulse until the ice is crushed and serve promptly for the best results

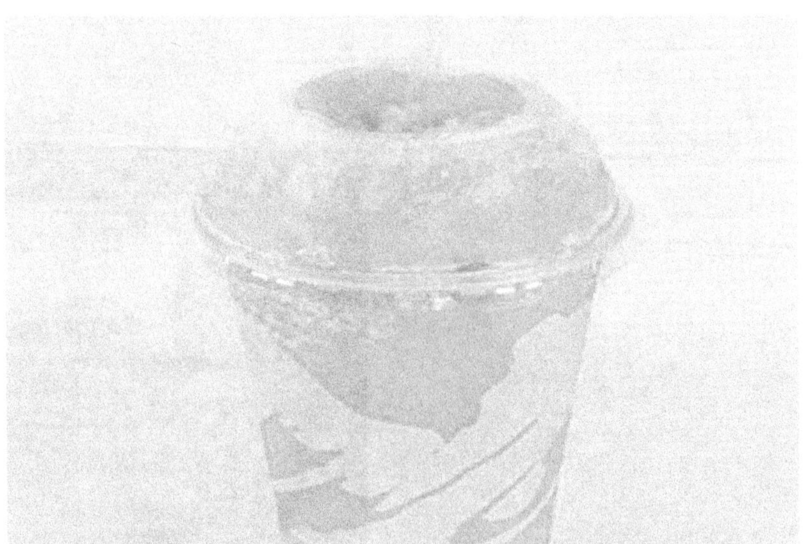

Nutrition

Calories: 414 Carbohydrates: 106g Protein: 0g Fat: 0g Sugars: 103g

Preparation Time: 5' *Cooking Time: 0'* *Serves: 1*

199. Chuy's Texas Martini Margarita

Ingredients

- ***2 ounces Tequila***
- ***1 ounces Patron Citronge***
- ***1 ½ ounces fresh lime juice***
- ***1 ½ ounce sugar water***
- ***Lime wedge & 2 jalapeno olive on a sword***
- ***Glass: Martini***

Directions

1. Fill ice in a shaker and using jigger pour alcohol in shaker bottom.
2. Add sugar water and lime juice and top with shaker top and shake vigorously.

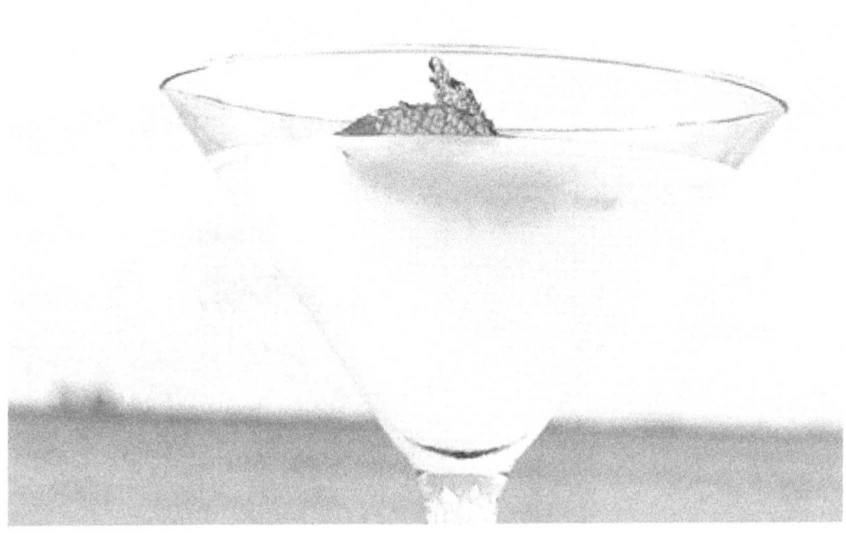

Nutrition

Calories: 112 Fat: 17 Carbs: 50g Sugars: 5g Protein: 7g

Preparation Time: 5' *Cooking Time: 0'* *Serves: 1*

200. Los Cabos' Mexican Spiked Coffee

Ingredients

- ***1 ounces Tequila Blanco***
- ***½ ounces Kahlua***
- ***6 ounces Black coffee***
- ***Whipped cream***
- ***Cinnamon powder***
- ***Sugar***

Directions

1. Wet the edge of the glass in water and coat with the sugar.
2. Caramelize the sugar rim.
3. Flame the tequila & Kahlua and serve in a glass with the sugar rim.
4. After that, add black coffee and whipped cream, and then top with cinnamon.

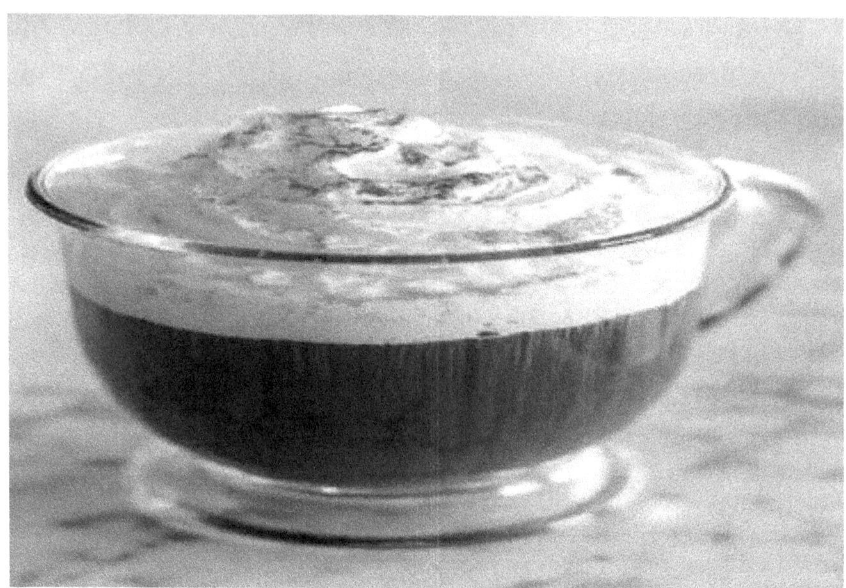

Nutrition

Calories: 120 Fat: 15g Carbs: 45g Sugar: 8g Protein: 14g

Conclusion

What prompted me to search for these so-called 'secret recipes' is the fact that once I found the one for my favorite dish, I could indulge in it whenever I wanted at home.

Another reason I wanted to find some copycat recipes for places to eat is that you can save a lot of money by cooking those dishes yourself. No transportation cost, no tipping, and you may enjoy the meal without getting all dressed up. Also, determining the length of my serving is great.

Without a doubt, eating well seems like a repetitive and exhausting activity. Yet, a solid eating routine assumes an essential job in keeping up your body weight, dealing with yourself, and maintaining a healthy lifestyle with the help of these recipes.

These copycat recipes are tested over and over again to make sure that you are creating precise dishes from the restaurant. Culinary Experts spend hours modifying those recipes to get the perfect flavor. These recipes are as near the real thing as sitting your favorite restaurant proper in your kitchen.

If you have your own family and like to go out to restaurants, but do not enjoy the awful service charge related to a terrific meal out, then these restaurant copycat recipes are for you.

You don't need to be a trained chef to prepare dinner your pleasant personal meals at home with restaurant copycat recipes. All you want are eating place copycat recipes, the components listed, and get admission to your kitchen.

Imagine impressing your friends and own family with food that they have most effectively enjoyed at sure restaurants, proper from the comfort of your very own domestic. They might imagine that to procure take out, and you could adorn that thought because simplest you'll recognize the truth—that you created these masterpieces within the comfort of your kitchen with restaurant copycat recipes.

While eating in a restaurant is a reward for some families, it has become a standard comfort for some individuals. You get benefits in the regions of nourishment, wellbeing and financial matters when you limit feasting out and start eating your own one of a kind copycat plans food.

Copycat food permits you to plan and adapt your meals, so you can utilize common fixings rather than unfortunate prepared nourishments. Handled nourishments, often served in restaurants or accessible at dinners prepared in the supermarket, in general, will be high in sodium, fat, and included sugars. As per the BBC, the World Wellbeing Association suggests enormously diminishing the admission of prepared nourishments.

This book aims to give you the knowledge and serve as a guide in your journey towards creating your favorite restaurant's recipe. I have given you many recipes that you can choose from. You can recreate recipes form Taco Bell, KFC, Red Lobster, and many more. You can create them for breakfast, dinner, lunch, drink, and desserts equipped with much nutrition.

I hope that this book is of a great help to you and that you would be able to do the recipes stated in this cookbook. This may serve as a guide for you and your family. Enjoy and have a happy meal!

CPSIA information can be obtained
at www.ICGtesting.com
Printed in the USA
BVHW011340061120
592698BV00010B/486